The Inside Story
of Medicines

The Inside Story of Medicines: A Symposium

editors

Gregory J. Higby

Elaine C. Stroud

American Institute of the History of Pharmacy
Madison, WI
1997

ISBN 0-931292-31-X (cloth)   0-931292-32-8 (paper)

American Institute of the History of Pharmacy
425 N. Charter St., Madison, WI 53706

Publication No. 16 (New Series)
Gregory J. Higby and Elaine C. Stroud, General Editors

Contents

FOREWORD, *Michael Harris* **vii**
INTRODUCTION OF KEYNOTE SPEAKER, *Robert A. Ingram* **1**
MEDICINES IN AMERICAN SOCIETY—A PERSONAL VIEW, *C. Everett Koop* **5**

Section 1. The History of Therapeutics

Old Drugs, Old and New History, *John M. Riddle* **15**
The Therapeutic Crisis of the Eighteenth Century, *J. Worth Estes* **31**
The Road to Twentieth-Century Therapeutics:
   Shifting Perspectives and Approaches, *Guenter B. Risse* **51**

Section 2. Case Studies of Drug Discovery

Alkaloids to Arsenicals: Systematic Drug Discovery
   Before the First World War, *John Parascandola* **77**
The Discovery of Insulin: The Inside Story, *Michael Bliss* **93**
M&B 693 (Sulfapyridine), *John E. Lesch* **101**
The Introduction of the Thiazides:
   A Case Study in Twentieth-Century Therapeutics, *Robert M. Kaiser* **121**
Planning and Serendipity in the Search for a Nonaddicting
   Opiate Analgesic, *Caroline Jean Acker* **139**

Section 3. The Disciplines of Medicine Making

The Recent History of Pharmacognosy, *Varro E. Tyler* **161**
Pharmacology: Current and Future Trends, *George A. Condouris* **171**
Current and Future Trends in Medicinal Chemistry, *John A. Montgomery* **185**
Recent Trends and the Future of Pharmaceutics, *George Zografi* **195**
Clinical Testing:
   New Developments and Old Problems, *Mark Parascandola* **201**

Section 4. From Medicines to Market and Patient

Recent Trends in Drug Development, *Louis Lasagna* **217**
Sure Cure: Public Policy on Drug Efficacy before 1962, *John P. Swann* **223**
Historical Perspectives on the Marketing of Medicines, *Mickey Smith* **263**
Physician-Pharmacist-Patient Interaction, *Paul L. Ranelli* **277**
The Global Impact of Medicines, *William H. Foege* **287**

Concluding Remarks, *Gregory J. Higby* **297**

NAME INDEX **299**

v

Foreword

THE symposium "Medicines: The Inside Story," held in Atlanta, Georgia, at the Carter Center on March 28-29, 1996, was the fourth and final part of an innovative project about medicines. The core of the *Medicines: The Inside Story* project is an interactive 4,000 square foot exhibition that travels the country presenting to several million people the in-depth messages of the project. In addition to the traveling exhibit, a second part of the project is a planetarium show called "InnerSpace" that employs a unique forum for visitors to learn about medicines and how they work in the body. A high school education program brings the visuals, interactives, and messages of the exhibition and planetarium show into the American classroom. This education program on CD-ROM was distributed free to teachers.

The Inside Story of Medicines: A Symposium presents the thinking and work of scholars, historians, health administrators, and the CEO of one of the leading pharmaceutical companies in the world, who participated in the symposium in 1996. These authors actively contributed to other segments of the *Medicines* project, and they were asked to present here a view of their discipline as it relates to medicines, giving the reader an overview as well as a view to the future. Periodically we need to assess where we are in the quest for medicines, and the cure of disease and suffering. I hope this book is a stepping stone in that process.

The past century has seen more advances in science and technology than in all the years that came before, and medical innovations have been among the most startling. While new discoveries continually increase the rate of progress, even the most revolutionary developments stand on the shoulders of their predecessors. For this reason, *Medicines: The Inside Story* is firmly rooted in an historical approach, looking to the past in order to give viewers a better sense of where they are in this rapidly changing picture.

Despite this steady progress in science and technology, however, society has not kept up with the changes in medicines. The news is filled with so many reports of medical advances that most people expect that there will always be fast, effective, and accessible cures for every condition. Although we have cured or prevented many diseases and are making remarkable strides

vii

against others, the fact remains that many challenges still lie ahead.

The *Medicines* exhibition lays out the wealth of our knowledge and illuminates the gaps that remain, empowering visitors to participate in taking care of their own health. But *Medicines* alone cannot provide all of the answers, and it is my hope that visitors will come away from the project wanting to know more. I hope that they will ask questions, read books and newspapers, and use the growing collection of electronic resources to find out more about their bodies and about the medicines that help keep them healthy.

We have chosen to focus on the medicines themselves in order to better understand what they are, how they work, how they are used, and the roles they play in people's lives. The project also looks at some pressing issues that have gained public attention: animal testing, clinical trials, quackery, and alternative systems of medicine. We have been scrupulous in our efforts to present a balanced view on these controversial topics, and visitors will find tools that allow them to explore and understand the issues for themselves.

It has been a privilege for me to create and direct *Medicines: The Inside Story,* and I would like to personally thank Glaxo Wellcome Inc. for offering me this unusual opportunity. Glaxo Wellcome provided not only the necessary funding, but the creative freedom to do the job right. Their flexibility and "hands-off" policy allowed us to stretch our imagination in what seemed like limitless directions, and ultimately led to the production of an extraordinary exhibition, planetarium show, education program, and symposium. The staff at Glaxo Wellcome continually responded to our needs with both their time and expertise.

A number of individuals at Glaxo Wellcome merit special mention. On behalf of the *Medicines* team, I would like to thank Charles A. Sanders, M.D., former CEO of Glaxo Inc., for giving the project initial approval and Dr. Margaret Dardess for overseeing the project with a gentle and supportive hand. Dr. Robert A. Ingram, CEO of Glaxo Wellcome Inc., has actively supported the project and helped it to develop far beyond its initial conception, and for that I am grateful. A special thank you goes to Dr. Elliott Sogol for his role in the creation of the project and for being a colleague, mentor, and friend to us all. For many of the visuals, thanks are due to Chig Wills and his talented design staff.

Hundreds of people and organizations have made this project possible, and are listed in the museum exhibit catalog. However, there are a few indi-

---

Michael Harris received his B.Sc. in Pharmacy from the Brooklyn College of Pharmacy in 1969 and his M.S. in the History of Pharmacy, from the University of Wisconsin-Madison in 1991. He specialized in the history of American pharmacy, particularly the artifacts and the practice of pharmacy. Mr. Harris directed the creation of the major traveling exhibit, *Medicines: The Inside Story.*

viduals who have been the foundation on which we stand, and we would like to acknowledge them here: Dr. John Parascandola for his truly valued advice and seemingly endless knowledge; Dr. Greg Higby for believing in us and for his and Dr. Elaine Stroud's excellent work on editing the symposium book. To our core advisers and readers: Dr. David Triggle, Dr. Phil Skolnick, and Dr. John Swann for their countless hours and free advice—a special thank you.

Special thanks go to Dr. Michael Heisler not only for his wise advice but for embracing the project and bringing it under the supportive roof of the Task Force for Child Survival and Development. Thanks also to Dr. William Foege and the Task Force Board of Directors for becoming a partner with us in health education.

I would also like to recognize our contractors, the partners who translated our ideas and images into reality. We would like to extend our thanks to Miles Fridberg Molinaroli for the exhibition design and graphics, to Image Communications for the interactives and videos, and to Sky-Skan for the planetarium show. Our appreciation also goes to Design and Production for fabricating the exhibition and to Artex for allowing it to travel gently around the country.

Finally, I have been extremely lucky in finding the unique group of people who became the *Medicines* staff. Their hard work and support are responsible for the creative quality and effectiveness of *Medicines* as a whole. All of the staff have given much of themselves and they have been singularly devoted to excellence in its every aspect. The group includes Patti Tuohy, Tom DiGiovanni, Katie Gray, Kathleen McRoberts, Teri Kestenbaum, Jane Ilsley, Abigail Porter, Deborah Pennington, Edwina Smith, Mark Parascandola, Katie Lynch, Bill Laffey, Gladys Johnson, and Marguerite Smith. There are the hundreds of teachers who made the education program a viable and useful tool for thousands of American teachers and millions of students. A special thanks are in order for the education managers of the exhibition, notably the first manager, Mary Rigger, and the planetarium directors who made the exhibition and planetarium show accessible to millions of visitors.

I hope you find the finished project every bit as exhilarating and eye-opening as it has been for us to bring it to you.

MICHAEL R. HARRIS
Project Director, Medicines: The Inside Story

Introduction of
Dr. C. Everett Koop

by Robert A. Ingram
President and CEO, Glaxo Wellcome, Inc.

T his symposium is one element in a four-part program called *Medicines: The Inside Story*, which also includes a museum exhibit, a planetarium show, and a classroom instructional manual that includes a CD-ROM of the exhibit. I don't know how many of you have seen our exhibit, *Medicines: The Inside Story*, but I hope all of you will take an opportunity to tour it. We're very proud of it. I am as proud of the exhibit as anything we have supported, and it represents a tremendous effort on the part of Michael Harris and the team that he has recognized.

I want to thank you all for taking time out of your schedules to be with us. At the symposium today we will explore the history, the present, and the future of pharmaceutical discovery, and more importantly, what pharmaceutical discovery means to all of us. I think everyone in this room recognizes that each of us either is or someday will be a patient. But we also represent the leading edge of succeeding generations of Americans whom I hope will come to view the medical miracles of today with as much commonplace interest as we view antibiotics or the polio vaccine.

We at Glaxo Wellcome are proud to sponsor this *Medicines* project, because ours is the business—ladies and gentlemen—of innovation. And innovation is what brings the medical breakthroughs that allow us to lead longer, healthier, and better quality lives. Those of you who have visited the *Medicines* exhibit will have seen what for me, among many impressive parts of that exhibit, is an unforgettable photo of the children lined up row upon row in iron lungs suffering from the plague of polio. As I said to my friend Dr. Koop this morning, I clearly remember those days, the days in the early 1950s when my mother wouldn't allow me to swim because of the dread fear of polio, when children were kept indoors for fear of infection. I remember several of my high school classmates attending graduation in iron lungs because of the polio epidemic. I think many of you in this room probably can remember those days as well.

Yet today polio and iron lungs are virtually a memory, preserved in museum exhibits and on the pages of history books. I have three sons; all of them are grown. The youngest is a college student, and none of them understands what I'm talking about when I mention iron lungs. That's a history made possible by the talent and insight of medical pioneers like Jonas Salk, Albert Sabin, and countless others who have dedicated their lives to the fight against disease. I would point out that we have with us today a giant in that field, Bill Foege. That fight continues today, building upon the stores of knowledge developed by earlier generations. The work that Salk did in the twentieth century clearly built upon the work of Pasteur in the nineteenth, which built upon the work done by Jenner in the eighteenth century. So too the scientists of today, working in government, in academia, and in private labs like ours at Glaxo Wellcome are building upon that strong heritage of innovation in order to discover tomorrow's cures for the diseases that we face today.

Ladies and gentlemen, that is why this symposium and the rest of the *Medicines* project are so important. It is our role—I would submit it is our responsibility—to encourage succeeding generations of young people not only to understand the miracles of the past made commonplace today, but also to take up the standard in our continuing battle against disease and to lead the fight against a foe that, sadly, will always be with us in some form. We must, I believe very firmly, awaken and nurture in these young people the spirit of discovery. We must light in them the spark of knowledge and feed that spark until it really does become a roaring flame. I came here from the Education Summit, where it was my privilege to represent business in North Carolina along with our governor. But I must say that as important and worthwhile as I felt that experience was, I had an experience just before we came into this room encountering some young students from here in Atlanta. They were very bright, very talented, very articulate young people who have, at an early age, identified science as their area of interest. Frankly speaking, folks, we don't have enough of them. We need to build that talent pool of young, bright people who are going to pursue the answers to HIV, to Alzheimer's, to cancer. And someday, there's no doubt, we will look upon those diseases, or our children will, with the same wonder that my own children look at polio and the iron lung. I think there's no more important thing we can do.

Today, it is my privilege—and it is a privilege and pleasure—to say that we have with us one of the great pioneers in the history of medicine and health, a man who has truly distinguished himself internationally, as a physician, scholar, and citizen/activist, but in my personal view, he is the best example I know of a public servant. As his many awards, 35 honorary doctor-

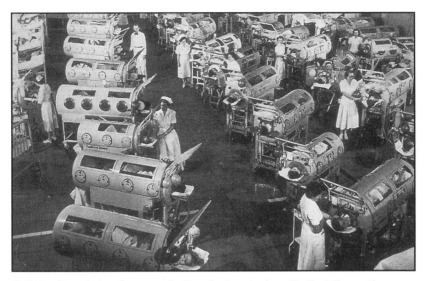

Polio patients in iron lungs, at the Rancho Los Amigos Medical Center, Downey, California, in 1952. (Center for Disease Control and Prevention.)

ates, and a lifetime of achievement will attest, our next speaker has dedicated his life to improving health and the quality of life not only for all Americans, but particularly for the children of both this country and around the world. As some of you who know him know, he was formerly a pediatric surgeon, who turned his talents from conducting operations in a surgical suite to directing the course of public policy in the halls of government, first as the Deputy Assistant Secretary for Health at the U.S. Department of Health and Human Services, and then, as I think all the world knows, as our Surgeon General, appointed by former President Reagan. As Chairman of the Safe Kids National Campaign, he served as an outspoken advocate for accident prevention, particularly those accidents that turn children into victims. No one is unaware, I think, of his launching an anti-smoking campaign with a zeal that captured the attention of the press, of policy makers, of consumers, and of industry alike. I must say I think we're seeing now just how right his effort in that area really is turning out to be. A prolific writer and thinker, he is the author of more than 230 articles and books on medicine and surgery, biomedical ethics, and health policy. The list of awards he has earned in honor of his achievements is too long to mention here this morning. Suffice it to say that he has been awarded the William E. Ladd Gold Medal of the American Academy of Pediatrics for his outstanding contributions to pediatric surgery; the Public Health Service Distinguished Service Medal in recognition of his extraordinary leadership of the U.S. Public Health service; and the Medal of the Legion of Honor from France. I think you also know he was recently awarded the well deserved Presidential Medal of Freedom. His energy, his determination, and I can tell you, his dedication, are both legendary and awe-inspiring to anyone who knows him.

My mother, who is 81, like most mothers, bores her friends talking about how proud she is of her son. But I must tell you, whenever my mother talks about me, I know from her friends that the thing she perhaps is as proud of as anything is that she can honestly say that her son knows and is a friend of Dr. Koop. I hope you will join me in welcoming a man, and I believe an American hero, who has been a friend of medicine, a friend of children, and a friend of health. There is no one, in my opinion, who is better to talk to us this morning about the importance of this whole endeavor. Please join me in welcoming Dr. C. Everett Koop.

Keynote Address: Medicines in American Society—A Personal View

by Dr. C. Everett Koop

I am delighted to be with you today, to have a few minutes to share with you some of my thoughts—and even a few recollections—of the role of medicines in the practice of medicine, in the science and art of healing.

This is an unusual speaking opportunity for me. As most of you know, since the day I left my post as your Surgeon General, I have devoted myself to the challenge of health care reform in the United States. During the last seven years, I have criss-crossed this nation many times, speaking out on the *ethical* imperative for health care reform, and offering concrete suggestions about what we need to do. I must admit I was disappointed by the inability of the President and the Congress and the American people to come to agreement on health care reform, disappointed, but not surprised. After a lot of high expectations generated by the Clinton Administration and others, the great health care reform juggernaut came to naught. So, this slow pace is nothing new.

I remember discussing the need for health care reform several years ago with that fine old gentleman, Claude Pepper, who really was the senior spokesman for all of us who shared concerns about our health care system even back then. A very elderly man, closer to 100 than most of us will ever get, Claude Pepper would often say that he was sure that we would eventually get health care reform, but not in his lifetime. After he died, I've been told, Mr. Pepper went to heaven, and the first thing he asked God was if there would ever be health care reform in the United States. I understand that God replied, "Yes, there will be . . . but not in my lifetime!"

We face sweeping changes, not all of them good. We face great challenges, not all of them bad. As Congress and the country have now learned, when it comes to all the problems associated with health care reform, there is

---

Dr. C. Everett Koop received his M.D. degree from Cornell Medical College in 1941. After serving an internship at the Pennsylvania Hospital, he pursued postgraduate training at the University of Pennsylvania School of Medicine, Boston Children's Hospital, and the Graduate School of Medicine, University of Pennsylvania, from which he received the degree of Doctor of Science (Medicine) in 1947. After promotions up the academic ladder, he was named Professor of Pediatric Surgery, School of Medicine, University of Pennsylvania in 1959 and Professor of Pediatrics in 1971. He is presently the Elizabeth DeCamp McInerny Professor at Dartmouth.

A pediatric surgeon with an international reputation, Dr. Koop became Surgeon-in-Chief of the Children's Hospital of Philadelphia in 1948 and served in that capacity until he left academia in 1981. He was the Editor-in-Chief of the Journal of Pediatric Surgery.

Dr. Koop was appointed Deputy Assistant Secretary for Health, U.S. Public Health Service (PHS) in March 1981, and sworn in as Surgeon General on November 17, 1981. Additionally, he was appointed Director of the Office of International Health in May 1982. As Surgeon General, Dr. Koop oversaw the activities of the 6,000-member PHS Commissioned Corps and advised the public on health matters such as smoking and health, diet and nutrition, environmental health hazards, and the importance of immunization and disease prevention. He also became the government's chief spokesman on AIDS. He resigned on October 1, 1989 and continues to educate the public about health issues through his writings, the electronic media, and as Senior Scholar of the C. Everett Koop Institute at Dartmouth.

The recipient of numerous honors and awards including 37 honorary doctorates, he was awarded the Denis Brown Gold Medal by the British Association of Paediatric Surgeons; the William E. Ladd Gold Medal of the American Academy of Pediatrics in recognition of outstanding contributions to the field of pediatric surgery; the Order of the Duarte, Sanchez, and Mella, the highest award of the Dominican Republic, for his achievement in separating the conjoined Dominican twins; and a number of other awards from civic, religious, medical and philanthropic organizations. He was awarded the Medal of the Legion of Honor by France in 1980, inducted into the Royal College of Surgeons of England in 1982, and the Royal College of Physicians and Surgeons of Glasgow. In May 1983, Dr. Koop was awarded the Public Health Service Distinguished Service Medal in recognition of his extraordinary leadership of the U.S. Public Health Service. After retirement, he was presented with the Surgeon General's Exemplary Service Medal and the Surgeon General's Medallion. In September 1995, Dr. Koop was awarded the Presidential Medal of Freedom.

Dr. Koop is the author of more than 230 articles and books on the practice of medicine and surgery, biomedical ethics, and health policy. He was awarded an Emmy in 1991 in the News and Documentary category for "C. Everett Koop, M.D.," a five-part series on health care reform. Two of the shows in this series were awarded Freddies in 1992: Best Film in the Category of Aging for "Forever Young," and Best Film in the Category of Family Dynamics for "Listening to Teenagers."

no panacea, no single magic bullet; there are no easy answers, only hard choices. That is because Americans have three demands for our health care: (1) immediate access to health care, (2) the latest high-tech medicine, and (3) a limited price. But now these three demands have become *incompatible*. We can usually supply any two of them, but it may be impossible to have all three. That is not a very pleasant diagnosis for our health care system, and not a very easy prognosis. That is why I say that this speaking opportunity is unusual for me. Instead of playing the role of stern diagnostician for the nation's health care system at the present, I will enjoy a time of celebration of what we have accomplished in the past, so we can take some cheer and confidence for the future.

A gathering like ours today is critical. We must be able to place the discovery and development of new medicines into a context that is worthwhile for both the health care professional and the public. As we go through the process of reforming our health care system—and, even though there was no legislative reform, the system is reforming itself, even as I speak—as we reform our health care system, we need to keep foremost in our mind the role that medicines play in medicine.

The earliest written documents of medical history, Egyptian papyri 4000 years old tell us of poppy seeds as a treatment for flatulence and iron as a treatment for baldness. As a glance at one evening's worth of television will show, we are still offering remedies—not cures—for these two ancient human afflictions. (From what I know of Egyptian art, all those images of bald pharaohs might indicate the severity of their problem!)

Closer to home, in our own history, we see the importance the first colonial physicians placed upon the drugs they extracted from the plants found in the new world. In their mainly-theological view of the world, they fully expected God to provide in each part of the world the natural plants needed to combat the illness of that part of the world. And while our world view may have become more secular, today many of us have faith in our god-given powers of discovery and intellect to derive what we need from the laboratory as well as from the natural world around us. But the complexities and mysteries of the modern scientific derivation of medicines can produce misconceptions about medicines among the public, and even among health practitioners.

This symposium, and the exhibition *Medicines: The Inside Story*—by addressing the history of therapeutics, by presenting case studies of drug discovery, by exploring the disciplines of medicine making, and by explaining how medicines get from market to patient—by these methods this symposium will indeed tell the inside story about medicines, a story that should be better known by all.

Although there are mornings that I *feel old* enough to have been around since the time of the pharaohs, I'm not quite that old. But, I am older than most people currently at work in our health care system and in health care industries. Actually I guess I could just say that I am older than most people, . . . period!!

My grandchildren frequently ask me questions like "did they have telephones when you were a boy?" or if there were trains when I was a little boy, or maybe even if I remembered the invention of the wheel. But my recollections of medicine and medicines do go back far enough to be appropriate to the subject of this conference.

When I was a college student on summer vacation, I worked in a small 50-bed hospital on Long Island, starting out doing scut-work, working my way up to doing blood counts and helping in autopsies, cutting thousands of sections on the microtome, and eventually catching the eye of the chief surgeon of the hospital, who also served as chief surgeon at a nearby 300-bed hospital for crippled children. This was in the days before sulfanilamide and before antibiotics. He took me under his wing, and gave me a rare experience. There were only four diagnoses in that hospital:

•Congenital defects of orthopedic nature,
•Aftermath of polio,
•Tuberculosis of the bone, and
•Osteomyelitis.

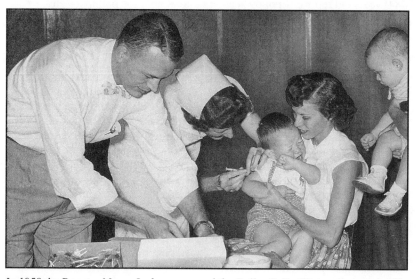

In 1958 the Decatur Moose Lodge sponsored the Dollar Polio Clinic, where over 400 shots were administered for a fee of $1 each. Daniel R. Freeby (left), a pharmacist in Decatur, Indiana, assists at the clinic, which was a community effort to protect area children from polio. (Drug Topics Collection, American Institute of the History of Pharmacy.)

One of my chores was to change all dressings on osteomyelitis patients, once a week. Some of these wounds stretched from ankle to hip, with bones exposed. It took me from 8 am Monday morning until 5 pm Friday afternoon to change all the dressings in the hospital; we really had very little to help these young patients. In the summer, the children were put outside in their purulent dressings. Often, when I uncovered the wound, I would find maggots in it. But that was good, because maggots ate away the decayed flesh, actually helping the patient by cleansing the wound. So we raised more maggots, by catching flies in a jar with a cover and a cheese cloth stretched halfway down, so the eggs would drop through the cloth, and we'd extract the maggots, and use them therapeutically.

The only medication I had was balsam of Peru. I would soak strips of gauze in that nice smelling but sticky compound, pack the wound and apply the dressings. In my senior year in college, a new drug appeared, called Prostalin, brand name for the first sulfanilamide. The nurses knew it was good for infections, and even worked against streptococcus, but they didn't know it required a steady dosage over a period of days, and used it like aspirin. There are very few physicians today who have had experience before sulfanilamides, so I am a rare bird.

Later, as a surgical resident at the University of Pennsylvania, I was the custodian for the entire city of Philadelphia for the new drug, penicillin. I doled it out to sick patients on the pleas of their physicians, between five and seven every afternoon. Even for the worst infection, we never gave any patient more than 100,000 units a day.

But my most poignant recollections of the differences that modern medicines can make are the recollections, not of a physician, but of a parent and grandparent. I never lost the sense of wonder when I saw a youngster's fever and infection controlled by an antibiotic. I will never forget my first walk through a colonial New England cemetery, where tiny gravestones mark the many young children "carried away by fever." In the world of medicines, these are the good old days. And now, I'd like to make a few remarks that will anticipate what follows in the symposium today and tomorrow.

This story that will unfold will be one of tradition, serendipity, systematic research, and compassion. A context will be provided for not only an historical understanding of the past and present, but also for the future of medicines.

This has been a century of great achievements in therapeutics—vaccines, hormones, antibiotics, analgesics, antihypertensives, antipsychotics, vitamins, and antineoplastics—among a host of new agents. To many people, these have all appeared to arise from nowhere, to be added to the armamentarium with ease. Like the drugs of old, however, this is not the case. One misconception is that the medicines of ancient times were all useless and inert. Instead, recent research has revealed that our ancestors had a sophisticated understanding of plant drugs and their utility. Although scores of drugs were carried along by tradition only, they were all placed within a Hippocratic and Galenic context that was shared by healers throughout the western world for centuries. *The Greek Herbal of Dioscorides*, from the first century A. D., provides hundreds of plant, animal, and mineral remedies for illness, and was used by European physicians for the next 1500 years.

Further advances came during the Middle Ages, when Arabic chemists discovered and cataloged many substances in the process of their search for a substance that would transform metal into gold . . . not the last instance of medicines being discovered by serendipity. Also during the Middle Ages, physicians used opium and alcohol as pain relievers, and employed a variety of emetics.

While the Renaissance brought great advances in anatomy—especially the work of Vesalius—the next great changes in medicines came in the eighteenth century, as Jenner began his work with inoculation and vaccination. New drugs upset old theories that had become fossilized, especially as scientists began the pharmaceutical assault upon micro-organisms.

By the 1800s, a greater understanding of the human body and its processes, the work of Pasteur and others, plus the concurrent development of scientific chemistry, set the stage for the modern era of drug exploration.

I greatly look forward to this afternoon's session when a group of historians will look at the modern process of drug discovery in more detail. Before the twentieth century, drugs either came from antiquity (such as opium), out of folk traditions (like digitalis), or were found by chance. Beginning in the late 1800s, men like Paul Ehrlich pioneered the scientific exploration for new drugs. Chance findings still yielded great results, as with penicillin, but as our century progressed, more drugs came out of well-organized research projects, typified by the efforts of scientists who worked on the sulfa drugs.

As we will learn as well from the insulin story, research is a human activity, fraught with egos and frailties. In the early 1800s, physicians and pharmacists alike acquired their knowledge of medicines in classes taught by professors of chemistry and materia medica. The roots of the modern sciences of medicine making can be traced to that time.

Tomorrow we will hear about some of the key disciplines of medicine making, what progress has been made during the recent past and where they are heading. These are exciting times. In medicinal chemistry, new technological developments are changing how drugs are discovered. In pharmacology, the explosive growth of the biological sciences has changed the disciplinary landscape. Pharmacognosy, the direct descendent of the old discipline of materia medica, is now in a renaissance, inspired by a combination of interest in folkloric knowledge about drugs and a widespread desire for milder, more "natural" medicines. And in pharmaceutics, the usually quiet science of drug delivery systems, new dosage forms hold significant promise for greatly improved medicine use with reduced side effects.

And yet, even with safe and well-designed medicines, problems loom on the horizon. During the final session of this symposium, some of the most difficult and important issues facing the future of medicines will be addressed: change is coming in the health care sphere, primarily in the area of managed care, which threatens to stifle drug discovery and development by removing essential incentives. The present system of regulation, which has made our medicines the safest in the world, is under scrutiny by congressional leaders who believe that less regulation is better for our nation.

The marketing of pharmaceuticals, which had been clearly different for prescription drugs and over-the-counter remedies, is now growing murky. The inter-professional relationships of physicians and pharmacists are being strained under the often contradictory pressures of consumerism, professionalism, and benefits management.

And finally, we must remember to look beyond our shores and consider the health of the world's community and how our work in health care research can benefit humanity as a whole.

Before concluding, I would like to suggest a few questions for discussion as the symposium progresses:

• In what areas of health have medicines had their greatest impact? And in what areas of health have they seemed to fail?

• Do the chronic diseases of the industrialized West attract more research attention than the acute illnesses afflicting much of the developing world?

• Are there limits to what medicines can do in theory, and if so, what are they?

• Are present health practitioners doing an adequate job to assure the proper use of medicines, and if not, what can they do to improve matters?

• What is the long-term future for medicines research in the United States and what can be done to improve its prospects?

I am honored to have been asked to take part in your symposium. I share your sense of pride in what medicines have done for humanity. I share your enthusiasm for what they can still do in the future. But we all also share a sense of human limitations.

I went into medicine for the same reason that folks pursue the discovery of medicines: to prolong life and to alleviate suffering. We have done a lot of both, but there comes a time when we reach our limits. There comes a time when life can no longer be prolonged, when suffering is inevitable. . . . We need to remember this. We need to remember what health care really means. We need to understand our limitations as well as our aspirations.

As I have said "health care" so often in the last minutes, how many of you translated that to health<u>cure</u>? We put too much emphasis on curing, too little on <u>caring</u>. We need to do more about the times we cannot provide the cure, but still can provide the care. Curing can cost billions, while caring comes from the heart and soul, and is always ethical.

Sometimes, when dealing with complex issues of curing and caring, with the role of medicine—and medicines—in society, the place of healing in life, the meaning of life itself, . . . sometimes an anecdote sums things up just right. This one has to do with a couple who died and went to heaven, and when they got there, as you might expect, they found things to be superb.

One day, they were sitting together, and the man said to his wife, "We should not be surprised about how wonderful things are here. Do you remember what the minister told us? Do you remember that the Bible said that the 'eye has not seen, nor has ear heard the wonders that God has prepared for those that love Him,' and look around you, is there anything upon which you could improve?"

He paused and added, rather pointedly, "you know, we could have been here three years ago if you hadn't discovered non-fat food!"

But, not to be dismayed, she said, "Three years ago! We could have been <u>five</u> years ago if you had only stopped listening to those health messages from C. Everett Koop!"

Thank you.

Section 1.

History of Therapeutics

<hr>

Medicines are among humanity's oldest tools. Some of the most ancient human settlements, such as Shanidar in modern Iraq, show evidence of prehistoric drug use dating back over 40,000 years ago. In the first section of *The Inside Story of Medicines*, the history of therapeutics before 1900 is addressed by three leading historians.

In John Riddle's view, the drugs used in ancient times should not be judged as inert out of hand. Instead, we should evaluate seriously those remedies taken to combat diseases we today diagnose as gout, atherosclerosis, benign prostatic hypertrophy, and cancer. For his test case, Riddle chooses that very old class of medicines, the laxatives, and places them in historical context.

The transition from traditional rational systems of therapeutics to the modern experimental approach began in the 1700s. J. Worth Estes takes us back to the era when conflicting explanations of drug activity broke down the dominance of Galen's theories of humoral balance. In addition to the usual figures discussed in this period—Boerhaave, Cullen, Brown, and Rush— Estes brings in the learned opinions of Thomas Jefferson.

During the 1800s the chaotic state of therapeutics gradually gave way to a more objective, physiologically-based approach. As Guenter Risse demonstrates, however, physicians still sought broad, holistic explanations for drug action despite the specific advances of pharmacology and pathology. Physicians regained their traditional respect for the healing power of nature and researchers looked for new ways to utilize the immune system through vaccines and antitoxins.

The history of therapeutics is a fascinating tale that shows what a large part medicines have played in the development of Western thought and science. This section reminds us as well of the debt we owe the unknown discoverers of cinchona, opium, and other drugs that are still in use or were important precursors of medicines that today improve the lives of millions.

Old Drugs, Old and New History

by John M. Riddle

T ODAY in the United States the number of persons incarcerated in prisons exceeds one million, with estimates as high as eighty percent being there for drug-related crimes. The political issue of drugs and related crime is at or near the top of most public opinion polls. Yet history courses or texts on American and western civilizations seldom mention drugs. When they do, the subject is shortly exhausted.

Hans Zinsser's *Rats, Lice and History* directed attention to diseases and plagues as being as historically important as wars. He decried the attention that historians paid to the latter while being nearly oblivious to the former.[1] Human discoveries, through trial, error, and serendipity, of substances that affect somatic chemistry, that combat microorganisms, regulate health, and promote healing are surely more ignored than either wars or diseases. Yet it can be demonstrated that the ancients discovered the contraceptive and abortifacient consequences of taking certain substances and were able to regulate effectively their reproductive rates. This occurred long before the science of endocrinology made us aware that plants and a few minerals could suppress and, in some instances promote, fertility. Unable to see how people regulated fertility, historians and demographers have chronicled devotedly long periods of relative population stability or decline without believing that the mysterious secrets attributed to the ancients resided in their medicine boxes and bottles.

God distributed natural resources unequally as a divine means of causing humans to interrelate and exchange goods and services, or so postulated Adam Smith and the liberal economists. In both the ancient and medieval worlds, a large part of international trade was in pharmaceuticals. Judging from trade records, drugs probably accounted for the greatest bulk and value

15

of trade items from Eastern Asia to Iceland, from Sweden to the Sudan. A theory of the fall of the Roman Empire was that its economic collapse was caused by a prolonged, irreversible unfavorable balance of trade with the East that exported drugs but imported little from the West. Let us not forget that the motivation for Columbus' discovery was trade with the East, specifically the Spice Islands, spice being a synonym for drugs. So long as malaria was endemic to central Africa, Europeans avoided its paths. Once cinchona bark or quinine was discovered, they walked its ways and colonized its land and people, an act made possible by a drug.[2]

Over the last decade of researching classical and medieval medicine, I became interested in whether the drugs prescribed might truly have had some effect. Were they, as leading pharmacologist Arthur K. Shapiro said, merely placebos?[3] Harry F. Dowling emphatically asserted that before 1700 fewer than two dozen drugs were effective.[4] Some doubt any effectiveness in ancient or medieval medicine. L. J. Henderson, a prominent sociologist, opined that prior to 1912 a random physician and a random patient with a random disease had no better than a 50-50 chance of benefiting from the encounter.[5] In other words, a sizable community of scholars regard pre-modern medicine as well-meaning attempts to positively influence health with as much harm as good, at best, and ignorant and largely folkloristic or philosophical nonsense, at worst.

Medicine is studied as a cultural system, but surely it is more than that. Viewing medicine merely within a cultural context provides no answer to the question about effectiveness, only about the capacity of people for self-delusion. Did those people who lived and suffered before our century find medicine largely ineffective in helping people with disease, pain and injury? As George Sarton said, in any given culture at any time there are probably more practitioners of medicine than all the other sciences together. Pharmacy often was extended to cover what we call nutrition, because the distinction between a food and a drug is ill-defined, with some peoples not making a distinction at

John M. Riddle is an Alumni Distinguished Professor at North Carolina State University, where he has been since 1965. As the author of seven books and many articles, he is Past-President of the American Institute of the History of Pharmacy. Fellowships and scholarships include the National Humanities Foundation, Fulbright, American Council of Learned Societies, and the Institute for Advanced Studies (Princeton). Among his more recent publications is *Contraception and Abortion from the Ancient World to the Renaissance* (Harvard University Press, 1992), which has been the subject of major articles in the *New York Times, London Times, Manchester Guardian,* and *Washington Post,* many of which were syndicated in national presses and of presentation on CNN, NPR, BBC, and CBC, and *Eve's Herbs: A History of Contraception and Abortion in the West* (Harvard University Press, 1997).

all. The Greek and Latin word, *diaeta*, meant, broadly, medical treatment that may include *pharmakon*. A *diaeteticus* was a medical practitioner who did not use surgery. Because past and present medicine is practiced more through drug therapy than through other available instruments (such as surgery, massage, and physical therapy), the question about drugs' effectiveness is absolutely central to medicine's role. Oliver Wendell Holmes was most emphatic: "I firmly believe that if the whole materia medica, *as now used*, could be sunk to the bottom of the sea, it would be all the better for mankind,— and all the worse for the fishes."[6]

Some years ago I compared the drugs mentioned in various writings ascribed to Hippocrates, all written between approximately 440 B.C.E. and 330 B.C.E., to four modern guides of pharmacy, pharmacognosy, and herbal medicine.[7] In all, the Hippocratic writings had 257 drugs.[8] All but twenty-seven were found in one or more of the four modern guides. Of the twenty-seven that were not, most were foods (*e.g.*, cucumber and lentil) and three were animal products (eggs, castoreum, and horn). One was water, which, of course, would not be found in a modern pharmacy guide. Nonetheless, in certain conditions, such as dehydration, water acts as a drug, inasmuch as it is a substance introduced to restore a healthy condition. In reversing the process, I looked at the natural-product drugs from resins and resin combinations currently being used, some eighteen named in Tyler, Brady, and Robbers, *Pharmacognosy* (1981). All the drugs that were found in the Mediterranean were contained in the Hippocratic Corpus and similar writings of the period. The same can be said of the plant alkaloids. Of the thirty-four found in the modern guide, all those from plants growing around the Mediterranean were found in ancient Greek works. In other words, all the drugs extant in the environment of the ancient Greeks that we know and use today as drugs had already been discovered.

Such an approach establishes a presumption that Greek pharmacy was rational, but there is no proof because these data do not show how the Greeks employed the drugs. Given their theoretical approach of balancing humors, we do not know if their applications were scientific, in our sense. Comparing ancient diagnostic words for afflictions, diseases, and symptoms is notoriously difficult. Words can be translated but precise meanings in differing contexts escape the combined approaches of medicine and linguistics.

As a means to address the question about whether the ancients used drugs in ways we consider rational, I propose to examine some examples of natural products used as drugs in ancient and modern times. To avoid arbitrary selection of modern drugs that skew the results, I selected Rudolf Fritz Weiss' *Herbal Medicine* (Beaconfield, U.K., 1988) as the modern reference, and looked at a group of drugs for which there is reasonable certainty as to the modern and ancient actions, namely, the laxatives. In this discussion the concern is how, not why, laxatives were used and, for present purposes, I make no distinction between laxative, purgative, and cathartic.[9]

Cassia

The first herbal laxative Weiss lists is senna, obtained from two species of *Cassia* , containing as active principles anthraquinone glycosides as active principles that act primarily on the colon.[10] It is marketed as an over-the-counter product under brand names such as Senokot, Laxagel, and Perdiem Granules.[11]

Cassia used as a laxative was unquestionably known to medieval people, but confusion arises in ascribing its use to the ancients. First, the word *casia* is Greek and Latin, but the name was also applied to a kind of cinnamon, possibly the same as Linnaeus gave to *Cinnamomum cassia*. Cinnamon in the form of bark or ground bark was imported to the Meterranean from Asia, the "Spice Islands," and one of its usages was as a laxative. Cassia, on the other hand, was native to southern and eastern Africa, the same region that cinnamon passed through on the trade route from Asia to Madagascar as the ships caught the monsoon winds. A low perennial shrub, cassia's leaves and fruit pod serve as a laxative product. The ancients were not familiar with the plants, however, only the products from them.[12]

The true cassia was described and distinguished from cinnamon by ibn Masawaih (d. 1015), the Arabic medical writer, on the basis of definitive descriptions of the plants.[13] Avicenna (ibn Sina, 980-1037) explained that *casia* (in Latin translation) is "casia," which he says is superior to cinnamamon. He also extols "casia's" expelling qualities.[14] Under "casia fistula," however, which definitely is what we call cassia, Avicenna praises its purgative qualities achieved through expelling phlegm and cholera.[15] The sixteenth-century French botanist, Charles de L'Ecluse (Clusius) asserted that it was the Arabs and not the Greeks who discovered cassia.[16] In contrast, Pietro A. Mattioli, a sixteenth-century commentator on Dioscorides, believed that Andromachus, a Greek writer about the same time as Dioscorides, knew of true cassia (*cassia fistula*).

By the late Middle Ages in the West, the possible confusion between cinnamon and cassia was clarified in the working vocabularies. Previous knowledge of the difference between the two is harder to discern, although it is quite possible that the ancients made the distinction that is unclear to us. However we can conclude that pre-modern people in the West had and used cassia as a laxative.

Rhubarb

Rhubarb (*Rheum offinale* Baill. + sp.) is the second natural-product laxative listed by Weiss.[17] Its roots supply anthraquinones that have laxative qualities; this product is sold now under the name of Grandel's Liver and Gallbladder Tablets. Cultivated rhubarb, however, does not have the same medicinal qualities as the medicinal rhubarb. Medicinal rhubarb has a long tradition of significance in trade and as a laxative. Clifford Foust in *Rhubarb* has recently written about the history of this plant whose value stimulated international trade. There is solid evidence that the ancients valued rhubarb and employed it as a laxative.[18]

Aloe

When I speak about ancient herbs, I often ask the audience, "How many of you have an aloe plant in your home?" The normal response is about half the audience. To the follow-up question about its use, most reply that they use it for burns. Aloe *is* good for burns and a variety of other skin afflictions. It is also the third herbal laxative listed by Weiss.[19] Ancient and medieval people employed aloe for burns, a variety of skin problems, and as a laxative, as well as other usages.[20] Dioscorides and Galen referred to its laxative qualities, and the medieval, pseudo-Galenic tract, *Properties of Simple Drugs*, listed aloe under purgatives.[21] The recommended ancient dosage was two spoons of aloe with water or warm milk.[22] Avicenna spoke of its ability to expel phlegm and bile from the body.[23] All purgatives but aloe are harsh on the stomach, said Paul of Aegina (sixth century).[24]

Modern medicine postulates that aloe's cathartic action is due to a stimulation of peristalsis, probably as a result of irritation of mucous membrane especially in the upper bowels. Kneipp Herbal Tablets contain aloe as

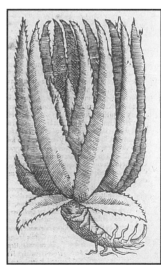

Drawing of Aloe, from Dioscorides (1566). (Courtesy National Library of Medicine.)

the principle ingredient for laxative action, but, by and large, aloe use for this action is more a product of the past than present pharmacy. Modern usage consists mostly of mixing aloe with other laxative preparations, but, then, that is exactly what Dioscorides said in the first century about aloe: "mixed with other laxative medicines (*kathartikos*) it makes them less harmful in the stomach."[25]

Buckthorn and Cascara Sagrada

Laxatives made from two species of buckthorn (*Rhamnus frangula*, or alder buckthorn; *R. catharticus*) are Weiss' next two entries.[26] The term cascara sagrada came from Mexico through the Spanish.[27] Today it is sold under proprietary names such as Caroid Laxative and as an ingredient in some brands of Milk of Magnesia, Kondremul (with mineral oil) and Ex-Lax (with phenolphthalein).[28]

There is no question that the cathartic qualities of the buckthorn were well-known from early modern times, but Alexander Tschirch, the great historian of pharmacy, attributed its earliest use as a laxative to the 9th century.[29] Avicenna clearly knew that it was a laxative.[30] The difficulty comes with interpreting the ancient evidence concerning the laxative properties of buckthorn, as separate from its dermal uses. The tree grows from north Africa to the British Isles, and Middle English medical works recommend its laxative qualities under the names of *thevethorne, thethorn, thebanthron, thethethron,* and *sisulap*.[31] Pliny spoke of its dermal effects especially as an applicant for various kinds of sores and wounds but did not directly mention a laxative effect.[32] Many of the same dermal qualities were ascribed to the buckthorn by Dioscorides and Galen, but, upon closer examination, these writiers seemed to know of its laxative qualities. Dioscorides describes two kinds of buckthorn: 1) *ramnos* called *spina alba* by the Romans and identified by Jacques André as *R. cathartica* L.; and 2) *lycium*, possibly referring to *R. petiolaris* and/or *R. lycoïdes*, and/or *R. punctata*. The only medicinal uses Dioscorides ascribed to *ramnos* were for erysipelas and herpes, two dermal afflictions.[33] On the other hand, *lycium*, also a buckthorn, was recommended for *koiliakos*, meaning "suffering in the bowels."

Galen repeats Dioscorides' usages.[34] However, a pseudo-Galenic work, *peri antemballomenon* or *Quid pro quo* (a guide to drug substitutes), reasonably confirms the use of buckthorn as a laxative, explaining that the substitute for aloe is buckthorn (*lycium*).[35] The appearance of buckthorn in this last work tells us far more than the mere listing of medicinal usages found in Dioscorides and Galen; it informs us of primary uses. Dioscorides listed over twenty medicinal uses for aloe. Conjecturally the average person on the Roman street would know all the applicaions but would associate it with just one or two main uses, just as people today know aloe for burns only. So what was the main use? Aloe was not recommended for erysipelas and herpes (unlike other dermal products), but both aloe and buckthorn were recommended as laxatives (so interpreting *koiliakos*). Therefore, with reasonable certainty, one can say that the ancients employed buckthorn (cascara sagrada). Also we learn that *koiliakos* likely meant constipation, and an important use for aloe was as a laxative.

Linseed from Flax

The same plant that produces fibers for textiles (*Linum usitatissimum* L.) also produces one of nature's best laxatives, linseed. Two factors combine in this one natural product to cause its laxative effects: the mucilage is a good bulking agent and the oil lubricates the intestines for mechanical stimulation.[36] The ancient Egyptians grew flax for cloth, and employed the oil from the seeds as a medicine, but apparently only for topical application.[37] There is no doubt, however, that the Greeks and Romans knew of linseed's laxative qualities. Dioscorides unambiguously said that it "draws out the excrement."[38] Other ancients spoke of its medicinal value for such action.[39] Today linseed is sold under such names as Linusit Gold and Linum Laxans Complex, although its use has declined in recent times.[40]

Psyllium Seed and Metamucil

Judging by the shelf space in my local pharmacy, perhaps the most widely employed laxative is psyllium seed from *Plantago pysllium* L., popularly known as Spanish psyllium, fleaseed, and fleawort. The generic name is plantain, the bane of homeowners with a lawn, where the broad leaves clutter the grass like dandelions. Its action is similar to linseed, with the active substance known as psyllium hydrophyllic mucilloid.[41] Psyllium is the last herbal laxative discussed by Weiss.[42]

The ancients knew of the medicinal properties from related species psyllium, of the same genus but perhaps not the exact *psyllium* species. Pliny, Dioscorides, Galen and Celsus describe it probably referring to two or more species.[43] Alhtough we are unable to identify the exact species, if any, to which Dioscorides referred, he said that plantain is both an antidiarrheal agent and a laxative (*koiliakos*).[44] The combination of the two actions was common in the medicinal products of the ancient world going back at least to the Ebers Papyrus (ca. 1550 B.C.E.).[45] The herbal of pseudo-Apuleius described psyllium's actions as "good for sickness of the belly" and explained that it "maintains health in the interior."[46] *Circa instans*, the popular herbal during the later Middle Ages, expressed its usage much closer to our vocabulary: contra constipacionem ventris.[47] Similarly, Avicenna spoke highly of it in his general discussion about purgative therapy.[48]

Weiss' Laxatives

The six laxatives above—from cassia to psyllium (as named by Weiss and in his order), from Senokot to Metamucil—are found in drugstores internationally. So too were they found in home drug chests, cupboards, and in the stock of drug sellers from classical antiquity. Critics may interject that my methodology is flawed because I used Weiss' *Herbal Medicine*, that a more scientific, main-line guide to modern medicine would yield different results. To answer this criticism, let us extend the list by comparing the discussion of laxative drugs in Goodman and Gilman's *Pharmacological Basis of Therapeutics*, a recognized authority on modern medicine, with what was known of them in early medicine. Goodman and Gilman classify laxatives as irritant cathartics, bulk cathartics, and emollient cathartics.

The first group among the irritant cathartics in *The Pharmacological*

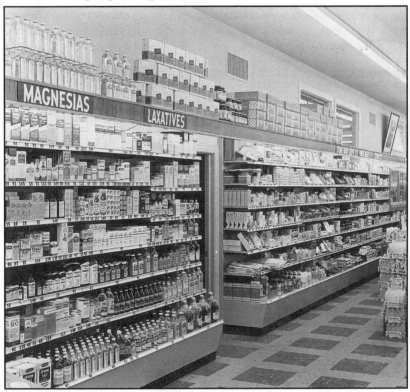

Some of the laxatives described by Dioscorides find their way in some form to pharmacy shelves. (Drug Topics Collection, American Institute of the History of Pharmacy, 1954.)

Basis of Therapeutics is the emodin cathartics: cascara sagrada, senna, rhubarb, and aloe, all already discussed. The resinous cathartics listed are jalap, colocynth, elaterin, and podophyllum, none of which was listed by Weiss.

The ancients did not know jalap, the dried root of the plant *Exogonium purga*, for a simple reason: it is product of the New World, having been imported to Europe from Mexico in the sixteenth century. Nicolas Monardes (1493-1588), a physician whose books made him the most widely-read Spanish medical writer in Europe, investigated new medicinal plants by talking with travelers on the docks at Seville. An English translation of Monardes' treatises on the drugs from the Americas by John Frampton (who was a merchant) in 1596 was entitled: "Joyfull Newes out of the New Founde Worlde." The joyful news included jalap.[49]

Colocynth, fruit of *Citrullus colocynthis*, and elaterin, from the fruit of *Ecballium elaterium*, are resinous cathartics. Ancient medical authorities testify to colocynth's purgative qualities. Dioscorides said that it was taken both orally and as an anal suppository to purge execrement.[50] The ancients were familiar with the drug named *elaterion* (Greek/Latin), which is a product manufactured from the plant in a carefully prescribed manner. Dioscorides said that the best product for laxative purposes was two years old and given in a dosage of one obol (equivalent to a modern dosage of from 3 to 6 mgm.), or about the same dose in both modern and ancient guides.[51] The last resinous laxative named in Goodman and Gilman is podophyllium, from mayapple (*Podophyllum peltatum*), a plant native to North America and probably introduced into European pharmacy through contacts with the American Indians.[52]

The last of the irritant cathartics mentioned in *Pharmacological Basis of Therapeutics* is a laxative all too familiar to the present author, castor oil. and its relative, croton oil. Castor oil comes from the *Ricinus communis* tree. It is sold as a laxative under such names as Alphamul, Emulsol, and Fleet Flavored Castor Oil. The oil is a bland emollient with a triglyceride that is hydrolyzed by the fat-splitting enzymes of glycerol and ricineolic acid, the latter stimulating through irritation of the intestinal membranes.[53] The explanation just given was not known to the ancients. Like my mother, they knew the oil and the consequencies of taking it.[54] The Egyptian Ebers papyrus expressed the consequence succinctly: it loosens the excrement.[55] Workmen at Deir el-Medîna were issued rations of castor oil at regular intervals, although it may have been for skin annointment or even lamp oil as well as a laxative.[56] The English author of an herbal, derived partly from Dioscorides, said that "croton wort" "is not a native of England," and praised its magical, not laxative, qualities.[57] Croton oil comes from the seeds of *Croton tigilium*, a tree from east Africa and southeast Asia. The Arabs introduced the drug to the Western Europeans.[58] It was unknown in the West until described by Cristoval Acosta in 1578, although it may have been introduced by the Arabs earlier.[59] The grounds for confusion lie in the fact that the Greek and Latin for castor oil (*Ricinius* plant) is *kroton* or *croton*. A Greek synonym was *kiki*, similar to the Coptic *kiki*, meaning the seeds of the plant. One can conclude, however, that the Western ancients knew it not.

Earlier in the twentieth century, mercurous chloride or calomel ($HgCl_2$) was a popular laxative. One recipe at mid-century mixed calomel with colocynth and jalap.[60] The ancients knew mercury and mercury ores as poisons and, with limited topical uses, as a medicine, but not for internal uses.[61] A pseudo-Dioscoridean alchemical tract found in the Leiden Papyrus describes the manufacture of a compound employing mercury and amonium salt.[62] A Syrian alchemical work of the eleventh or twelfth century attributed to Zosimus described the manufacture of mercurous choloride or calomel (a *vitriol*).[63] Albertus Magnus described a process of combining quicksilver (mercury) with "salt," thereby producing a white chloride, that is, calomel.[64] Ibn Sina's (Avicenna) writings on minerals, possibly based on a lost Aristotelian work on minerals, described the manufacturing of mercury compounds including their combination with salt.[65] Calomel appears as a product of the alchemists' laboratories called *mercuris dulcis*. The term salt included not only neutral salts but alkalis and acids as well.[66] Pseudo-Mesue's treatise on purgatives says that a number of laxatives come from salts of minerals.[67]

The name calomel probably derives from the same root, *mel* for "honey", *cal* from Greek *kalos*, thus "beautiful honey."[68] Geber or Jabir ibn Haiyan, the legendary alchemist (ca. tenth century), spoke of medicines as a product of mercury compound manufacture.[69] The *Pharmacopeia Londinensis* of 1618 included *mercuris dulcis*, despite a distrust of mercury and antimony compounds by apothecaries of the period.[70]

The same thing said about calomel can be ascribed to magnesium salts, which are the next class of laxatives in Goodman and Gilman: the saline cathartics.[71] The mechanism of action is complex and, without going into more detail, a number of ions in these compounds are absorbed into the intestinal wall for stimulation. Two important modern laxatives are magnesia magma (Milk of Magnesia) and potassium and sodium tartrate (Compound Effervescent Powders). While the ancients were familiar with the basic minerals, they did not manufacture them as saline compounds and administer them as laxatives.[72] A magnesium salt was the product of alchemical research during the Middle Ages.[73] Geber wrote of liquid compounds "flowing" from metallic preparations as "milk."[74] In commenting on Pseudo-Mesue's treatise on cathartics, De' Luzzi Mondino (d. 1326), a physician whose father and uncle were apothecaries, spoke of a lotion made from the mineral magnesia.[75] Therefore, through a long history of evolution the "milk of magnesia" from a late medieval pharmacy has come to be found on our shelves today.

The final class of cathartics or laxatives is called colloidal, fiber and emollients: bran, agar and tragacanth, psyllium seed, and liquid petrolatum (mineral oil). We have already discussed psyllium seed. Bran is the by-product of the milling of wheat. Dioscorides said that bran (*piturias*) of wheat benefits those with stomach cramps (*strophoumenos*, i.e., constipation).[76] In general the ancients thought that various cereals aided digestion in various ways and, of course, their grain was less refined than ours.

Agar is a species of algae, a hydrophilic colloidal substance. Dioscorides wrote of *agarikon* (which is unidentified in most guides), that is, a laxative.[77] Although many modern authorities thought that his word applies to a type of fern, it may refer to our agar. According to the method of arranging medicines by physiological effects, Dioscorides began Book Three with *agarikon* and followed it with rhubarb, both of which were, he said, laxatives.[78] *Agarikon*, he said, was taken orally in amounts of one to two obols with honeywater. Whether Dioscorides' *agarikon* is our agar is unlikely, since Galen described it as a laxative (*kathartikon*) taken from the root of a plant.[79] The great historian of pharmacognosy, Alexander Tschirch argues that agar from algae (our modern agar) is a discovery of modern times and described first in the nineteenth century.[80] The Pseudo-Mesuean treatise *On purgatives* (ca. tenth century) described *agaricus*, however, as two kinds, one from from a tree and another a fungus.[81] Similarly Petrus Matthiolus described Dioscorides' *agarikon* as: "Agaricum fungus est in arboribus nascens."[82]

Tragacanth was widely known among the ancient and medieval peoples, but it was not known as a laxative.[83] It was not listed as a laxative by Nicolaus (*Antidotarium* in Mesue, *Opera* (Venice, 1623), p. 162). Pietrus Matthiolus, however, commented that Dioscorides failed to mention tragacanth's purgative qualities, perhaps because he did not know the form (gum) in which it was taken.[84]

The last laxative on the Goodman and Gilman list is mineral oil, and it is the last historically to be discovered. Mineral oil (liquid petrolatum) is a petroleum distillate and was employed topically in the mid-ninteenth century.[85] In Germany it was given for tapeworms, but its mild laxative qualities were recognized. Mineral oil now has its place on our shelves as a laxative.[86] Interestingly, it was once mixed with agar for enhancement.[87]

Conclusions

Almost all the laxatives that appear on our pharmacists' shelves today were also found on our ancestors' shelves. In most cases they were also known to the ancients; a few (cassia, croton oil, and, possibly, tragacanth and agar) were medieval discoveries. Calomel was a product of alchemical laboratories, and mineral oil an early chemical product development whose laxative qualities were serendipitously learned, as with all the laxatives discovered. Doubtlessly it was anonymous people long ago who noted that when a certain substance was taken they had a bowel movement four to twelve hours later.

The example of laxatives as a category to test the efficacy of ancient drugs is more easily demonstrated than, say, analgesics, anodynes, and drugs for mental disturbances (psychodelics and tranquilizers, for instance). Such research will establish, I believe, that ancient medicine was rational. When that point is proved, however, many more steps need to be taken to understand the context of early medicine. Certainly, the questions are more complex than the pure empiricism of taking this-or-that for such-and-such.

Many more laxatives were known to the ancient and medieval peoples than we have discussed here. Our method has been to restrict the laxatives to those that were named in leading authorities on herbal medicines and in modern pharmacology: Weiss, and Goodman and Gilman. For example, Valerius Cordus, who wrote a leading pharmaceutical text in the sixteenth century, recorded a compounded laxative called "Electuary of Psyllium According to Mesue" that contains twenty-three herbs, including psyllium seed and rhubarb.[88] The index to Pseudo-Mesue's *De purgantium medicamentorum* classifies laxatives in two broad categories, mild (*clementer*) and strong (*valenter*) and under each according to their humoral actions, thus, *chologoga* (evacuates bile), *phlegmagoga*, and *melanogoga*.[89] Listed are forty-nine herbs and four minerals including *salis genera*.

In general, the ancients believed that good health depended to some degree on daily evacuations of the bowels and urine in amounts commensurate with the quantity of food and drink. Generally people ought not to take laxatives, but should the body need assistance, mild laxatives may be necessary.[90] Galen rejected the teachings of Erasistratus, who argued that each medicine produces juices that convert into specific body humors, thus a melanogogue converts into a fluid that expels melancholic fluids through attraction.[91] For specific ailments where one or more humors are in excess, stronger laxatives, purgatives as it were, are necessary. The ancient and medieval physicians administered specific laxatives and/or purgatives for a long list of diseases and ailments, such as erysipelas, gout, melancholy, cancer, and elephantiasis.

Because laxatives of the ancients were effective, one cannot easily persuade that the administration was rational from our perspective until one can determine the syndromes constituting ancient disease and judge whether a particular laxative would be helpful. Only when we can better understand ancient medicine in both the context of their and our sciences can we determine whether ancient medicine is rational *from our perspective*. I suspect that most people did not take medicines that they did not perceive as benefiting them. Modern scholars assert that because ancient medicine could not effectively deal with diseases, physicians administered laxatives for most ailments because there was a certain result from it, and this positive act gave people confidence that physicians knew what they were doing.[92] Whereas the hypothesis may seem to have justification, I suspect that basically it is incorrect. Can one generalize about our laxatives being beneficial within the context of our medical science? Effective, yes, but beneficial only as perceived by the individual. Certainly a laxative *qua* laxative is not a placebo. Certainly, too, their laxatives worked. How they worked in the context of their medicine should be the subject for future research. In the end, we shall learn and marvel that our ancestors were as intelligent and clever as we are.

Notes and References

1. Hans Zinsser, *Rats, Lice and History* (New York, 1996; repr. of 1935 ed.).
2. Daniel R. Headrick, *The Tools of Empire. Technology, and European Imperialism in the Nineteenth Century* (New York, 1981), pp. 66-76.
3. Arthur K. Shapiro, "The Placebo Effect in the History of Medical Treatment: Implications for Psychiatry," *American Journal of Psychiatry* 116 (1959): 298-304.
4. Harry F. Dowling, *Medicines for Man* (New York, 1973), p. 14.
5. Bernard Barber, *Drugs and Society* (New York, 1967), p. 4.
6. Oliver Wendell Holmes, *Currents and Counter-currents in Medical Science with Other Addresses and Essays* (Boston, 1856), p. 39.
7. Varro E. Tyler, Lynn R. Brady, and James E. Robbers, *Pharmacognosy*, 8th ed. (Philadelphia, 1981); *United States Dispensatory*, 25th ed. (Philadelphia, 1955); Walter Lewis and Memory Elvin-Lewish, *Medical Botany* (New York, 1977); and George Edward Trease and William C. Evans, *Pharmacognosy*, 11th ed. (London, 1978).
8. John M. Riddle, "Folk Tradition and Folk Medicine," in *Folklore and Folk Medicines*, John Scarborough, ed. (Madison, 1987), pp. 36-39.
9. The study of why laxatives were taken is a subject requiring more research because categories do not coincide readily in modern and pre-modern usages. Why laxatives are taken is well discussed by Avicenna, *Canon of Medicine*. Bk. 1, fen 4, chaps. 5-7 (Basel, 1556, pp. 139-141); and Pseudo-Mesue, *De medicamentorum purgantium...libro duo* in: Mesue, *Opera* (Venice, 1623).
10. Rudolf Fritz Weiss, *Herbal Medicine*, A. R. Meuss, trans.(Beaconfield, U.K., 1994), pp. 107-8.
11. *Physicians' Desk Reference*, 47th ed. (Montvale, N.J., 1993),*s.v.*
12. John M. Riddle, *Dioscorides on Pharmacy and Medicine* (Austin, 1985), pp. 98-104. The woman pharoah, Hapshepsut (ca. 1450 B.C.E.), brought back *kdy-kdt* (which is generally translated as cassia) from the land of Punt, somewhere in the Sudan-Somalia region where cassia grew. See J. Innes Miller, *The Spice Trade of the Roman Empire, 29 B.C. to A. D. 641* (Oxford, 1969), pp. 144, 154.)
13. Wolfgang Schneider, *Lexikon zur Arzneimittelgeschichte*, 7 vols. (Frankfurt, 1968-1975) 5/ 1: 248-51.
14 Avicenna. *Canon* (n. 9),2. 2. 154 (Basel, 1556, p. 213).
15 Avicenna. *Canon* (n. 9) 2. 2. 196; also as *cassia fistula* in Yuhanna ibn Serapion, *Practica* (Venice, 1530), fol. 63v.
16. Alexander Tschirch, *Handbuch der Pharmakognosie*, 3 vols.(Leipzig, 1910) 1/2: 629.
17. Pietro A. Mattioli, *Commentarii in sex libros Pedacii Dioscoridis* (Venice, 1565), p. 47.
18. For example, see Dioscorides. *De materia medica* 3. 2 (Wellmann, ed.); Avicenna. *Canon*.(n. 9) 2. 2. 585 ("reubarbarum," according to Gerard of Cremona, the Latin translator).

19. Weiss, *Herbal Medicine* (n. 10), pp. 109-110.
20. John Scarborough, "Roman Pharmacy and the Eastern Drug Trade. Some Problems as Illustrated by the Example of Aloe," *Pharmacy in History* 24 (1982): 137-143.
21. Dioscorides. *De materia medica* (n. 18), 3. 22; Galen. *De simplicium medicamentorum temp. ac. fac.* 6. 23 (Kühn ed., 11: 821-822); pseudo-Galen in Cambridge, Gonville and Gaius College, MS 379, 12th c., fol. 57.
22. Dioscorides. *De materia medica* (n. 18), 3. 22.
23. Avicenna. *Canon* (n. 9) 2. 2. 66 (Basel, 1556, p. 191).
24. Paul. *Seven Books of Medicine*. 1. 43, 7. 4 (Francis Adams, ed.).
25. Dioscorides, *De materia medica* (n. 18), 3. 22.
26. Weiss, *Herbal Medicine* (n. 10), pp. 110-112.
27. Tschirch, *Handbuch* (n. 16), 2/ 2: 1406.
28. *Physicians' Desk Reference*, 47th ed.(n. 11), p. 2074; *The United States Pharmacopeia*, 18th rev. ed., pp. 100-102; the Caroid Laxative I found on my local pharmacist's shelves.
29. Tschirch, *Handbuch* (n. 16), 2/ 2: 1402; Schneider, *Lexikon* (n. 13), 5/ 3: 162. The statement is also found in Friedrich A. Flückiger and Daniel Hanbury, *Pharmacographia. A History of the Principal Drugs of Vegetable Origin met with in Great Britain and British India*, 2nd ed. (London, 1879), p. 157.
30. Avicenna. *Canon* (n. 9), 2. 2. 586 (Basel, 1556): s. v. "ramech."
31. Tony Hunt, *Plant Names of Medieval England* (Cambridge, 1989), p. 131; Peter Bierbaumer, *Der botanishche Wortschatz des Altenglischen*, 3 vols. Grazer Beiträge zur englischen Philologies 1-3 (Bern/ Frankfurt, 1975-1979) 3: 236; R. J. Stracke, *The Laud Herbal Glossary* (Amsterdam, 1974), p. 1268.
32. Pliny, *Natural History*. 24. 76. 124- 77. 127 (W. H. S. Jones, ed., 7:90-92).
33. Dioscorides *De materia medica* (n. 18), 1. 90.
34. Galen. *De simplicium medicamentorum temp. ac fac.* 7. 11. 20, 17. 1 (Kühn ed., 12: 64, 111).9.
35. Pseudo Galen, *De succedaneis liber* [in Latin trans.] (Kühn ed., 19: 724).
36. Weiss, *Herbal Medicine* (n. 10), pp. 112-114; Louis S. Goodman and Alfred Gilman, *The Pharmacological Basis of Therapeutics*, 2nd. ed. (New York, 1955), p. 1019.
37. Lise Manniche, *An Ancient Egyptian Herbal* (London and Austin, 1989), p. 116.
38. Dioscorides, *De materia medica* (n. 18) 2. 103.
39. Galen. *De alimentorum facultatibus*. 1. 32 (Kühn ed. 6:549; Pliny *Natural History* (n. 32), 24. 91. 142; cf. other refs. in Schneider, *Lexikon* (n. 13), 5/2: 257-259; Tschirch, *Handbuch* 2/1: 314-328, esp. 325-7.
40. Weiss, *Herbal Medicine* (n. 10), pp. 113-114.
41. Goodman and Gilman, *Basis for Therapeutics* (n. 36), p. 1059.
42. Weiss, *Herbal Medicine* (n. 10), p. 114, who also names isapaghua or spogel seed from *Plantago ovata*, that grew in India, and came later to the West.
43. Pliny, *Natural History* (n. 32), 25. 39. 80; Dioscorides *De materia medica* (n. 18), 2. 126; Galen, *De methodo medendi*, 14. 10 (Kühn ed. 10, 981); and Celsus, *De medicina*, 6. 18. 10, cf. Jacques André, *Les noms de plantes dans la Rome antique* (Paris, 1985), p. 202.
44. Dioscorides, *De materia medica* (n, 18), 2. 126.
45. J. Worth Estes, *The Medical Skills of Ancient Egypt* (Canton, MA., 1989), p. 101.
46. *Herbarius*. 1 (Howalt and Sigerist ed.), p. 22.
47. Platearius, *Circa instans*, fol. 89 (Hans Wölfel ed.), p. 94.
48. Avicenna. *Canon* (n. 9), 1. 4. 5 (Basel, 1556, p. 140).

49. Nicolas Monardes, *Herbolaria de Indias*, Xavier Lozoya, ed. and comm. (Sevilla, 1574; repr.[Mexico?], c. 1990), p. 105; ———, *Joyfull newes out of the new-found worlde...* John Frampton, trans. (London, 1596), fol. 27v.
50. Dioscorides, *De materia medica* (n. 18), 4. 176; Galen. *De simpl. med. temp. ac fac.* 7. 38 (Kühn ed., 12: 34).
51. Dioscorides, *De materia medica* (n. 18), 4. 150; Goodman and Gilman, *Basis for Therapeutics* (n. 36), p. 1051; Avicenna, *Canon* (n. 9), 2. 2. 130 (Basel, 1556, p. 206); Tschirch, *Handbuch* (n. 16), 3/1: 821-822 for use by the ancient Egyptians, see Estes, *Medical Skills* (n. 45), p. 101.
52. Goodman and Gilman, *Basis for Therapeutics* (n. 36), pp. 1052-1053; see also Schneider, *Lexikon* (n. 13), 5/3:95-96; John Crellin and Jane Philpott, *Herbal Medicine Past and Present*, 2 vols. (Durham, N.C., 1990) 2: 301-303.
53. Goodman and Gilman, *Basis for Therapeutics* (n. 36), pp. 1053.
54. Dioscorides *De materia medica* (n. 18), 1.32, 4. 161; the ancient Mesopotamians knew the plant, as expressed in the Sumerian words, *AG.PAR* and *AT.KAN*, and the Akkadian word, *vgabegalzu.*
55. Estes, *Medical Skills* (n. 45), p. 102.
56. Manniche, *Egyptian Herbal* (n. 37), p. 143.
57. Herbarium. 171 (published in *Leechdoms, Wortcunning and Starcraft of Early England*, Thomas Oswald Cockayne, ed., 3 vols. [London, 1961 repr.], 1: 309).
58. Tschirch, *Handbuch* (n. 16) (1909), 2/1: 584.
59. Flückiger, *Pharmacographia* (n. 29), p. 565; Schneider, *Lexikon*, 5/1: 389—who says Arabs; Al-Kindi used castor oil, apparently not croton oil, in his *Medical Formulary*, Nos. 140, 143, 146 (Martin Levey trans., *Medical Formulary* [Madison, 1966] p. 238).
60. *Dispensatory of the United States of America*, 25th ed. (Philadelphia, 1955), p. 816.
61. Dioscorides, *De materia medica* (n. 18), 5. 94-5; Pliny, *Natural History* (n. 32), 33. 41. 123-42. 125; Theophrastus. *Peri lithon.* 58. 60 Caley and Richards, eds.) and discussed in the edition and translation by Earle R. Caley and John F. Richards, *Theophrastus On Stones* (Columbus, Ohio, 1956), pp. 203-205; al-Kindi (*Medical Formulary* (n. 59), 147, Levey ed.) put pure mercury in a compound as a clyster into the urethra for urinary problems.
62. Leiden Papyrus. 90 (M. Berthelot, ed., *Collection des anciens alchimistes grecs*, London, 1963, p. 47.)
63. Zosimus 3. 5-6, and identified as calomel by Edmund O. von Lippmann, *Entstehung und Ausbreitung der Alchemie* (Berlin, 1919), p. 393.
64. Albertus Magnus. *De mineralibus.* 4. 2 (Dorothy Wyckoff ed., pp. 206-208).
65. Avicenna, *De congelatione et conflutinatione lapidum* (E. J.Holmyard and D. C. Mandeville, eds., in Arabic and Latin, pp. 34, 38-40).
66. Maurice P. Crossland, *Historical Studies in the Language of Chemistry* (London, 1962), p. 77.
67. Pseudo-Mesue, *De medicamentorum purgantium* (Venice, 1623), fols. 66v-67.
68. According to Leonard Goldwater (*Mercury. A History of Quick silver* [Baltimore, 1972], p. 168) the name may be attributed to Turquet de Mayenne (1573-1655) who experimented with mercurial salts. Goldwater says correctly that the *OED* (s.v.) is incorrect in tracing its etymology to *melas*, meaning black.
69. Gerber, *Of the Sum of Perfection.* 16 (E. J. Holmyard, ed.[London, 1928], pp. 111, 113).
70. Maurice Crosland, *Historical Studies in the language of Chemistry* (Cambridge, MA, 1962), p. 95.

71.   Goodman and Gilman, *Basis for Therapeutics* (n. 36), pp. 1056-1058.
72.   Dioscorides, *De materia medica* (n. 18), 5. 143 (*serpentine*, a magnesium silicate); 5. 106 (*stupt-ria*, a sulfate compound that includes potassium); Theophrastus, *Peri lithon* (n. 61), 41 (magnesia).
73.   M. Berthelot, *Collection des anciens alchimistes grecs* (London, 1963), p. 256.
74.   *Of the Invention or Verity, or, Perfection* (E. J. Holmyard, ed., London, 1928, p. 207.
75.   Mondino, "Commentary," to Pseudo-Mesue, *De medicamentorum purgantium*, in: *Opera* (Venice, 1623), fol 14v.
76.   Dioscorides, *De materia medica* (n. 18), 2. 85.
77.   Dioscorides, *De materia medica* (n. 18), 3. 1.
78.   See the discussion of the identification of *agarikon* in Riddle, *Contraception*, p. 182, n. 60.
79.   Galen. *De simpl. med. temp. et fac.* 6. 5 (Kühn ed. 11: 813-814).
80.   Tschirch, *Handbuch* (n. 16) (1909), 2, pt. 1: 304-314.
81.   Pseudo-Mesue, *De medicamentorum purgamentorum* (Venice, 1623), fol. 51
82.   Mattioli, *Commentario* (Venice, 1565), p. 637.
83.   Theophrastus. *Enquiry into plants.* 9. 15. 8; Dioscorides, *De materia medica* (n. 18), 3. 20; Paul of Aegina. *Books of Medicine.* 7. 3. s.v.; Galen. *De simpl. med. temp. ac fac.* 8. 19. 8 (Kühn ed. 12:143; Pliny. *Natural History* (n. 32), 26. 87. 140; see discussion by Tschirch, *Handbuch* (n. 16), 2/ 1: 404-405.
84.   Mattioli, *Commentario* (Venice, 1565), p. 677.
85.   *The Pharmacopoeia of the United States of America.* 6th ed. (New York, 1882), p. 248; cf. *The Dispensatory of the United States of America*, 7th ed. (Philadelphia, 1847), p. 534.
86.   *Dispensatory of the United States*, 25th ed. (Philadelphia, 1955), pp. 1027-1028.
87.   *Dispensatory of the United States*, 25th ed. (n. 86), p. 1028.
88.   Valerius Cordus, *Dispensatorium, Hoc Est, Pharmacorum Consiciendorum Ratio* (Venice, 1556), pp. 150-151.
89.   Pseudo-Mesue's *De purgantium medicamentorum* in Mesue, *Opera* (Venice, 1623) fol. 23v.
90.   Galen. *Comm. Hippocr. de humor.* 1. 12 (Kühn ed. 13: 105-149), for broad context of purging in various forms; Paul of Aegina, *Seven Books of Medicine.* 7. 4 (Francis Adams, ed., pp.480-485); Celsus. *De medicina.* 5. 5.
91.   Galen. *De purgantium medicamentorum facultate.* 1 (Kühn ed., 11:324-325).
92.   This assertion I have heard from time to time at conferences but I know no one who has said it in print.

The Therapeutic Crisis of the Eighteenth Century

by J. Worth Estes

Most drugs discussed in this volume were created in the twentieth century, and most are known to act selectively at specific physiological and biochemical target sites. Seldom does a modern physician prescribe a drug that affects the entire body, the "system," as it was called in the eighteenth century. But at that time, most drugs did exactly that, as far as anyone could tell, although some parts of the body might be affected more than others by any given remedy. Moreover, the number of explanations of drug actions grew throughout the century until, by 1800, doctors faced a possible crisis when making their therapeutic decisions.

Humoralism

The pathophysiologic concepts used by eighteenth-century physicians were unlike our own ideas of specific diseases with specific causes and specific treatments. The primary concept that dominated medical therapeutics between about 500 B.C. and A. D. 1850 held that the maintenance or restoration of health required stabilizing the equilibria among the four putative liquid "humors" of the body: blood, which was associated with heat and moisture; phlegm, associated with moisture and cold; black bile, with cold and dryness; and yellow bile, with dryness and heat. When any of the humors increased or decreased in quantity or quality, from whatever cause, the resulting destabilization of the system led to the production of correlative symptoms.

This explanation of illness provided satisfactory explanations of eighteenth-century doctors' bedside observations, permitting them to conclude that unbalanced humors could be rebalanced by drugs with appropriately opposite properties. For instance, because bilious fevers were associated with dryness and increased body heat, they should be treated with cool, moist drugs, to restabilize the blood and yellow bile, the humors that were most seriously disturbed in such patients.

Solidism

The first major new theory of disease to achieve prominence in the eighteenth century followed from the medical hypotheses popularized by Friedrich Hoffmann of Halle from about 1695 and by Hermann Boerhaave of Leiden from 1708, and further developed by William Cullen of Edinburgh from 1776.[1] Although each gave different emphasis to the involvement of the nerves and blood vessels in the manifestation of disease, their theories shared the underlying premise that symptoms were the consequences of disturbed, or unbalanced, irritability of the solid fibrous components of those two tissues, as expressed by their tone—their innate strength and elasticity, disturbances that could secondarily disturb the humors. Historians have since labelled this concept as the "solidist theory," to distinguish it from the older humoral theory, based on the body's fluid components.

Hoffmann and others expanded the operational definition of humors to include all the different secretions and excretions of the body. In effect, they thought of both vessels and nerves as hollow tubes that propel their contents through the body with forces proportional to the tone of their constituent fibers, and producing humors characteristic of the organs that manufacture them. Boerhaave, for instance, argued that disease occurs when a patient's fibers are either too weak or too stiff, and that such imbalanced fibers, in conjunction with the content of the patient's diet, can secondarily alter any of his multiple humors. That is, the body is healthy when blood or the supposed "nerve fluids" can circulate freely, or when sweat, urine, and feces can be expelled freely, and so forth. As Hoffmann wrote, "whoever eats well, digests well, and excretes well, is healthy."[2]

J. Worth Estes, M.D., is Professor of Pharmacology at the Boston University School of Medicine, where his research specialty is the history of therapeutics. He is the author of many books and papers on the history of drugs, including *Hall Jackson and the Purple Foxglove: Medical Practice and Research in Revolutionary America, 1760-1820* (1979) and *Dictionary of Protopharmacology: Therapeutic Practices, 1700-1850* (1990). His most recent essay is "Changing Fashions in Therapeutics," which appears in *Caduceus* 11(1995): 65-72. Dr. Estes is also Secretary-Treasurer of the American Association for the History of Medicine.

    Solidist theorizing led to the development of two major approaches to
therapy.[3] If a patient's symptoms indicated that they were caused by
hyperirritability of his system, manifested chiefly by a rapid heart rate, the
physician's immediate goal was to lower the pulse, which would indicate that
he had corrected the excessive irritability. Thus, the first step in the conventional treatment of such illnesses consisted of the so-called "depletive,"
"evacuant," or "sedative" regimen, using remedies thought to be directly
antispasmodic or indirectly sedative, to remove or neutralize the symptoms
produced by increased body tones. The major depletive drugs were emetics,
cathartics, diuretics, narcotics, refrigerants, and blisters; the blisters were assumed to counterirritate underlying pyrogenic inflammatory processes. These
agents were most important as the initial steps in the standard regimen prescribed for fevers, the most prevalent illnesses of the eighteenth century.
Similar reasoning also led doctors to rely on bleeding to reduce tension and
tone in the arteries, as well as to remove foul humors from the blood, in the
early stages of febrile illnesses. Standard depletive regimens also involved
avoiding whatever would "feed" the internal fires of the inflammation, such
as meat and exercise. Other therapies designed to reduce the force of the fevered circulation included externally applied heat and diaphoretic drugs,
which stimulated the release of heat as sweat; both measures were thought to
dilate and relax blood vessels on the surface of the fevered body, to facilitate
the loss of pathological heat. Thus, a decreased heart rate was the principal
criterion of drug efficacy in fevers.
    By contrast, the second major therapeutic mode relied on stimulating
measures to increase the tone of a debilitated heart and arteries, inducing
them to contract more forcefully, thus speeding the removal of whatever
pathogenic factors had weakened the patient. This became the standard second step in fever therapy. Stimulating the nerves was assumed to secondarily
increase the activity of cardiovascular tissues as well as that of the brain, but
stimulants were also used to strengthen, say, the nerves in paralyzed limbs or
the arteries in poorly functioning kidneys. Drugs classified as "tonics" were a
principal simulating method, although cold water or electricity from a static
electricity generator were occasionally used for the same purposes. Tonics
were thought to be particularly valuable for speeding the recuperation of patients who had been weakened by fever. In addition, some drugs used as
evacuants could be interpreted simultaneously as stimulants of specific tissues; emetics, for instance were said to stimulate the stomach, just as diaphoretics were assumed to stimulate the arteries that supply the sweat glands.
    Few of the drugs used in either evacuant or stimulant therapeutic regi-
mens were new to medical practice in the eighteenth century. For instance,
ancient humoralism had originally encouraged the use of emetics to remove
pathogenic materials or foul humors—especially yellow bile—via the stomach. Solidism permitted the additional conclusion that emetics diverted

pathogenic irritations from deep within the body to the gastrointestinal arteries, whence the excess heat generated by the feverish pulse would be freely dissipated into the stomach cavity and then eliminated from the body as it passed on out into the ambient air. At the same time, the act of vomiting was evidence that an emetic had strengthened the stomach's fibers, giving them added tone that would then be transmitted to the rest of the body via the nerves that connect the stomach with the central nervous system.

Chemical Therapeutics

Chemical concepts of pathophysiological processes had entered medical thinking in the mid-sixteenth century, but even chemically adept physicians, such as Boerhaave and Cullen, could not fully exploit such ideas until Antoine Lavoisier's experiments permitted the conclusion that the carbon and hydrogen in food "burn" when they combine with oxygen in the body, to form carbon dioxide.[4] By the 1790s, physicians could begin adding his chemical concepts to their humoral and solidist medical thinking, partly because the new information made it easier to interpret a fast respiratory rate as one more manifestation of increased combustion within the fevered body, along with a fast pulse. That is, they thought that rapid breathing was necessary for replacing the oxygen that was being burned up in febrile patients. Indeed, followers of Lavoisier, especially Antoine Fourcroy, argued that oxygen itself was an appropriate remedy, although he was unable to provide convincing proof of its efficacy. Others interpreted Lavoisier to fit their own theories. For instance, Christoph Girtanner of Göttingen postulated that the degree of irritability manifested by the fibrous components of the "system" was directly proportional to the amount of oxygen to which they were exposed. His reasoning helped explain the efficacy of standard depletive remedies, including bleeding, as the result of removing excess, pathogenic, oxygen, while others tried to show that oxidants can restore irritability to normal.

The new "pneumatic" chemistry of respiratory gases also helped explain older notions about acidic and alkaline remedies, by noting that, for instance, when carbon dioxide dissolves in water, it forms carbonic acid, which can form neutral salts when it reacts with certain bases. Since the sixteenth century the most important aspect of pathological acid-base imbalance had been physicians' assumption that sites of inflammation were characterized by their alkalinity. Therefore, fevers and related diseases should be curable with acid remedies. By the end of the eighteenth century, then, chemical notions of therapeutics had provided new rationales for therapeutically balancing the body's acids and alkalis.

Keep in mind that these theories—humoral, solidist, and chemical—were not competing explanations of patients' symptoms. Instead, doctors relied on all three simultaneously to explain their clinical observations at the bedside.

Brunonianism and other Notions

Other new ideas must have added to the potential for confusion in medical thinking. For instance, in the 1770s John Brown of Edinburgh began arguing that life is not an inherent property of the body, but, rather, that the phenomena of life depend on the degree to which the body, or its tissues, can be excited by external stimuli. If a patient, or some part of him, was insufficiently excitable, Brown classified his illness as "asthenic;" if the patient was hyperexcitable, his illness was called "sthenic." To a much greater extent than was possible in the humoral and solidist traditions, he thought the degree of a patient's illness could be precisely quantified on an eighty point scale.

Brown concluded that therapy should be directed toward restoring the patient's excitability to normal with the only appropriate remedies—stimulants (see **Table 1**). First, he said that appropriate therapy for sthenic diseases—those characterized by excessive excitability—required remedies with only weakly stimulating properties. Most such remedies were already in routine use as depletive or evacuant remedies in humoral and solidist regimens. By contrast, patients who had been weakened by asthenic diseases required even stronger stimulants, including methods that were also used in ancient restorative regimens. The one major difference was Brown's conviction that four drugs—musk, camphor, ether, and opium, in that order of increasing potency—were the best stimulants for asthenic patients. Because his system was based on the notion that disease occurs when the body's excitability reaches either of the extremes on his eighty point scale, he argued that health would be restored when the disturbed excitability was returned to its normal twenty point range at the center of his scale. Thus, Brown's concept, like the humoral, solidist, and chemical approaches to therapy, relied on the notion of balancing the body's "system."

Table 1. Remedies suitable for treating sthenic and asthenic illnesses.

STHENIA	ASTHENIA
Bleeding, if pulse is fast	Exercise
Cold	Heat
Vegetable diet	Meat diet
Water, Beer	Strong wine, Spirits
Emetics	Musk
Cathartics	Camphor
Diaphoretics	Ether
	Opium

According to John Brown, *The Elements of Medicine* [1795 rev. ed.] (Portsmouth, N.H.: William & Daniel Treadwell, 1803), chs. 9-10

Some aspects of Brown's therapeutics had been in conventional use long before he developed his theory, and some of his novel ideas were assimilated into standard regimens throughout Europe. However, his system failed to win general acceptance as a guiding principle, not because of its unprovable premises, but because it became apparent that it was virtually impossible to measure the degree of a given patient's excitability with the accuracy he demanded, which precluded choosing a suitable remedy in the precise dose his system required.[6]

The last significant therapeutic novelty of the Enlightenment was Benjamin Rush's hypothesis—his certainty—that all disease is attributable to generalized debility, which produces a compensatory increase in pathological irritability. Although his idea may have been inspired by verifiable bedside observations,[7] it gained few adherents even among Rush's friends and colleagues in Philadelphia. Indeed, the patients he treated with multiple bleedings and large doses of mercury, in the form of calomel, must have had their own reservations about Rush's methods—unless, of course, they survived his prescriptions.

A few other theories were only ludicrous, even at the time. For instance, Franz Anton Mesmer advocated treating patients with disturbances in what he termed their "animal magnetism" by transferring, via a hand-held metal rod, the pathogenic forces that afflicted them into a foul-smelling tub filled with "magnetized water." The controversy engendered by what appeared even then to be charlatanry led to the appointment of a French commission (Benjamin Franklin and Lavoisier were among its members) that used reason and experiment to demolish Mesmer's lucrative fad in 1784. And then there was Johann Kämpf's "doctrine of the infarctus," which postulated that all disease was attributable to fecal impaction,[8] but his theory probably benefited only the sellers of cathartics and enemas. Thus, although the thinking of the majority of eighteenth-century physicians could encompass two or more unproven pathophysiological concepts simultaneously, they were able to reject others.

The Problem of Establishing Efficacy

While physicians adhered to drugs that had been in common usage for some time—centuries, in most cases—several writers realized that it was the theories that changed, not the drugs. One of the most acute observers of medical theorizing was Thomas Jefferson. In 1807 he wrote to Dr. Caspar Wistar in Phildelphia:

> . . . the adventurous physician goes on, and substitutes presumption for knowledge. . . . He establishes for his guide some fanciful theory of corpuscular attraction, of chemical agency, of mechanical powers, of stimuli, of irritability accu-

mulated or exhausted, of depletion by the lancet and repletion by mercury, or some other ingenious dream, which lets him into all nature's secrets at short hand. On the principle which he thus assumes, he forms his table of nosology, arrays his diseases into families, and extends his curative treatment, by analogy, to all the cases he has thus arbitrarily marshalled together. I have lived myself to see the disciples of Hoffman[n], Boerhaave, Stahl, Cullen, Brown, succeed one another like the shifting figures of a magic lantern. . . .The patient, treated on the fashionable theory, sometimes gets well in spite of the medicine. The medicine therefore restored him.[9]

Jefferson recognized that the circulation, which Harvey had discovered nearly two hundred years earlier, and the more recent discoveries of respiratory gas exchange, were observable facts, while humoralism and solidism were insupportable conjectures that should be abandoned. As he said, "The only sure foundations of medicine are, an intimate knowledge of the human body, and observation of the effects of medicinal substances on [it]."[10]

But what criteria could his contemporaries use when choosing substances for their patients? Why did doctors continue to prescribe the 1300 remedies they did,[11] and why had many of those drugs remained in use for centuries? And, why did patients continue to take those drugs, many of which had famously unpleasant effects, when only a tiny handful of them could have had any truly beneficial effect?

One of the most frequently prescribed drugs was the Peruvian bark, or cinchona. Imported from South America since at least the 1650s, it had been found to be nearly always effective in the treatment of the malarias (then called "intermittent fevers"), characterized by shaking chills, followed by a febrile period, occurring at regular intervals.[12] But by the late eighteenth century, Peruvian bark was being prescribed for the majority of patients with any fever.[13] Indeed, its remarkable therapeutic success rate in the intermittent fevers led doctors to prescribe it for patients with the "continued fevers" that included most other febrile illnesses. Over the years physicians almost always found that, after initial evacuant or depletive therapies had put fever patients on the road to recovery, the subsequent administration of Peruvian bark, while the patient was still debilitated, strengthened and thus restabilized the body.

Most physicians probably inferred that Peruvian bark was a tonic because debilitated patients regained their strength after taking it. Cullen explained that it is a strengthening remedy whose powers are transmitted via the nerves from the stomach to the rest of the body. He argued that it was indicated for patients who had been weakened by fever, regardless of its type, and whose inflammatory symptoms had been removed by conventional depletive measures.[14] Moreover, the astringent properties of the bitter quinine in the bark must have facilitated the conclusion that the drug contracted—that is, strengthened—the body's tissues.

Experimental Evidence of Efficacy

The widely accepted efficacy of many fever remedies might have been explained by a series of experiments performed by the Rev. Stephen Hales.[15] He is remembered today chiefly for his pioneering measurements of blood pressure in a horse, published in 1733, but buried away in the same book are his studies of the effects on arterial diameter of several drugs that had long been used to treat fevers.

Hales probably invented the novel method he used for studying the effects of drugs on arteries. After exsanguinating a dog, he slit its small intestine opposite the side penetrated by the mesenteric arteries. Then he inserted a copper tube into the descending aorta, and measured the time required for fixed amounts of fluids poured into the tube to run out of it as they passed into the gut lumen. He found that heat dilates arteries, and that cold, as well as tonic drugs like oak bark, camomile flowers, cinnamon, and Peruvian bark were vasoconstrictors. This explained why the latter could correct the debilitating weakness that characterized most serious fevers after the crisis had passed. So did alcohol and mineral waters, especially those that contained substantial amounts of iron.[16]

Hales's conclusions were consistent with contemporary solidist concepts of drug actions. However, these experiments are not cited in the later clinical literature, although doctors did cite other parts of the same book. That is, physicians probably simply read about these experiments, nodded their agreement with Hales's conclusions, and then moved on to the next chapter. Nevertheless, Hales's mesenteric artery preparation was an innovative experimental approach to understanding drug action, which eighteenth-century practitioners equated with efficacy.

Several British and Continental investigators devised animal and human experiments to explore the sites and mode of action of opium, which was unarguably effective in controlling bowel movements, pain, and wakefulness. **Table 2** summarizes the results of several series of experiments designed to determine how opium produces its most obvious effects on the nervous system and the heart. Some of the frog experiments foreshadowed Claude Bernard's classical experiments in which he demonstrated the effect of curare on the neuromuscular junction in the mid-nineteenth century. By

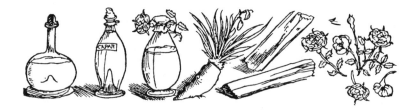

contrast, these earlier experiments did not reveal, at least to the satisfaction of impartial commentators, whether opium affects nerves directly or via the circulation. Neither did similar experiments on animal and human subjects lead to any firm conclusions about opium's effect on the heart. Indeed, there was no agreement as to whether opium increased or decreased heart rate, or whether that effect, whatever it was, was associated with the drug's effect on nervous tissue, or with its clearcut effect on gut motility. But at least several investigators were trying to answer important questions about one of the century's few truly effective medicines.

Table 2. Summary of conclusions of experimental attempts to ascertain how opium affects the nervous system and the heart.

Freind, *et al.* (1711 ff.):	Dog & cat vessels *in vivo* & *in vitro*	rarefied blood → ↑ arterial diameter → compressed nerves → ↓ neural function
Whytt (1756)	Frogs w/o brain or cord	↓ neural function directly
Monro II (1761):	Frog, exposed sciatic nerve & microscopic study of blood flow in small vessels	↓ neural function directly & via circulation
Fontana (1781)	Frogs (>300), sciatic nerve preparation	↓ neural function via circulation
von Haller (1752)	Frogs, dogs	↓ peristalsis, ↓ contractility
von Haller & Sproegel (1751)	Frogs *in vivo* & frog hearts *in vitro*	↓ heart rate, cardiac arrest
Garthshore (1764)	Self	↑ heart rate; ↓ irritability, sleep
Bard (1765)	Self, 3 friends, & 6 convalescent patients	↓ heart rate
von Haller (1776)	Self	↑ heart rate

Collated from Andreas-Holger Maehle, "Pharmacological experimentation with opium in the 18th century," in Roy Porter and Mikulás Teich, eds., *Drugs and Narcotics in History* (Cambridge: Cambridge University Press, 1995), pp. 52-76.

In one famous eighteenth-century clinical trial, naval surgeon James Lind evaluated six methods for curing scurvy at sea. **Table 3** outlines the protocol in which he administered six different treatments to six groups of two patients each. The only men who recovered fully were the two who received oranges and lemons until Lind's supply of the fruits ran out after six days.

Table 3. Lind's clinical trial of antiscorbutics.

REMEDY	DAILY DOSE
CIDER	1 quart
ELIXIR VITRIOL (H_2SO_4)	25 drops
VINEGAR	2 spoonfuls
SEA WATER	1/2 pint
ORANGES & LEMONS	2 oranges, 1 lemon
ELECTUARY (of garlic, myrrh, mustard, etc.), with tamarinds, barley water, & creme of tartar	One (?)

From, James Lind, *Treatise on the Scurvy,* 3rd ed. (London: S. Crowder, D. Wilson and G. Nicholls, T. Cadell, T. Becket and Co., G. Pearch, and W. Woodfall, 1772), pp. 191-93

Eighteenth-century physicians regarded scurvy as a form of febrile inflammation, which meant that it was associated with alkalinity. Thus, it was perfectly reasonable to treat scurvy with acids such as these. Moreover, according to solidist thinking, some acids were regarded as stimulating tonics that would strengthen the body's fibers when they had been weakened by disease, and scurvy was characterized clinically by serious weakness.

Although today Lind is often said to have compared his test therapy, citrus fruits, with five negative control groups, he did not know—he had no *a priori* reason to know—that five of these six acids were not truly effective. He only set out to compare the relative merits of six acids in treating a presumed fever associated with alkalinity, and, sure enough, one of them worked better than the other five. In short, his experiment merely validated current explanations of the pathogenesis of scurvy and its appropriate treatment. Indeed, Lind himself did not recommend citrus fruits more than other classical antiscorbutics, so it was another fifty years before the Royal Navy adopted limes as standard issue on its ships. That is, Lind's clinical trial merely validated the therapeutic *status quo*, as had Stephen Hales's experiments in the 1730s.

The one major new remedy to burst on the eighteenth-century medical scene was the purple foxglove, digitalis. Used for many years without any remarkable therapeutic effect, it had been abandoned earlier in the century after it was found to be toxic to two French turkeys. In 1775 William Withering of

Birmingham, England, began a ten-year clinical trial of its efficacy and toxicity in the treatment of dropsy in about 158 patients.

One of the problems he faced was the choice of an optimally effective pharmaceutical preparation of digitalis. His data, summarized at the top of **Table 4**, showed Withering that three common methods of preparing digitalis—the decoction, dried leaf, and infusion—were about equally effective as remedies. However, the decoction proved to be more toxic than the others, presumably because it contained a number of impurities leached from the container in which it was prepared, so he abandoned the decoction.[17] Other investigators also found the new drug to be effective, although, for unknown reasons, two of them—Quin and Ferriar—achieved substantially lower cure rates. At any rate, Withering's exemplary experimental study, bolstered by his use of historic controls, directly stimulated the use of digitalis for dropsical

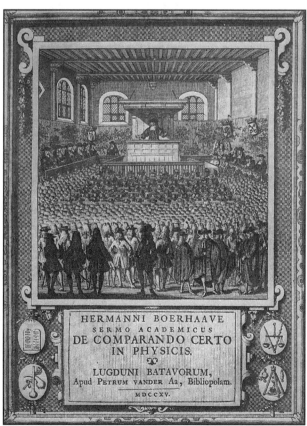

The medical hypotheses popularized by Hermann Boerhaave at Leiden led toward the solidist theory of disease. The title page of his 1715 text shows the popularity of Boerhaave's lectures.

HERMANNI BOERHAAVE
SERMO ACADEMICUS
DE COMPARANDO CERTO
IN PHYSICIS.

LUGDUNI BATAVORUM,
Apud PETRUM VANDER Aa, Bibliopolam.
MDCCXV.

patients for the next fifty years.[18]

Table 4. Early clinical trials of digitalis.

INVESTIGATOR	PREPARATION (N)	CURES (%)	TOXICITY(%)
Withering, 1785	Decoction (15)	80 %	55 %
	Dried leaf (35)	77 %	14 %
	Infusion (78)	69 %	19 %
Jackson, 1790	Infusion (11)	73 %	9 %
Quin, 1790	Infusion (11)	46 %	18 %
Maclean, 1810	Infusion (94)	83 %	16 %
Ferriar, 1816	Unknown (29)	45 %	21 %
Blackall, 1818	Infusion (35)	71 %	17 %
Beller, *et al.*, 1971	Leaf & pure glycosides (135)	100 %	23-29 %

From, Estes, *Hall Jackson and the Purple Foxglove* (see n. 18 below), p. 183.

A clinical trial of several established diuretics in the treatment of dropsy was carried out around 1780 (see **Table 5**). Digitalis did not produce nearly as many cures as current oral reports of Withering's work had prob-

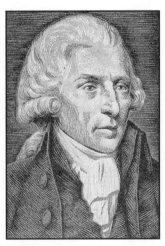
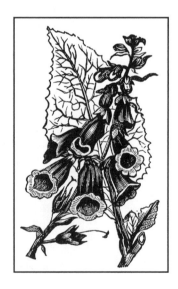

William Withering and the foxglove.

ably led the unidentified investigator to expect, but three standard diuretics—cream of tartar, calomel, and Becher's Tonic Pills (made with black hellebore, myrrh, and blessed thistle) were as effective as others had found digitalis to be (see **Table 4**).

Table 5. Summary of comparative clinical trials of eight modes of treating dropsy in the late eighteenth century, probably at Edinburgh.

Treatment	No. of Courses	No. Cured or Relieved	No. Not Cured or Relieved *
DIGITALIS	25	12	13
Cream of Tartar	11	10	1
Calomel	6	5	1
Becher's Tonic Pills	6	5	1
Nicotiana	2	1	1
Squills	1	0	1
Dover's Powder	1	1	0
[Abdominal tap]	2	0	2
	54	34	20

* includes 9 deaths (= 19% of all patients)

See n. 19 below.

Even if most physicians agreed that digitalis was effective in the treatment of dropsy, they argued over its mechanism of action. Withering assumed that digitalis removes the excess fluid associated with dropsy by acting primarily on the kidneys to produce diuresis. Others were not so sure. Because the pulse was usually rapid in dropsy, some doctors classified it as a fever, caused when blood vessels became too weak to reabsorb normal tissue fluids. Therefore, since the pulse almost always returned to its customary range when digitalis was administered, many physicians considered the new drug a sedative of the vascular system.

Other physicians performed experiments they hoped would settle the matter, by measuring the pulse rates of patients, themselves, and their friends, after administration of digitalis. The pulse first rose in some of these experiments, confirming the hypotheses of those who assumed the drug was a stimulating tonic with an effect on the heart that resembled Withering's hypothesis that it affected the kidneys. But experimenters who observed that the pulse fell concluded that it was, indeed, a sedative. The solution to the paradox would not be reached until the early twentieth century.[20] Nevertheless, digitalis continued to be prescribed for patients with dropsy until the 1830s, when it disappeared from general medical practice, although for reasons that had nothing to do with its efficacy in dropsy.[21]

Clinical Evidence of Efficacy

Eighteenth-century doctors continued to use drugs and analogous measures to adjust, to fine-tune, the body's internal equilibria, its balances, regardless of just what they thought had disturbed its humors or tones or acidity in the first place. Several academic physicians, notably at Edinburgh, occasionally subjected newly imported drugs to clinical evaluation, but not as systematically as Withering had studied digitalis, and with virtually no negative or even historic controls. Nevertheless, they did manage to reject a few new drugs, but only because they appeared to be no better than those already available.

If physicians did not rely on experimental evidence in making their therapeutic choices, and if they seldom carried out explicit clinical trials, what evidence did they use when deciding whether to prescribe any given drug? Because catharsis, vomiting, sweating, diuresis, blistering, or bleeding usually did occur when the physician intended them to, or because the pulse and respiratory rates decreased, doctors and patients alike thought they had sufficient evidence that the remedies had done something beneficial for the patient's body.[22] But was there some other, less presumptive, reason why patients—and their doctors—tolerated the unpleasantnesses associated with their favorite remedies? And, how did they deal with the uncertainties of drug efficacy?

Table 6 shows the discharge status of a large sample of Edinburgh Royal Infirmary patients in the eighteenth century. About 81% of all patients were discharged as completely or partially cured, and 73% of all teaching ward patients recovered to some extent. Although Dr. Andrew Duncan thought that only about 60% of his teaching ward patients had recovered to any degree, he concluded that nearly one fourth of them would have recovered without any treatment.[23] The higher death rates among teaching patients are not surprising, since they were among the sickest in the hospital. Moreover, because they came from lower socio-economic brackets, they were probably less well nourished or otherwise prepared for eventual recovery.

Clinical results for substantial numbers of patients at the Philadelphia Dispensary over seven years beginning in 1786 are abstracted in Table 7. The overall death rate was nearly 4.5%, about the same as at Edinburgh. It is instructive to examine the death and recovery rates for patients with the various categories of disease listed. The death rate was about 5% for infectious diseases, by far the most prevalent of all the diagnoses made at the Dispensary and elsewhere on land and sea. By contrast, deaths were far more frequent among patients with conditions—like dropsy—that are now known to affect the heart, about 20%. That is, cure rates and death rates varied with diagnosis, as suggested by these data, and probably with socio-economic status, as suggested by the Edinburgh data. Mortality rates among other eighteenth-century adult patient populations were in the same range, about 2.7% to 6%, except when a major epidemic disease, like small pox or yellow fever, occurred. But on the whole, the eighteenth-century records that have been studied so far show that about nineteen out of twenty adult patients survived their illnesses.[24]

Table 6. Selected therapeutic results at the Edinburgh Royal Infirmary in the eighteenth century.

	All Patients* 1770-1800	Teaching Ward Patients, 1771-1799	Dr. Duncan's Ward Patients, Feb-Apr 1795
(N)	(3047)	(808)	(65)
Completely cured	70.8 ± 7.8 %	55.9 %	38.5 %
Partially cured	10.5 ± 3.8	16.8	21.5
Not cured	0.3	0.2	29.1
Died	4.0 ± 1.3	7.8	6.2
Discharged self	5.5 ± 2.7	9.7	4.7
Other disposition	8.9	9.6	———

* Mean + S.D. for every fifth year

Collated from data in Guenter B. Risse, *Hospital Life in Enlightenment Scotland* (n. 3).

Conclusions

Many, if not most, eighteenth-century physicians acknowledged the operation of what they called the *vis medicatrix naturae*, the healing power of nature, even if they seldom relied on it alone. Still, many drugs were presumed to assist nature in restoring the body to normal. Not until the publication of Jacob Bigelow's celebrated *Discourse on Self-Limited Diseases* in 1835 did the notion that many diseases tend to disappear without medical treatment begin to attract widespread professional recognition.[25]

Today we know that few remedies used during the Enlightenment could have provided much in the way of true cures. But doctors thought they were providing effective treatments; after all, the vast majority of their adult patients survived. What neither doctors nor patients could have known at that time is that the survivals were really evidence of the efficacy of the body's normal repair mechanisms, such as the immune and inflammatory response systems, without which recovery rates would probably have been minimal. Recovery rates even as high as 95% would surely not be taken as proof of efficacy today.

Table 7. Dispositions of 9683 adult patients treated at the Philadelphia Dispensary in 1786-1792.

Modern Disease Categories	Death Rate (%)	"Cure" Rate (%)	% of All Diagnoses	% of All Deaths
Cardiovascular	23.2	42.1	2.5	12.8
Central nervous system	3.6	47.1	1.4	1.1
Genitourinary	2.0	63.3	0.5	0.2
Musculoskeletal	1.0	70.1	6.4	1.4
Female reproductive tract	0	82.8	2.9	0
Infectious	5.5	84.0	65.1	79.2
Eye, Head, and Neck	0.5	84.8	2.3	0.2
Gastrointestinal (non-infectious)	1.1	89.5	8.4	2.1
Accidents	0.7	91.9	5.6	0.9
Other	1.9	62.3	4.9	2.1
ALL PATIENTS	4.5	62.3	(100)	(100)

From: J. Worth Estes, "Making therapeutic decisions with protopharmacologic evidence," *Transactions & Studies of the College of Physicians of Philadelphia*, n.s. 1 (1979): 116-37.

Eighteenth-century doctors could not know that measures such as catharsis, vomiting, sweating, diuresis, blisters, or bleeding were unable to affect their patients' recoveries. They lacked the data, which are optimally collected only in negatively controlled double-blind trials, that would have permitted them to infer that most of their medicines had not truly helped their patients. They could only conclude that they had preserved their patients' lives. Some may have been frustrated by competing pathophysiological theories, and a few may have recognized, along with Jefferson, the intellectual confusion implicit in the number of possible interpretations of how drugs affected their patients' bodies, but they—and their patients—could continue to be confident in their empirically validated therapeutic methods. We can recognize that most of their drugs—with the exceptions of Peruvian bark, opium, and digitalis—could not have contributed substantially to recovery from illness, and even then only in the short run.

Jefferson accepted the supremacy of the *vis medicatrix naturae* when he summarized what he and most academically-oriented regular physicians perceived to be the usual practice:

> We observe nature providing for the re-establishment of order, by exciting some salutary evacuation of the morbific matter, or by some other operation which escapes our imperfect senses and researches. She brings on a crisis, by stools, vomiting, sweat, urine, expectoration, bleeding, &c., which, for the most part, ends in the restoration of healthy action. Experience has taught us, also, that there are certain substances, by which, applied to the living body, internally or externally, we can at will produce these same evacuations, and thus do, in a short time, what nature would do but slowly, and do effectually, what perhaps she would not have strength to accomplish. . . . Where, then, we have seen a disease . . . relieved by a certain natural evacuation or process, whenever that disease recurs under the same appearances, we may reasonably count on producing a solution of it, by the use of such substances as we have found produce the same evacuation or movement. . . . Having been so often a witness to the salutary efforts which nature makes to re-establish the disordered functions, [the physician] should rather trust to their action, [than] hazard the interruption of that, and a greater derangement of the system, by conjectural experiments on a machine so complicated and so unknown as the human body.[26]

In short, neither Jefferson nor the majority of practitioners acknowledged that there was a crisis in medical care so long as it was based on observations of what appeared to "work" in any given illness, although they might have agreed that there was a therapeutic crisis implicit in the multiple explanations of disease and, therefore, its cures.[27] The major therapeutic principle was simply that because most patients survived, their remedies could be judged to have been effective. The irony is that doctors may not have been uncomfortable in the face of so many explanations of disease and its cures, since they could always cite their patients' high recovery rates, no matter what therapeutic rationales they exploited. It would not be until after pharmacists began to make purified therapeutically effective extracts of ancient botanical remedies in the early nineteenth century, and after investigators such as François Magendie, Claude Bernard, Rudolf Buchheim, and their followers were able to demonstrate the benefits possible from experimental pharmacology later in the century, that the unrecognized crisis could be resolved.

Notes and References

1. For an effective synthesis of these teachings, see Lester S. King, *The Medical World of the Eighteenth Century* (1958; rprt. ed. Huntington, N.Y.: Robert E. Krieger Publishing Co., Inc. 1971), 59-93, 214-219. Also see Friedrich Hoffmann, *Fundamenta Medicinae* [1695], trans. Lester S. King (London: Macdonald, 1971).

2. Hoffmann, *Fundamenta* (n. 1), pp. 41, 48.
3. Guenter B. Risse, *Hospital Life in Enlightenment Scotland: Care and Teaching at the Royal Infirmary of Edinburgh* (Cambridge: Cambridge University Press, 1986), chapter 4, pp. 177-239, and J. Worth Estes, Appendix D: "Drug usage at the infirmary: the example of Dr. Andrew Duncan, Sr.," pp. 351-384. For other illustrations of what was, essentially, solidistic medicine superimposed on humoralism, also see: Guenter B. Risse, "'Typhus' fever in eighteenth-century hospitals: new approaches to medical treatment," *Bulletin of the History of Medicine 59* (1985): 176-195; Guenter B. Risse, "Hysteria at the Edinburgh Infirmary: the construction and treatment of a disease, 1770-1800," *Medical History 32* (1988): 1-22; and J. Worth Estes, "Quantitative observations of fever and its treatment before the advent of short clinical thermometers," *Medical History 35* (1991): 189-216.
4. The best discussion of the therapeutic consequences of Lavoisier's work is: Frederic L. Holmes, "The chemical revolution and the art of healing," *Caduceus 11* (1995): 103-126. Also see: King, *Medical World* (n. 1), p. 78, and J. Worth Estes, "The medical properties of food in the eighteenth century," *Journal of the History of Medicine and Allied Sciences 51* (1996): 127-154.
5. John Brown, *The Elements of Medicine* [1795 rev. ed.] (Portsmouth, N.H.: William & Daniel Treadwell, 1803); King, *Medical World* (n. 1), pp. 143-147.
6. Guenter B. Risse, "Brunonian therapeutics: new wine in old bottles?," *Medical History*, Supplement No. 8 (1988): 46-62.
7. J. Worth Estes, "The yellow fever syndrome and its treatment in Philadelphia, 1793," in: J. Worth Estes and Billy G. Smith, eds., *"A Melancholy Scene of Devastation": the Public Response to the 1793 Philadelphia Yellow Fever Epidemic* (Canton, Mass.: Science History Publications), in press.
8. Frank A. Pattie, "Mesmer's medical dissertation and its debt to Mead's *De Imperio solis ac lunae*," *Journal of the History of Medicine and Allied Sciences 11* (1956): 275-287; Stephen Jay Gould, "The chain of reason vs. the chain of thumbs," *Natural History* (July 1989), pp. 12-21; Fielding H. Garrison, *An Introduction to the History of Medicine*, 4th ed. (Philadelphia: W. B. Saunders Company, 1929), p. 315.
9. Saul K. Padover, ed., *The Complete Jefferson* (New York: Tudor Publishing Co., 1943), p. 1062.
10. Ibid .
11. For this number, see J. Worth Estes, *Dictionary of Protopharmacology: Therapeutic Practice 1700-1850* (Canton, Mass.: Science History Publications, 1990.
12. Saul Jarcho, *Quinine's Predecessor: Francesco Torti and the Early History of Cinchona* (Baltimore: Johns Hopkins University Press, 1993), passim.
13. John Huxham, *An Essay on Fevers* (1757; rprt. ed. Canton, Mass.: Science History Publications, 1986), pp. 29, 35, 37, 47, 65; W. F. Bynum, "Cullen and the study of fevers in Britain, 1760-1820," in: *Medical History*, Supplement No. 1 (1981): 135-147; J. Worth Estes, "Naval medicine in the age of sail: the voyage of the *New York*, 1802-1803," *Bulletin of the History of Medicine 56* (1982): 238-253.

14. William Cullen, *First Lines of the Practice of Physic*, new ed., 4 vols. (Edinburgh and London: 1789), I, 245-247.

15. Stephen Hales, *Statical Essays: Containing Haemastaticks; or, an Account of Some Hydraulick and Hydrostatical Experiments Made on the Blood and Blood-vessels of Animals*, 2 vols. (London: W. Innys, R. Manby, & T. Woodward, 1733), vol. 2, pp. 48-63, 126-139.

16. Estes, "Quantitative observations" (n. 3).

17. J. Worth Estes and Paul Dudley White, "William Withering and the purple foxglove," *Scientific American 212* (June 1965), 110-119.

18. J. Worth Estes, *Hall Jackson and the Purple Foxglove: Medical Practice and Research in Revolutionary America 1760-1820* (Hanover, N.H.: University Press of New England, 1979), pp. 182-185.

19. These data are extracted and rearranged from their presentation in a printed table tipped into the Boston Medical Library's copy of Francis Home's *Clinical Experiments, Histories, and Dissections*, 3rd ed. (London and Edinburgh: J. Murray and William Creech, 1783). The table does not accompany any text in the book, although it is set in the same type and printed on the same paper stock; it belongs in some other book, but I cannot ascertain which. The author—or experimenter—is unknown, but it seems most likely that he was at the Royal Infirmary at Edinburgh.

20. Estes, *Hall Jackson* (n. 18), pp. 175-182, 189-198; Estes, "Drug usage" (n. 3), pp. 360-361.

21. Estes, *Hall Jackson* (n. 18), pp. 229-231.

22. Charles E. Rosenberg, "The therapeutic revolution: medicine, meaning, and social change in nineteenth-century America," *Perspectives in Biology and Medicine 20* (1977): 485-506.

23. Collated from Estes, "Drug usage" (n. 3), p. 385

24. Similar data, for other adult populations, appear in: "Some memoirs of [John Coakley] Lettsom," *Transactions of the Medical Society of London 110* (1995): 112-114; Estes, *Hall Jackson* (n. 18), pp. 100-109; and Estes, "Naval medicine" (n. 13); the latter includes additional data which portray graphically the natural history of several major diseases of the eighteenth century.

25. Jacob Bigelow, *Discourse on Self-Limited Diseases* (Boston: Nathan Hale, 1835).

26. Padower, *Complete Jefferson* (n. 9), p. 1062.

27. King, in *Medical World* (n. 1), p. 57, says that late eighteenth-century physicians found it necessary to achieve a "synthesis" of the various theories that assailed them. I'm not sure that they did anything quite so positive, although it is possible that my word "crisis" is too strong.

The Road to Twentieth-Century Therapeutics: Shifting Perspectives and Approaches

by Guenter B. Risse

T HIS essay sketches successive transformations in the therapeutic rationale based originally on holistic notions of the human body and a strong belief in nature's healing powers. I would like to deviate from traditional approaches enshrined in both the popular and specialized literature stressing the deplorable state of earlier therapeutics—sometimes considered hopelessly backward and even dangerous in relation to modern standards of efficacy. Among the representatives of such a progressive viewpoint was Lewis Thomas, a physician and successful writer, who asserted that all treatments before his time had been "the most frivolous and irresponsible kind of human experimentation."[1] The educated public, moreover, generally shares this negative perception about past treatment efforts, periodically devouring one more ghoulish story of medical vampirism—bloodletting killed George Washington but may have saved mad George III of England. Museum visitors, in turn, shudder at the sight of phlebotomy knives and cauterizing irons depicted as barbarous instruments of therapeutic torture.

Erwin Ackerknecht, one of the most prominent historians of this subject, admitted that "the history of therapeutics has always been particularly unsatisfactory from the point of view of logic."[2] Whose logic? That of a modern physician? As several authors have recently pointed out, therapeutics is primarily a social process, imbedded within broader cultural contexts and particular time periods. Moreover, popular notions of bodily function, the shifting nature of medical knowledge and experience, and transformations in the patient/healer relationship play important roles in therapy, together with location—home, office, hospital or clinic— financing, and more recently, medical technology. The task of this essay, then, is to discern some of the fundamental shifts in therapeutic strategies. What follows is a succinct presentation of basic views—as expressed by physicians—that guided their therapeutic approaches before the advent of the twentieth century.[3]

The Contours of Classical Humoralism

The theoretical principles that guided classical Graeco-Roman therapeutics were based on a number of popular notions about human functioning in relation to environment, presumably derived from domestic and folk views of bodily behavior in health and disease. Within such a framework, the human body was said to be composed of a number of inextricably mixed and blended elements and humors, each endowed with particular qualities. Whether in health or disease, the body responded as a single entity, with a natural tendency toward balancing its various components through the formation of new humors and the elimination of waste products. Such constant renovation was achieved through sources of food and drink, and the organism was conceived as acting like a veritable cooking vessel capable of boiling and blending the ingested ingredients properly so as to renew the bodily flesh and fluids. In addition, all persons were believed to possess a particular humoral blend that defined their individual bodily constitution. Nature, indeed, was destiny since this mix not only dictated bodily form, but also mental status and susceptibility to particular imbalances and diseases.[4] Since Hippocrates, such humoral imbalances were seen as the results of complex interactions occurring between the body's individual constitution, and the "non naturals": behavior, diet, and environment.[5] Air and climate, food and drink, sleep, exercise, and mental activity, were all considered essential for supporting life and the preservation of a healthy balance, and thus needed to be constantly monitored. Health management was part of the what ancient physicians called the "regimen," with dietary items given the primary responsibility to sustain the essential humoral harmony.[6]

Guenter B. Risse, M.D., Ph.D., is Professor and Chair, Department of the History of Health Sciences, University of California, San Francisco. A physician-historian, he has written extensively on the history of medicine and therapeutics, winning in 1988 the Welch Medal of the American Association of the History of Medicine for his book *Hospital Life in Enlightenment Scotland* (Cambridge, 1986). Dr. Risse is a contributor to the recent *Cambridge World History of Human Disease* (1993) and the *Companion Encyclopedia of the History of Medicine* (Routledge, 1993) as well as author of a forthcoming book on the history of hospitals.

In turn, classical disease concepts were largely predicated on models of internal poisoning and the behavior of external wounds. Physicians believed that all substances introduced into the human body were capable of behaving like poisons, altering the healthy humoral balance. They could be either inhaled, ingested, or otherwise acquired through direct contact. In the latter instance, these disease-causing substances sometimes collected under the skin, creating discrete local swellings. Among the internal effects of poisons were humoral stagnation and putrefaction. Under such circumstances, the body frequently sought to return to a healthy state by selectively discharging unwanted humors, many still in their "raw" or "uncooked" stage.

Indeed, based on such observations, the ancients described the presence of a natural healing force within the human body, immediately activated if the healthy balance was threatened by a poison or other noxious influence.[7] Natural healing could occur through a process of selective humoral pepsis or cooking, with the body driving out all excess or corrupted humors during critical moments of the disease process. Such drainage was usually accomplished through the body's natural outlets—by derivation—including vomiting and diarrhea, bleeding, sneezing, coughing, sweating, and voiding urine, as well as through menstrual and vaginal flows.[8] At other times, nature also tried to rid the body of dangerous wastes by creating alternative exits, pushing the poisons and impurities towards the surface of the skin to avoid excessive humoral accumulations near the vital organs. All natural efforts followed particular evolutionary paths towards slow and gradual "lysis" and recovery, or they ended in so-called crises, sudden and dramatic humoral discharges that could end in death.

Based on this model, therapeutic interventions sought to duplicate natural healing efforts. The ancient physicians feared that if the body's natural efforts appeared to fall short or their timing was off, sickness could permanently establish itself through poisonous deposits, leading to chronic conditions and death. Practitioners, therefore, were encouraged to imitate the natural healing actions without causing additional bodily harm. This cautious approach characterized the therapeutic rationale of ancient Greek healing craftsmen and their descendants. It consisted in the medicinally assisted expulsion of all poisons through the usual excretory organs by the employment of emetics, purgatives, cathartics, enemas, expectorants, and diuretics, as well as bloodletting. If some of these agents could accomplish more than one or two of these expulsive functions, they would assume the category of a *panacea* or cure-all. In antiquity there were also searches for specific antidotes (*theriacs*) to neutralize poisons based on their emetic and purgative qualities.[9] Some of these compounds were created by combining viper flesh or scorpions with other ingredients. Indeed, the selection of antidotes or medicines was frequently guided by notions of sympathy and signature, whereby plants, animals, and minerals were believed to disclose their healing qualities

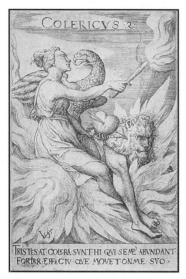 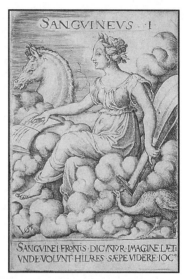

The influence of the four humors of ancient medicine extended to artistic imagery, as shown in the sixteenth-century work shown here, from Virgilius Solis the Elder. Choleric personality traits are represented on the left, and a sanguine temperament on the right.

through physical clues or signs linked to disease manifestations.

At other times, alternative routes for such an expulsion were chosen. If the natural outlets for noxious humors appeared blocked, insufficient, or considered dangerous, practitioners followed nature by creating diversions. Particular areas of the skin were chosen as substitute passages for the expulsion of the poisons and uncooked humors. To accomplish the discharges, healers massaged, irritated and scarified the skin, employed cups or leeches, produced new blisters and running sores, as well as localized burns through cautery irons or moxibustion. All these procedures sought to displace the offending poisons from the vicinity of vital internal organs. The expectation was that, once herded into discrete but far less dangerous patches of pustules and abscesses near the surface of the skin, the poisons became visible and amenable to draining by the practitioner.[10]

In sum, classical therapeutics were based on a coherent humoral framework of bodily functioning in health and disease. This theory was quite simple and easily understandable to both healers and patients. Holistic in approach, it lent itself to individualized adjustments based on diet and life style, mostly executed within the sick person's home environment by employing domestic resources and family networks. Respectful of natural developments, such ancient treatments expected to imitate or follow the spontaneous evolution of self-limited disease processes. In doing so, humoral therapy frequently claimed success, thus confirming the healers' clinical knowledge, judgment, and skill. The humoral approach remained quite popular throughout the Middle Ages and Renaissance in Europe, contributing to the creation of a growing number of professional physicians whose identity, status, and income were closely linked with this paradigm.[11]

Recasting Humoralism: Seventeenth and Eighteenth Centuries

As the European medical marketplaces expanded in the seventeenth century following the establishment of modern national states and a stronger mercantile economy, competition among would-be healers intensified. There were also shifts in world view among elite populations and new models of bodily function in health and disease that created challenges for the classical schemes. Still, most medical practitioners continued to adhere to the basic concepts of humoralism in spite of challenges by Paracelsus and his followers. They introduced a number of new chemical preparations in the form of tinctures, essences, and extracts into the established pharmacopoeia.[12] Vindicated by William Harvey's new circulatory schemes, practitioners now went through a process of recasting the traditional humoral scheme according to mechanical, chemical, and eventually neurophysiological principles.[13] Humors were now envisioned as composed of small particles. Humoral transformations, in health and disease, were reinterpreted as mechanical actions or chemical processes of fermentation, under the direction of the nervous system.[14] Most physicians, however, including Thomas Sydenham, remained strong advocates of the healing power of nature.[15]

By the eighteenth century, a number of medical systems developed new theories and therapeutic rationales that were grafted onto the traditional humoral scheme. William Cullen, for example, based his ideas on neuromuscular physiology and pathology. A proper degree of excitement or tension in the nerves assured the normal transmission of impulses for normal bodily activities, including both solid and fluid components. Disease resulted from alterations of excitement. An increase caused vascular spasms, increases in circulation, and chemical abnormalities. A decrease produced generalized debility and collapse of functions.[16] Thus, the therapeutic rationale shifted toward regaining a balanced excitement in the sick body through a combination of traditional depletion measures—if there was too much nervous excitement—or with stimulating agents if there were deficiencies. Among the former remained the emetics and purgatives, antispasmodics and sedatives, and of course, bloodletting. Characterized as stimulants were tonics, opium, warm baths, meat, and alcoholic beverages. Traditional drugs were recast into these two major categories, although others such as diaphoretics, diuretics, expectorants, and astringents were retained for their specific actions.[17]

This therapeutic reasoning was merely superimposed on the existing humoralism. It meant that physicians focused their primary efforts on the workings of the nervous system that guided the rest of the body. In 1803, James Gregory, an Edinburgh professor, succinctly summarized the process by declaring that "the greater part of a physician's practice consists in exciting, promoting, restraining, and sometimes irritating by art the various operations of nature in the human body."[18] This approach stressed that nature was primarily in charge, and practitioners were merely following and assisting. Questions such as why should one use Peruvian bark if it interfered with the "natural working" of a fever illustrated the tensions between an expectant approach and the employment of newer drugs that could prove efficacious and thus provide a critical edge to physicians competing for patients in the medical marketplace.

An additional challenge to traditional humoralism occurred towards the end of the eighteenth century, when another medical system appeared in Scotland, created by Cullen's former student, John Brown. His doctrine accepted the existence of one fundamental vital principle, excitability, normally in balance within all living beings, and constantly generated by stimulation from

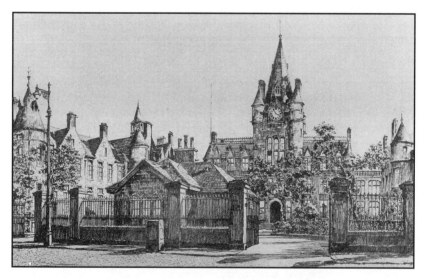

The main entrance to the Royal Infirmary of Edinburgh. (The etching by Wilfred C. Appleby appears on the frontispiece of A. Logan Turner, Story of a Great Hospital: The Royal Infirmary of Edinburgh 1729-1929 *(Edinburgh, 1937).)*

environmental and internal sources. With disease representing in most cases an imbalance from a lack of stimulants, *asthenia*, or occasionally the opposite *sthenia*, Brown went further than Cullen. Based on a simplified stimulation system, the new rationale demanded that the physician support the diseased body with the aid of stimulating foods and medicines. This approach also remained holistic and individualized, seeking a natural balance.[19]

Eighteenth-century hospitals, meanwhile, only played a limited role in such therapeutic shifts. Hospital physicians believed themselves to operate at a disadvantage for a number of reasons. First, they were ignorant about the health background, life-style, and constitutional character of their new patients. Second, the hospital patients came from different social classes, occupations, and geographical locations than their usual private clientele. How could these modifiers be factored in? Were country folk really healthier than city dwellers? Moreover, patients were admitted to institutions some time after the onset of illness, often late in the evolution of a disease. In addition, they usually provided incomplete accounts, thus creating diagnostic and management difficulties for hospital physicians who wished to ascertain earlier developments.[20] Finally, both the institutional setting and its routine operations tended to limit physicians' therapeutic choices. In-house formularies were a first step toward a universal rather than an individual approach. Such considerations diminished somewhat the importance of eighteenth-century hospitals as sources for new medical knowledge regarding therapeutics. Clinical experiments with several drugs weeded out ineffective items of the materia medica and helped establish lower dosages for drugs still considered useful.[21] By the end of the century, this new approach based on a neurophysiological humoralism came under increased pressure because of a strong resurgence of empiricism in medicine. Although closely linked to the identity and social standing of Europe's contemporary medical profession, an expanding range of clinical observations began to question the validity and need for medical systems, together with the value and success of the traditional depletive practices imbedded in these rational systems. Natural recovery became, once again, fashionable.

French Skepticism and the Numerical Method

By the early nineteenth century, numerous, improved, and sustained clinical observations ushered in a period of growing therapeutic restraint. In France, the leading figures of the Paris Medical School, Pierre J. G. Cabanis and Philippe Pinel, sought to pursue methodologies designed to improve the certainty of medical activities, including treatment. Medical systems and the bases of their rationality came under attack, now perceived as harmful strictures to empirical advances at the bedside.[22] But how much of disease evolution was natural instead of caused by the physician's art? Both authors still supported the notion of the physician-qua-artist, using his intuition, instincts, and talent to sympathize with patients and devise personalized therapeutic plans. However, a more solid foundation for making such judgments was needed, including better and repeated clinical observations, regular recording of the witnessed events, and a quantitative comparison of the collected data.

At first, older therapeutic rationales based on constitutional and holistic views of the body survived. In the true spirit of Hippocratic empiricism, French physicians were urged to modestly recast their roles as nature's helpers, reinforcing natural healing tendencies and thus assuming an expectant posture that simply sought to provide nourishment and proper environmental hygiene. Medical systems and the bases of their rationality came under attack since they were now perceived to be harmful straitjackets. hampering empirical advances at the bedside. While expressing ignorance concerning the causes of disease, Pinel, for example, questioned the usefulness of traditional treatments such as purging and bleeding, preaching instead therapeutic caution and skepticism.[23]

At the same time, autopsies designed to localize lesions in various bodily organs and ascribe the manifestations of clinical disease to the dynamics between complex organ systems, created a much more fragmented image of the human body. Much of this took place in Paris, where physician-surgeons primarily observed the sick poor sheltered in large hospitals, and carried out systematic dissections of those who died there. Under the circumstances, both the severity and universality of the bodily lesions and high death rates suggested preventative rather than curative efforts. Given the seriousness and extent of the pathology thus uncovered, only palliation loomed as the treatment of choice. Laennec, for example, in treating tuberculosis in 1819, adopted such a therapeutic stance, producing diversionary blisters and local burns on the chest, prescribing cough suppressants and expectorants, and creating an artificial marine environment with the help of fresh seaweed spread around the hospital wards.[24]

Gradually, the French physicians' professional reputation and social standing no longer came to depend on individualized therapeutic recommendations, but on their knowledge regarding the nature and evolution of individual diseases through physical diagnosis and pathological anatomy. Some diseases had inexorable and fatal outcomes, others were self limited. The new approach was to detect the presence of particular disease entities and study their natural evolution. The previously shared knowledge about disease between patients and their physicians, so useful in forging a trusting relationship and negotiating therapeutic strategies for more than two thousand years, was shattered. For treatment, patients now became much more dependent on their physician's knowledge and judgment.[25]

By the 1820s, traditional depleting measures such as purging and bloodletting continued to be practiced without more rigorous attempts to record and tabulate their clinical effects. At this point, another French academic, Pierre Louis, tried to draw further attention to this matter (including the bloodletting excesses of another contemporary colleague, Broussais), by proposing the employment of a "numerical method" to study the tabulated information and draw inferences from it, including those necessary for the treatment of disease.[26] In successive publications, Louis challenged practitioners to collect their clinical data and subject it to mathematical analyses. Rhetorically, he challenged the entire medical profession, declaring that "without statistics, therapeutics is nothing more than a jumbled heap of banal and doubtful recipes."[27]

This new quest for medical certainty was predicated on the belief that, in the preceding decades, clinical knowledge had achieved such critical levels that practitioners could now establish average evolutionary pathways for many disorders and discard a range of unusual individual variations. This notion may have resulted from the influence of hospital medicine and its universalizing tendencies. "Suppose that you have some doubts as to the efficacy of a particular remedy: how are you to proceed? Will you compare two cases in which the remedy has been employed? Surely not, you would take as many cases as possible of as similar a description as you could find, and count how many recovered under one mode of treatment and how many under another; in how short a time they did so, and if the cases were in all respects alike, you would have some confidence in your conclusions."[28]

Louis's construction of a numerical therapeutic rationale caused a great stir in France and prompted a series of academic debates about its merits during the 1830s. Some physicians argued that the inherent complexity and variability of clinical conditions doomed all efforts at calculation. Others focused on the individuality of patient and disease, postulating that they battled each other under particular physical and environmental conditions impossible to universalize. "Individuality," concluded Louis's major opponent, François J. Double, "is an invariable element in pathology. A disease is not a simple, fixed, and uniform entity," adding that "therefore every absolute method is repugnant to therapeutics."[29] This was especially true for internal therapies, more complex and nuanced, providing inconclusive results difficult to quantify. As Double remarked, "were it [numerical method] ever effected, medicine would cease to be either a science, an art, or even a profession, it would become as mechanical as the employment of the shoemaker."[30]

Louis's approach to therapeutics was grounded in early nineteenth-century French hospital medicine. Indeed, hospitals had gained in importance as sources of new medical knowledge through extensive clinical and pathological studies, not therapeutic approaches, although the "numerical method" now tried to do just that. Quantification was believed to override individual clinical judgments, creating the danger that therapeutic decisions would be made by the application of predetermined formulas arrived at through statistical calculations. Such a change in the decision-making process of the medical profession was perceived as a great threat to the physicians' identity and social standing. However, the appeal of a statistically informed therapy remained somewhat restricted to a small elite of academic Parisian physicians primarily active in institutional environments where more universalizing tendencies flourished naturally. It made less sense in private medical practice contexts where therapeutic specificity was still essential in supporting professional identity.

The role of hospital medicine in fostering therapeutic skepticism was acknowledged by Double, who observed during the debates that "one evil of the present state of medicine [is] that our experience is too exclusively that of hospitals. We thus only see one condition of life and the disease already established, and can seldom retain the patient long enough to see all the steps by which health is gradually reestablished."[31] In the end, Louis's challenge failed to persuade the medical profession to accept statistical information for determining a therapeutic rationale. However, these debates managed to advance the existing caution and skepticism, forcing practitioners to face the notion that qualitative physiological functions needed to be better understood before planning selective therapeutic interventions.

In the United States, meanwhile, practitioners at first continued to apply the notions of the Edinburgh systematists, undoubtedly influenced by Benjamin Rush who considered the origin of most illnesses to be excessive stimulation. Thus, they prescribed a traditional antiphlogistic regimen. Others, influenced by their new Parisian teachers, increasingly turned away from rationalism to empiricism.[32] In their view, acute diseases were either self-limited or serious enough to kill. With the help of nature, people afflicted with the former recovered spontaneously or in spite of treatment, while the latter merely qualified for palliation. Professional fragmentation, therapeutic skepticism, and a split between popular and medical views of bodily functioning fostered a yearning for a return to traditional, holistic approaches.[33] After all, was not the relief of suffering the cardinal obligation of a healer?

Sectarian Holism

In the meantime, effectively combining mind and body, traditional and popular holism found a home in so-called sectarian or fringe approaches to treatment, including homeopathy and hydropathy. In fact, the rise of homeopathy in the 1820s and 1830s occurred precisely as skepticism about traditional medical treatments was spreading. The founder of this alternative healing system, Samuel Hahnemann, formulated his famous *similia similibus* axiom, by which he meant that in the human body, every effective drug provoked a sort of disease. Imitating nature, practitioners would cure various ailments by simply administering the appropriate medication that caused a similar disease.[34]

The strategy of a rational homeopathic therapy rested on the principles of similarity and dilution. As noted, similarity involved the specific employment of those drugs that could be experimentally proven to produce in healthy volunteers a particular configuration of symptoms mimicking those of the disease to be treated. In Hahnemann's view, if a perfect fit could be made, the drug-induced disease would cancel the real one and return the patient to health. On the basis of these assumptions, Hahnemann after 1796 began sending his own children into the fields to collect medicinal plants. From dried flowers and various roots he prepared his own extracts or infusions and started testing them on himself, his family, and his friends. They all had to report every discomfort or symptom they experienced while under the influence of these medicines. The result of these experiences was a six-volume *Materia Medica Pura*, still considered the bible of homeopathic therapeutics.[35]

Not surprisingly, homeopathy represented a continuation of the classical approach to therapeutics: it presumed to follow nature, the natural world not constructed on the basis of perennial tensions between opposites locked in constant battle, but one in which similars could interfere, inhibit, or even cancel each other out. Moreover, homeopathy also viewed the human organism as indivisible, reacting as a whole through the total sum of clinical symptoms and signs. Likewise, health remained a dynamic balance ever to be maintained or restored. Patient uniqueness was an expression of individual constitution and susceptibility. In an era of depersonalized hospital medicine, when long rows of sick people were being analyzed and dissected for the sake of establishing precise pathological entities, and where treatment was only incidental or nonexistent, Hahnemann's therapeutic rationales provided a welcome alternative. Homeopathic patients were treated as individuals, not just merely viewed as examples of known diseases. Their complaints were to be carefully elicited, and special treatment plans were provided on the basis of unique symptomatic combinations.[36]

A separate therapeutic movement, hydropathy, began in the small Silesian village of Graefenberg during the 1820s, led by Vincent Priessnitz. This son of a local farmer had made some observations concerning the efficacy of cold spring water, first on minor trauma, then on internal diseases of the chronic variety such as rheumatism, gout, and digestive, and respiratory problems. Spearheaded by the chemical revolution, a growing interest in the medicinal effects of certain waters had been present in Europe since the eighteenth century. Friedrich Hoffmann, a professor of medicine at the University of Halle, had already played a prominent role through his chemical analyses of German springs. For Hoffmann, mineral waters were veritable panaceas, since they contained tonics, purgatives, astringents, collagogues, and diuretics, all designed to either eliminate or neutralize disease-causing humors. By the middle of the eighteenth century, chemists began to produce the salts present in spring waters, thus allowing consumers to make their own synthetic mineral water. Better yet, numerous springs simply bottled theirs, a practice that led to an extraordinary worldwide consumption of such products.[37]

In less than a decade, Priessnitz received official approval for operating his hydropathic institution. By mid-century, Graefenberg had become an international healing center, spawning a series of similar institutions both in Europe and in the United States. The basic treatment combined frequent baths and showers in cold spring water, alternating with periods of sweating in wool blankets, followed by lengthy walks in the surrounding hills. Water had to be drunk in great quantities. The diet was quite simple and wholesome, consisting of cold milk and dark bread for breakfast and supper, with a more abundant lunch of raw vegetables and some meat, even baked goods.[38]

To legitimize his wet and spartan routines in the eyes of the medical profession, Priessnitz formulated the theoretical underpinning of his hydropathy. Health was the natural condition of the human body and disease occurred through the introduction of foreign substances that disturbed the normal humoral mix. To restore proper balance, such poisons had to be flushed out of the human body with the help of baths, drinking of water, sweating, and exercise in fresh air. All these activities were aimed at displacing the *materia peccans* from vital internal organs to the periphery, as the cold water kept stimulating the entire system, including the skin.[39]

Like the ancients, Priessnitz postulated the existence of a high point in the battle between the healing powers of nature and the disease-causing humors. The hydropathic "crisis" was at hand when the patient's fever peaked, or spontaneous vomiting or diarrhea removed some undesirable matter from the body. The same was true if blood escaped from the nose or from hemorrhoids. Most importantly, while patients received hydropathic treatments, their skin could break out into a series of rashes, even pustules, which signaled that nature was ready to expel the disease-causing humors. As in ancient times, rubbing, massage, and sweating would now eliminate these poisons. As with homeopathy, the therapeutic rationale guiding hydropathy stressed similar holistic notions of the human body in health and disease, and basically went back to classical humoralism, albeit with a stronger emphasis on the role of water. Moreover, Priessnitz and his successors made sure that the water treatments were carefully tailored to the individual patient. Initially, prospective patients had to write to him giving a history of their health problems and previous treatments, and not all were invited to come to the institution. Later, preliminary evaluations and therapeutic plans formed part of each admission. As one British medical visitor admitted in 1843, "the patient very naturally cares not for the absence of scientific explanations, but renders his faith to fact and the long list of extraordinary cures which have been performed after the failure of the regular medical art."[40]

Therapeutic Nihilism

Before the mid-nineteenth century, some leading medical authorities considered the old "art" of medicine that sought to individualize and make particular sick people whole again to be outdated. A new strategy was called for. Instead of targeting the entire sick body, treatments were to be directed against the multiple manifestations of a disease. Within a framework that retained the notion of unique bodily constitutions, therapy had to be specifically applied with the intention of influencing abnormal processes believed to be implicated in the creation of bodily lesions. As before, the most important goal was to support the vitality and natural healing force of every sick body against the onslaught of disease, preferably through the use of stimulants or tonics.

This new rationale was inextricably bound up with political struggles within the prevailing European and American professional hierarchies. It implied a need for reform in which the traditional medical art was portrayed as linked to dogmatism, individualism, and professional elitism. In its place, reformers now urged adherence to the laws and facts of science, which were universal, verifiable, and democratic. According to Joseph Dietl, a representative of the Vienna School and an ally of the pathologist Karl Rokitansky and the clinician Josef Skoda in 1845: "As long as medicine remains an art, it cannot be a science. Art is the property of an individual, it is rooted in feelings and imagination. Science is an open discipline which everyone can join, part of the common property of the human spirit."[41] While Dietl's wish for medicine to adopt a scientific epistemology could be seen as laudable for the professional future of his colleagues, it seemed unclear what it would do for patients. Therapeutics traditionally had not been merely the logical inference and application of available medical knowledge, but a complex, idiosyncratic, and emotional interaction between the sick and their healers based on common understandings of the body.

Like his earlier French colleagues, Dietl stressed the importance of pathological anatomy and diagnostic accuracy through the employment of physical methods. In his view and that of the Paris Medical School, the goal of medical certainty had shifted from therapy to diagnosis.[42] Dietl also reacted against remaining notions of traditional humoralism and sought to simplify the existing materia medica, adopting an expectant and skeptical approach for his empirically-driven therapeutics. As their European counterparts elsewhere, Dietl and other Austrian physicians retained traditional beliefs in the healing power of nature, stressing that vital forces should be allowed to act unfettered by medical intervention. Such a hands-off posture at the bedside earned Dietl and others the characterization of "therapeutic nihilists," a pejorative label that has survived into our day.[43] This more extreme posture, primarily employed in teaching hospitals—Dietl was employed in a suburban Vienna institution—was widely decried by opponents as "meditations on death," the very antithesis of professionally-assisted healing. In the end, the would-be reformers hoped for a scientifically-grounded pharmacology and medical theory based on firm notions of causality.[44]

Within this new framework, the therapeutic rationale could no longer remain entirely holistic. Treatments now merely aimed to prevent, as well as selectively alleviate, some of the cardinal pathological processes while keeping the whole body strong enough to withstand the natural course. Since there were few specific remedies available at the time to stem the natural tide, only a few empirically proven measures should be employed. Depleting efforts, Dietl observed, continued to be utilized by those practitioners who did not perform extensive diagnostic examinations and were ignorant about the pathological anatomy and physiology of a disease. He, in turn, treated victims of typhoid fever with rest and a milk diet, as well as body washings with water and vinegar.[45]

Engaged in formulating a pathological physiology based on his cellular theory of disease, Rudolf Virchow sought to remedy this deficiency. Disease was no more than a series of living phenomena occurring under abnormal circumstances. Therefore, treatment had to be specifically directed against the altered conditions when they continued to change in the course of a disease. In a 1849 article, Virchow asked whether a scientifically-informed therapeutics derived from a thorough understanding of the disease process was actually feasible. Yes, there was a profusion of remedies and uncertainties about their actions as described in existing pharmacopoeias. And, yes, clinicians still possessed only limited clinical knowledge and large hospitals provided limited opportunities for therapeutic observations. Worst of all, experimentally acquired physiological and chemical knowledge was not always applicable in therapeutics. Virchow was opposed to therapeutic skepticism, and also discarded the numerical method. The hope was that an empirically driven therapy would eventually become a science.[46]

At about the same time, another German medical leader, Carl Wunderlich, complained that in spite of assurances that medicine had joined the exact sciences, there still was therapeutic anarchy. Patients kept demanding useless medicines from the old materia medica. These items had to be prescribed because of "the superstition of the patient and to strengthen his confidence," Wunderlich told his audience in 1851.[47] On the other side of the professional divide were the physiologists, busy studying the functioning of the human body, focusing on organic processes, and explaining them exclusively in chemical and mechanical terms. They shared a strong belief that science would eventually explain everything. "Physiological" therapeutics aimed to correct some of these processes but only with drugs whose actions could be satisfactorily explained.[48] Wunderlich explained that a truly rational therapy could only be built with the help of a science such as chemistry, since the effectiveness of particular compounds could then be explained through their structures and actions. So far, he lamented, this theoretical approach had not been successful.[49]

Wunderlich argued against a therapeutic rationale that took its initial cues from the clinical nature of an illness. He suggested that it be replaced by an approach focused on the pharmacological actions of a particular remedy. Departing from a standardized product with certain proven qualities, particular drugs could then be employed in a number of clinical conditions to determine their degree of efficacy. In this way, and with the help of statistical calculations, one could gradually arrive at a more precise set of therapeutic indications. The results were to be provided to local associations of physicians for distribution to all their members.[50]

Virchow and Wunderlich's ideas were readily echoed by Claude Bernard in his 1865 *Introduction to the Study of Experimental Medicine*. Bernard also viewed therapeutics as a basic component of a gradually evolving scientific medicine. In his view, the therapeutic effects of medicines on the human organism could only be understood on the basis of physiological actions responsible for all vital phenomena.[51] Wrote Bernard: "Experimenting physicians are Hippocratics and empiricists at one and the same time, in that they believe in the power of nature and the efficacy of drugs; only they want to know what they are doing; it is not enough for them to observe and act empirically, they want to experiment scientifically and to understand the physiological mechanism producing disease and the medicinal mechanism effecting a cure."[52] In the meantime, however, practitioners could ill afford to appear idle at the bedside: "we must resign ourselves to practice conjectural or empirical medicine" until experimenting physicians " would exert their influence successively on diseases one by one," determining their causes, declared Bernard.[53]

The first phase of a physiologically informed therapeutic strategy was to employ a few drugs with demonstrated pharmacological actions to change and reverse certain disease processes, such as quinine for malaria, and morphine for pain. The prescribed focus on discrete chemical compounds and study of their physiological actions bore fruit with the employment of salicylic acid—an antipyretic—by Kolbe (1860) and with the introduction of chloral hydrate—a hypnotic—by Liebreich (1869). The modest goal was to make individual patients comfortable through the employment of chemical compounds capable of influencing certain clinical manifestations without significantly changing the course and outcome of a disease process itself. During the next few decades, a veritable wave of new antipyretics—eight in seven years—and hypnotics—four new drugs in six years—hit the pharmaceutical market, creating problems for the hapless practitioners who tried to evaluate them.[54]

Informed by experimental physiology and pharmacology, this empirical therapeutic approach benefited from the growing quantification of clinical observations, especially after the 1860s, when a number of bodily functions such as temperature, respiration, and pulse could be actually measured and charted. Moreover, blood, urine, and other fluids were now subjected to standardized chemical and microscopical examinations, thus allowing for a much closer monitoring of particular disease processes. While the existence of constitutional factors was still acknowledged, reliance on universal scientific criteria tended to diminish the importance of an individual patient's social and moral status on the evolution of disease. Such a shift had fundamental implications for medical theory, epistemology, and professional medical identity. "Medicine is after facts, it has become objective. It does not matter who is at the bedside, the sick person has become a thing" lamented one German physician in 1870. " Since everybody must understand this, all 'Hippocratics' disappear. Naturally, this approach removes the comfort of the healer's house-visits, personal relationships loosen, and physicians are being changed and selected according to the nature of the disease."[55]

Beyond the Classical Model: Etiology and Specific Drugs

A second phase of the new scientifically-informed therapeutic strategy began with the employment of agents that had proved capable of specifically neutralizing or destroying causal agents of a disease. Joseph Lister's example with antisepsis in the 1860s, based on the early work of Louis Pasteur, demonstrated the possibility that certain new chemical compounds, the phenols, could poison and selectively destroy ferments, later the germs presumed to be present at the surface of wounds, and in the body's interior in numerous infectious diseases. By the late 1870s and early 1880s, technical improvements in the cultivation and study of bacteria under the leadership of Robert Koch confirmed the role of germs in the genesis of many infectious diseases. This raised hopes that the bacteriological paradigm could be useful for a causally-driven approach to therapeutics. As Claude Bernard had predicted, "diseases that have their seat in the outer organic environment such as epidemic diseases, are the easiest to study and analyze experimentally. These diseases will more quickly reach the stage that their causation is known and their treatment scientific."[56] Unlike in earlier historical periods, a therapeutic rationale aimed at destroying the perceived causes of a given disease became even more critically dependent on diagnostic precision. In this search for etiological agents, conducted largely in the laboratory, individual human factors became secondary.

This therapeutic stance assumed a life-threatening struggle within the body between two purposeful beings, the bacteria-produced disease and its human host. While the latter desperately sought to maintain control, the disease—personified and represented as a parasite or as the "other"— cruelly snatched that control away, causing a number of sudden functional disorders and symptoms. In the eyes of patients and practitioners, these manifestations were caused by a foreign invader.[57] Indeed, to dramatize the frightful new biological ontology, physicians freely resorted to military metaphors. Words like battle, combat, targets, defeat, and destruction began to appear in both the popular and medical literature. Therapeutic rationales, in turn, were constructed as wars against an resourceful enemy, employing specific weapons. "Antidotes" in the classical poison model became so-called "magic bullets."[58]

The early direction, based on Pasteur's studies, pointed toward the use of vaccines as specific preventatives, and sera as treatments. The concept of sero-therapy involved the employment of substances obtained from immunized animals, designed to selectively neutralize or destroy the causal germs.[59] But could each disease require for its cure a specifically prepared blood serum or should one also conceive of other bodily materials or chemical compounds capable of producing similar results? Unfortunately, events surrounding the failure of Koch's tuberculin in 1890 to cure tuberculosis led to skepticism about achieving such a goal. Referring to the discredited lymph, one author asked "how can one presume to pass to the clinic with the results of laboratory research in the naive thought of achieving the same results under very different biochemical conditions, which, moreover, cannot be possibly determined?"[60] Another editorial about the limits of bacteriological therapeutics was more optimistic: "it is fondly hoped that safe "specifics" will yet be found with which to oppose every malignant microbe." Citing the use of quinine in malaria and mercury in syphilis as the only two internal diseases in which such a desideratum had been achieved, the author observed that "it is quite possible that in the future we may be able to combat other internal diseases with equal directness, but it is nonsense for anyone to assert that we have any such therapeutic weapons now at our command."[61]

Two specific examples of the state of medical therapeutics before the end of the nineteenth century illuminate the contemporary uncertainties. Claude Bernard had already observed more than two decades earlier that hospitals were to become integral parts of the new scientific medicine. However, their future role would be restricted to clinical observation and verification while the true sanctuary for medical science was to be the laboratory.[62] Based on Koch's pathogenic notions, the causal approach suggested a need to neutralize or remove the cholera bacilli and their toxins from the body, possibly employing a serum.[63] In imitation of Koch's experiments with tuberculin, his disciple, Edwin Klebs prepared and tested in animals an emulsion of killed cholera vibrios, naming the product "anticholerin." He then proceeded to inject it subcutaneously in patients at Hamburg's Eppendorf Hospital during the 1892 epidemic. Said to have a specific toxic action on live bacilli, the results of treatment with anticholerin were not favorable, with Klebs' ward reporting a mortality rate of 67%.[64]

A second causal approach was to achieve intestinal antisepsis through the use of disinfectants specifically designed to kill the cholera and typhoid bacilli and to neutralize putrefactive processes and their poisons in the gut.[65] Recommended were enemas containing local antiseptics, from traditional eucalyptus and turpentine oil, carbolic acid, and iodoform, to the newer naphthol mixed with bismuth salicylate. Again, the results were poor, both in Hamburg and at Baltimore's Johns Hopkins Hospital. So what to do? Since causal therapy seemed rather dubious and ineffective, the Hopkins and Eppendorf physicians returned to the traditional antiphlogistic approach, symptomatic treatments designed to make their patients more comfortable while nature took its course. In both typhoid and cholera, fever, thirst, pain, nausea, diarrhea, and dehydration seemed to be most common. Antipyretics were ruled out by William Osler and others, since they seemed to intensify respiratory and cardiovascular symptoms. With the antiseptic and antipyretic approaches discredited, traditional hydrotherapy seemed indicated.

More importantly, the Hopkins physicians initiated periodic coldwater bath treatments in an effort to stimulate the flagging cardiovascular system.[66] Eppendorf physicians, in turn, attempted to rehydrate their cholera patients through subcutaneous infusions of 4% salt solutions. Plunging patients into the baths every three hours around the clock and providing them with a drink of whisky was Osler's approach.[67] Infused at Eppendorf with little discomfort under the right abdominal skin, warm saline solutions—usually two liters—seemed to act almost as life-savers, restoring pulse and peripheral circulation. There was, however, general agreement that the saline solutions, increasingly administered intravenously, were not really a cure for the disease. They acted merely as a cardiac stimulant and an agent facilitating the dilution of the poisons introduced by the cholera bacillus into the blood. Rest and food in a ventilated and clean environment would do the rest. In the end, physicians such as Osler in Baltimore and Rumpf in Hamburg simply attempted to strengthen the bodies of their charges in an attempt to guide the natural evolution of both typhoid fever and cholera. Thus, in the early 1890s, the promises of scientific medicine were still overshadowed by empirical schemes traditionally designed to foster natural recovery.[68]

Epilogue

In sum, I have tried to take you along on the protracted voyage traveled by medicine to arrive at a new scientifically-constructed rationale for therapeutics. For most of this trip, we stayed within a traditional and holistic framework of bodily functions based primarily on humoral theories deeply imbedded in many cultures. With great respect for the wisdom of our bodies, all we dared to do was to closely watch the natural evolution of our illnesses to their frequently successful endings, helping to reduce a bit our suffering along the way with measures designed to cleanse the innards and deflect the pain. The vigor with which these healing procedures were pursued, of course, was constantly renegotiated based on the anxieties of those who fell ill and their practitioners' professional knowledge, identity, and zeal for intervention. Wrote Alexander of Tralles circa A. D. 550, "the physician should look upon the patient as a besieged city and try to rescue him with every means that art and knowledge place at his command."[69] Seen from this perspective, most medicines were given to supplement, imitate, or lessen natural bodily reactions, and only a few—notably those for pain—shared our contemporary indications for a specific symptomatic control of human suffering. Thus, the mostly unflattering comparisons continuously made between us and physicians practicing before our century completely miss their mark.

If the holistic humoralism of yore proved to be epistemologically very stable before 1800, especially in its mechanical, chemical, and neurophysiological garb, the advent of pathological anatomy and then experimental physiology shattered traditional notions of bodily functions in health and disease commonly shared by patients and their physicians. For nineteenth-century practitioners, the notion of an increasingly fragmented human body composed of discrete organs and systems selectively afflicted by disease suggested new and specific targets for therapeutic intervention. After 1850 and beyond, the emergence and popularity of alternative medical systems such as homeopathy and hydropathy with their holistic therapies can be interpreted as reflecting the profound disillusionment with the growing therapeutic skepticism of mainstream medicine.[70]

Eventually, a new fiduciary relationship based on scientifically established frameworks began to take shape, although, as one frustrated German physician admitted as late as 1884, "ninety percent of the population has no understanding concerning the tasks of physicians."[71] Confused by the claims of newfangled scientific panaceas, large sectors of the German public supported a return to "natural therapy." A "physiologically"-informed rationale for therapy sought to selectively battle disease processes while attempting to bolster the natural healing forces now under siege by an implacable enemy, soon identified as armies of micro-organisms. Until the dawn of our century, the promise of specific therapeutic agents targeted to neutralize the very causes of certain diseases remained just that, a promise, and physicians such as Osler had recourse to some traditional agents such as cold water. The success story of our twentieth-century magic bullets,[72] however, could not and will not erase the perennial yearning for individuality and holism in therapy, a fact attested to by the impressive scope and popularity of contemporary alternative healing methods. I hope that in traveling with me on the twisting road to twentieth-century therapeutics, you have come to appreciate the shifting landscapes and points of interest on our historical journey.

Notes and References

1. Lewis Thomas, "Medical lessons from history," in *Medusa and Snail* (New York: Viking Press, 1979), p. 159.
2. E. H. Ackerknecht, "Aspects of the history of therapeutics," *Bull. Hist. Med.* 36 (1962): 389.
3. This contextual approach to the history of therapeutics can be found in G. B. Risse, "The history of therapeutics," in *Essays in the History of Therapeutics*, ed. W.F. Bynum and V. Nutton (Amsterdam: Rodopi, 1991), pp. 3-11. See also W. E. Mitchell, "Changing others: the anthropological study of therapeutic systems," *Man* 8 (1977): 15-20.
4. V. Nutton, "Humoralism," in *Companion Encyclopedia of the History of Medicine*, ed. W. F. Bynum and R. Porter, 2 vols. (London: Routledge, 1993), vol 1, pp. 281-91. For a recent summary, see I. W. Müller, *Humoralmedizin: physiologische, pathologische und therapeutische Grundlagen der galenischen Heilkunst* (Heidelberg: K. F. Haug, 1993).
5. The classical roots of the non-naturals are explained by L. J. Rather, "The six things 'non-natural," *Clio Med.* 3 (1968): 337-47, and P. H. Niebyl, "The non-naturals," *Bull. Hist. Med.* 45 (1971): 486-92.
6. I. M. Lonie, "A structural pattern in Greek dietetics and the early history of Greek medicine," *Med. Hist.* 21 (1977): 235-60.
7. Max Neuburger, "An historical study of the concept of nature from a medical viewpoint," *Isis* 35 (1944): 16-22 and also his *The Doctrine of the Healing Power of Nature thoughout the Course of Time*, trans. by L. J. Boyd (New York: Homeopathic Medical College, 1926).
8. S. Kuriyama, "Interpreting the history of bloodletting, *J. Hist Med.* 50 (1995): 11-46.
9. For details, see Gilbert Watson, *Theriac and Mithridatium. A Study in Therapeutics* (London: Wellcome Historical Medical Library, 1966).
10. William Brockbank, "Cupping and leeching," and "Counterirritation," in *Ancient Therapeutic Arts* (Springfield, Ill.: C.C. Thomas, 1954), pp. 67-102 and 105-34.
11. See J. M. Riddle, "Theory and practice in medieval medicine," in *The Town and State Physician in Europe from the Middle Ages to the Enlightenment*, ed. A. W. Russell (Wolfenbütel: Herzog August Bibliothek, 1981), pp. 47-61, and P. Gil-Sotres, "Derivation and revulsion: the theory and practice of medieval phlebotomy," in *Practical Medicine from Salerno to the Black Death*, ed. L. Garcia Ballester et al. (Cambridge: Cambridge University Press, 1994), chap 4, pp. 110-55.
12. One of the most lucid treatments of Paracelsus' theories is Lester S. King, "The philosophic approach: Paracelsus," in *The Growth of Medical Thought* (Chicago: University of Chicago Press, 1963), pp. 86-138.
13. A. B. Davis, "Some implications of the circulation theory for disease theory and treatment in the seventeenth century," *J. Hist. Med.* 26 (1971): 28-39.
14. For details, see Lester S. King, *The Road to Medical Enlightenment, 1650-1695* (London: Macdonald, 1970), and A. G. Debus. "The chemical philosophy and the scientific revolution." in *Revolutions in Science*, ed. W. R. Shea (Canton, Mass: Science History Publications, 1988) pp. 27-48.
15 . L. S. King, "Empiricism and rationalism in the works of Thomas Sydenham," *Bull. Hist. Med.* 44 (1970): 1-11.
16 . G. B. Risse, "Medicine in the age of Enlightenment," in *Medicine in Society,* ed. A. Wear (Cambridge: Cambridge University Press, 1992), pp. 149-95.
17. William Cullen, "Therapeutics," in Institutes of Medicine, lecture notes, Edinburgh, 1772,

vol. 7, p. 6 , MSS Collection, National Library of Medicine, Bethesda, Maryland. For a sample of Cullen's practice see G.B. Risse, "Cullen as clinician: organization and strategies of an eighteenth-century medical practice," in *William Cullen and the Eighteenth-Century Medical World*, ed. A. Doig et al. (Edinburgh: Edinburgh University Press, 1993), pp. 133-51.

18. James Gregory, *Additional Memorial to the Managers of the Royal Infirmary* (Edinburgh: Murray & Cochrane, 1803), pp. 412-13.

19. G. B. Risse, "The Brownian system of medicine: its theoretical and practical implications, *Clio Med.* 5 (1970): 45-51, and also "Brunonian therapeutics: new wine in old bottles?" in *Brunonianism in Britain and Europe*, ed. W. F. Bynum and R. Porter (London: Wellcome Institute for the History of Medicine, 1988), pp. 46-62.

20 . G. B. Risse, "Typhus fever in eighteenth-century hospitals: new approaches to medical treatment," *Bull. Hist. Med.* 59 (1985): 176-95. For more details, consult by the same author "Hospital care: state of the medical art," in *Hospital Life in Enlightenment Scotland* (New York: Cambridge University Press, 1986), chap 4, pp. 177-239.

21. J. W. Estes, "Making therapeutic decisions with protopharmacologic evidence," *Trans. Stud. Coll. Phys. Phila.* 1 (1979): 116-37. For an overview. see E. Lesky, "Klinische Arneimittelforschung im 18. Jahrhundert," *Beitr. Gesch. Pharmazie* 29 (1977): 17-20. A good reference work for eighteenth-century remedies is J. W. Estes, *Dictionary of Protopharmacology. Therapeutic Practices, 1700-1850* (Canton, Mass.: Science History Publications, 1990).

22 . G. B. Risse, "The quest for certainty in medicine: John Brown's system of medicine in France," *Bull. Hist. Med.* 45 (1971): 1-12.

23. P. Pinel, "Expectation," in *Dict. Sc. Med.* 14 (1815): 247-56. See also Erwin H. Ackerknecht, "Therapeutics," in *Medicine at the Paris Hospital, 1794-1848* (Baltimore: Johns Hopkins University Press, 1967), chap XI, pp. 129-38.

24. René T. Laennec, *Traité de l'Auscultation Médiate et des Maladies des Poumons et du Coeur*, 2 vols, (1819; repr. Paris: Masson, 1927), vol 1, p. 717.

25. J. Duffin, "Private practice and public research: the patients of R. T. H. Laennec," in *French Medical Culture in the Nineteeenth Century*, ed A. La Berge and M. Feingold (Amsterdam: Rodophi, 1994), pp. 118-48.

26. Pierre Louis, "Research on the effect of bloodletting in several inflammatory maladies," transl. W. J. Gaines and H. G. Langford, *Arch. Int. Med.* 106 (Oct 1960): 571-79

27. Quoted in George Weisz, "Academic debate and therapeutic reasoning in the mid-nineteenth century," in *The Medical Mandarins* (New York: Oxford University Press, 1995), p. 165 See also T. D. Murphy, "Medical knowledge and statistical methods in early nineteenth-century France," *Med. Hist.* 25 (1981): 301-19.

28. "Medical statistics," *Am. J. Med. Sci.* 21 (1837): 525. For details, see J. R. Matthews, *Quantification and the Quest for Medical Certainty* (Princeton, NJ: Princeton University Press, 1995).

29. Ibid., 250.

30. Ibid., 247.

31. The quoted text in English translation can be found in *Am. J. Med. Sci.* 21 (1837): 249. Also A. J. Bollet, "Pierre Louis: the numerical method and the foundation of quantitative medicine," *Am. J. Med. Sci.* 266 (Aug 1973): 92-101.

32. R. B. Sullivan, "Sanguine practices: a historical and historiographic reconsideration of heroic therapy in the age of Rush," *Bull. Hist. Med.* 68 (1994): 38-44, and C. Rosenberg, "The therapeutic revolution: medicine, meaning, and social change in nineteenth-century America,"

Persp. Biol. Med. 20 (1977): 485-506.

33. J. H. Warner, "The selective transport of medical knowledge: antebellum physicians and Parisian medical therapeutics," *Bull. Hist. Med.* 59 (1985): 213-31. For more details, consult John H. Warner, *The Therapeutic Perspective* (Cambridge, Mass.: Harvard Univ Press, 1986).

34. Samuel Hahnemann, *Organon of Medicine,* transl. from 5th German ed. by R. E. Dudgeon (Chicago: Hanemann Publ Co, 1896. See Lester S. King, "Similia similibus," in *The Medical World of the Eighteenth Century* (Chicago: University of Chicago Press, 1953), chap 6, pp. 157-91.

35. Samuel Hahnemann, *Materia Medica Pura.,* 2 vols, transl. and ed. C. J. Hempel (New York: Radde, 1846).

36. R. Jütte, "Professionalization of homeopathy in the nineteenth century," in *Coping with Sickness. Historical Aspects of Health Care in a European Perspective,* ed. J. Woodward and R. Jütte (Sheffield: Eur. Ass. Hist. Med. Health, 1995), pp. 45-66. For Germany, R. Witten, "The origins of homeopathy in Germany," *Clio Med.* 22 (1991): 51-63.

37. See articles in *The Medical History of Waters and Spas*, ed. R. Porter (London: Wellcome Institute for the History of Medicine, 1990).

38. R. T. Claridge, "Hydropathy or cold water cure as practiced by Vincent Priessnitz at Graefenberg, Silesia, Austria," *Edinburgh Med. & Surg. J.* 58 (1842): 155-86.

39. Vincent Priessnitz, *Priessnitz Manual of the Water Cure*, ed. and tranl. F. Graeter (New York: Radde, 1843).

40. Charles Scudamore, *A Medical Visit to Graefenberg* (London: Churchill, 1843), p. 39.

41. Josef Dietl, "Praktische Wahrnehmungen nach den Ergebnissen im Wiedner-Bezirkskrankenhause," *Zeitschr. Ges. Aerzte Wien* 1 (1845): 12

42. G. B. Risse, "A shift in medical epistemology: clinical diagnosis, 1770-1828," in *Proceedings of the 9th Symposium on the Comparative History of Medicine-East and West,* ed. Y. Kawakita (Osaka, Japan: Tanaguchi Foundation, 1987), pp. 115-47.

43. E. Lesky, "Von den Ursprüngen des therapeutischen Nihilismus," *Sudhoffs Archiv* 44 (1960): 1-20.

44. For details, see Claudia Wiesemann, *Josef Dietl und der therapeutische Nihilismus* (Frankfurt: B. Lang, 1991).

45. J. Dietl, "Zur Diagnose und Therapie des Typhus," *Wiener med.Wochenschr.* 5 (1855) No 44: 697-701, 716-20, 766-70. See also L. G. Stevenson, "Joseph Dietl, William Osler, and the definition of therapeutic nihilism," in *Festschrift Erna Lesky,* ed. K. Ganziger et al. (Vienna: Hollinek, 1981), pp. 149-52.

46. Rudolf Virchow, "Scientific method and therapeutic standpoints," (1849) in *Disease, Life and Man*, selected essays, transl. by L. J. Rather (Stanford: Stanford University Press, 1958), pp.40-66.

47. Carl A. Wunderlich, *Handbuch der Pathologie und Therapie* (Stuttgart, 1852), p. 75.

48. See Hermann E. Richter, *Organon der physiologischen Therapie* (Leipzig: O. Wigand, 1850).

49. C. Wunderlich, "Ein Plan zur festeren Begründung der therapeutischen Erfahrungen," *Schmidt's Jahrbücher* 70 (1851): 108.

50. Ibid., 110-11.

51. Claude Bernard, *An Introduction to the Study of Experimental Medicine*, transl. H.C. Green, reprint with new forward by I. B. Cohen (New York: Dover Publications, 1957), p. 2.

52. Ibid., pp. 209-10.

53. Ibid., pp. 214-15.

54. H. Schulz, "Neue Arzmittel und ärztliche Praxis," *Deutsch. med. Wochenschr.* 15 (1890): 12-

4. See J. R. McTavish, "Antipyretic treatment and typhoid fever: 1860-1900," *J. Hist. Med.* 42 (1987): 486-506.

55. Robert Volz, *Der ärztliche Beruf* (Berlin: Lüderitz, 1870), pp. 32-33. The passage was translated into English and appears in G. B. Risse, "Patients and their healers: historical studies in health care," in *Who Decides? Conflicts of Rights in Health Care,* ed. N. K. Bell (Clifton, NJ: Humana Press, 1982), pp. 27-45.

56. Bernard, *Experimental Medicine* (n. 51), p. 215.

57. For details, see S. L. Montgomery, "Codes and combat in medical discourse," *Science as Culture* 2 (1991): 341-90. See also A. Windrath, *Die Medicin unter der Herrschaft des bacteriologischen Systems* (Bonn: Otto Paul Verlag, 1895).

58. See C. Habricht, "Chemotherapy in Germany in the 20th century," in *History of Therapy,* Proceedings 10th International Symposium Comp. Hist. Med. East and West, ed. Y. Kawakita et al. (Tokyo: Ishiyaku Euro America, 1990), pp. 225-59.

59. See for example, P. Weindling, "From medical research to clinical practice: serum therapy for diptheria in the 1890s," in *Medical Innovations in Historical Perspective*, ed. J. V. Pickstone (London: Macmillan, 1992), pp. 72-83.

60. Quoted in *Therap. Gazette* 15 (Mar 16, 1891): 182-83.

61. Editorial, "The limitations of bacteriological therapeutics," *Therap. Gazette* 15 (Jun 15, 1891): 397.

62. Bernard, *Experimental Medicine* (n. 51), pp. 146-47.

63. E. Klebs, "Zur Pathologie und Therapie der Cholera Asiatica," *Deutsch. med. Wochenschr.* 18 (Oct 27, 1892): 975-78 and 18 (Nov. 3, 1892): 999-1003.

64. C. Manchot, "Ueber die Behandlung der Cholera mit dem Klebs'schen Anticholerin," *Deutsch. med. Wochenschr.* 18 (Nov 11, 1892): 1050-52, and F. Reiche, "The cholera in Hamburg in 1892," *Am. J. Med. Sci.* 105 (Feb 1893): 118.

65. A. von Genersich, "The complete washing-out of the intestinal tract as a treatment for cholera and allied conditions," *Lancet* 2 (Oct 14, 1893): 926-27.

66. The procedure is best described in W. Osler, "The cold-bath treatment of typhoid fever," *Medical News* (Phila) 61 (Dec. 3, 1892): 628-31.

67. Osler's approach to the treatment of typhoid fever and the importance of this disease in shaping nineteenth-century therapeutics has been analyzed by L. G. Stevenson, "Exemplary disease: the typhoid pattern," *J. Hist. Med.* 37 (1982): 159-81.

68. Under Osler, even bloodletting returned to the treatment of pneumonia. See G. B. Risse, "The renaissance of bloodletting: a chapter in modern therapeutics," *J. Hist. Med.* 34 (1979): 3-22. For a contemporary historical review, see S. Baruch, "The evolution of modern therapy," *Therap Gazette* 23 (1899): 369-77, and 448-54.

69. The quotation is taken from Maurice B. Strauss, ed., *Familiar Medical Quotations* (Boston: Little, Brown & Co, 1968), p. 442.

70. For a recent historical analysis of alternative medicine, consult K. B. Alster, "The origins of modern holistic thought," in *The Holistic Health Movement* (Tuscaloosa: University of Alabama Press, 1989), pp. 7-45, and Robert Jütte, *Geschichte der Alternativen Medizin* (Munich: C. H. Beck, 1996).

71. Heinrich Schmidt, *Streiflichter über die Stellung des Arztes in der Gegenwart* (Berlin, 1884), p. 32.

72. J. Parascandola, "The theoretical basis of Paul Ehrlich's chemotherapy," *J. Hist. Med.* 36 (1981): 19-43

Section 2.

Case Studies
of Drug Discovery

DRUG discovery excites the imagination. Through the application of science, a new substance arises to cure or ameliorate disease. It might not take more than a pinch of the new medicine to make people's lives longer and happier.

Despite the romantic images portrayed in movies like "Dr. Ehrlich's Magic Bullet," most drug discovery has resulted from mundane laboratory work and patient attention to detail. John Parascandola opens section two of the *Inside Story* with an overview of the search for new therapies from 1800 up through Ehrlich's 1910 announcement of salvarsan's efficacy against syphilis.

According to Michael Bliss, the "story of insulin's emergence is a splendid verification of the maxim that chance favors the prepared mind." In the case of insulin, the prepared minds often did not see things eye to eye. The insulin history also demonstrates the importance of "scaling up" the manufacture of new medicines to meet the enormous demand of a waiting public.

Sometimes, as John Lesch points out, drugs appear more as a technological innovation than a pure discovery. His case study, May and Baker (M & B) 693 or sulfapyridine, was developed through a team effort to search methodically through many possible sulfa candidates, plus a bit of serendipity. The popular press, however, tends to apply its praise for scientific developments to only one or two individuals. Although introduced with some fanfare in 1938, M & B 693 received great attention in 1943 when it saved the life of Winston Churchill. The importance of who discovered what and when suddenly came to the forefront.

In sharp contrast to M & B 693, the thiazide diuretics have no great fame. Instead, they have been used quietly for almost forty years to lower blood pressure in an effort to forestall stroke, heart disease, and kidney failure. As Robert Kaiser argues, they symbolize well the shift towards corporate research that had begun in the years between the World Wars and culminated

75

in the 1950s. And their rapid clinical acceptance shows as well how far the marketing of medicines had progressed from the turn of the century.

With new diuretics, like the thiazides, testing for efficacy is relatively simple. Physical measurements of kidney output and blood pressure can be taken before and after administration of the medicine. When the goal is pain relief, however, testing becomes a subjective matter. This issue is at the center of Caroline Acker's telling of the search for potent, yet nonaddicting, pain relievers.

This search continues on and shows how drug discovery and development can influence the way we understand how the body functions. Drugs continue to serve not only as tools for healing but as tools for exploring the inner workings of life itself.

Alkaloids to Arsenicals: Systematic Drug Discovery Before the First World War

by John Parascandola

Drug therapy in the twentieth century has been characterized by an increasing reliance upon single-entity chemical substances, generally isolated and often even created or modified in the laboratory. At least this has been the case for orthodox medicine in Western countries. Even when we derive a drug from a natural product, such as a plant or microorganism, our goal is to isolate a chemically pure ingredient that is responsible for the pharmacological activity of the substance. We then strive to synthesize the compound in the laboratory, and investigate whether we can improve on nature by enhancing the efficacy or reducing the toxicity of the drug through molecular modification. This paper will focus on the origins and early development of this systematic science of drug design.

If there is one image that has dominated the process of drug discovery in the twentieth century, it is probably that of the "magic bullet," the chemical compound that specifically eliminates the cause of a disease while leaving the patient essentially unharmed. In modern terms, we explain this specificity of action in terms of drug receptors in the cells of organisms. Although the magic bullet idea originated with infectious diseases, it has come to serve as a metaphor for drug therapy in general. In fact, the metaphor of the magic bullet has been commonly applied to problems far beyond the boundaries of medicine. People speak of the hope for "magic bullets" that can solve particular economic and social problems. Not infrequently, especially when applied to complex socioeconomic problems, the reference is in the negative, i.e., to the fact that a proposed solution is <u>not</u> a magic bullet.[1]

The use of the term "magic bullet" in medicine can be traced back to the work of Paul Ehrlich, the German physician and scientist, who first spoke of "Zauberkugeln" ("magic bullets") to combat pathogenic microorganisms around the turn of the twentieth century.[2] The general idea that drugs may exert a selective action on specific organs has long been recognized empirically and expressed vaguely in the traditional designation of certain remedies as cordials, hepatics, etc.[3] Even the concept of specific medicines that can seek out and destroy pathogens without doing undue damage to the host predates Ehrlich.[4] Ehrlich was also not the first to use a metaphor of a projectile weapon to represent the concept of drug specificity. The famous English biologist Thomas Huxley used the image of a torpedo in 1881 to describe how pharmacologists would be able to provide physicians of the future with drugs capable of affecting physiological functions in any desired way.

> It will, in short, become possible to introduce into the economy a molecular mechanism which, like a very cunningly contrived torpedo, shall find its way to some particular group of living elements, and cause an explosion among them, leaving the rest untouched.[5]

Nevertheless, it was Ehrlich who introduced the specific concept of the magic bullet, an image that served as one of the theoretical driving forces behind his research program for the development of chemotherapeutic agents. At the time that he introduced the organic arsenic compound Salvarsan into clinical practice in 1910, it did indeed appear to be a magic bullet for the treatment of syphilis. Undoubtedly Paul de Kruif's 1926 best-selling book, *Microbe Hunters* (which included a chapter entitled "Paul Ehrlich: The Magic Bullet"), and the 1940 Warner Brothers feature film starring Edward G. Robinson, *Dr. Ehrlich's Magic Bullet*, helped to popularize the magic bullet image in the United States.[6]

Ehrlich's theories of magic bullets, experimental chemotherapy, and drug receptors have greatly influenced drug design and development in the twentieth century. His ideas have formed an important part of the foundation

John Parascandola is Historian for the United States Public Health Service. He received his Ph.D. in History of Science from the University of Wisconsin-Madison in 1968, and then spent a postdoctoral year at Harvard University. From 1969 to 1983, he taught history of pharmacy and history of science at the University of Wisconsin-Madison, also serving as Director of the American Institute of the History of Pharmacy from 1973 to 1981. In 1983, he became Chief of the History of Medicine Division of the National Library of Medicine, a position that he held until moving to his current job in 1992. Dr. Parascandola's research interests have focused on the history of modern pharmaceutical and biomedical science. His book on *The Development of American Pharmacology: John J. Abel and the Shaping of a Discipline* (Johns Hopkins University Press, 1992) was awarded the George Urdang Medal.

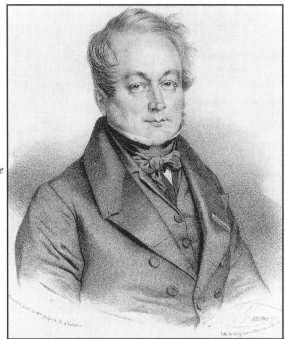

Françoise Magendie, one of the founders of experimental pharmacology, published a formulary promoting the use of pure chemical drugs such as the alkaloids. (Courtesy of the National Library of Medicine.)

on which modern efforts to make the process of drug discovery more systematic have been built, and I shall discuss his work in some detail. Ehrlich will not represent the starting point of my paper, however, but rather the end point. I will begin by considering those developments of the previous century that culminated in Ehrlich's approach to drug discovery.

The Discovery of the Alkaloids

The beginnings of modern systematic drug development, which is an interdisciplinary field based upon the interaction of sciences such as chemistry and pharmacology, can be traced back to the early nineteenth century. The laboratory sciences on which our current biomedical research is based largely emerged as specific disciplines in the nineteenth century, although their roots in some cases go back further in time. Chemistry has been, and remains, a key science in the process of drug design. Although some chemical processes had been used in preparing pharmaceuticals for centuries, it was not until after chemistry was established as a modern science under the influence of Antoine Lavoisier and his contemporaries at the end of the eighteenth century that its full impact began to be felt in pharmacy. Similarly, although physiological processes had long been of interest to physicians, it was not until physiology and pharmacology developed as experimental sciences, beginning especially with the work of François Magendie in the early nineteenth century, that these subjects came to play a significant role in drug development.

It was the interaction of chemistry with physiology and pharmacology that led to a major turning point in drug development in the early part of the nineteenth century, i.e., the discovery of the alkaloids. In many ways, the beginnings of a more systematic approach to drug development begins here, as implied in the title of my paper. It was necessary to understand something about the chemical composition and structure of drug molecules and the relationship of those factors to physiological activity before one could begin to develop new chemical therapeutic agents by a more rational process than trial and error. First, however, one had to isolate the active constituents of crude drugs so that their chemical and pharmacological properties could be studied. The alkaloids played a key role in this process.

As chemistry began to evolve into a modern science, pharmacists played a significant role in the process. Pharmacists possessed chemical knowledge and chemical equipment used in the preparation of certain pharmaceuticals, and some of them became involved in the teaching of chemistry and in chemical research. Using the back room laboratories of their pharmacies for their research efforts, some European pharmacists made important chemical discoveries. Not surprisingly, one area of interest to them was chemical analysis of the plant substances that made up so much of the materia medica of the day. One of the most skilled of the pharmacist-chemist investigators, Carl Scheele of Sweden, discovered several new acids in plants in the late eighteenth century, including tartaric acid and citric acid.[7]

Far more important from a therapeutic standpoint was the discovery of the plant bases known as alkaloids, another development in which pharmacists played a key role. This class of drugs includes many important therapeutic agents, such as the opiates and quinine. The field of alkaloid chemistry was opened by the isolation of morphine from opium in the early years of the nineteenth century. It was a young German pharmacist, Friedrich Sertürner, who first isolated morphine in 1805. It was not until he expanded and refined his studies in an 1817 paper, however, that his work had a significant impact. In this paper, he named the physiologically active principle of opium "morphium," after the god of dreams. He demonstrated its pharmacological powers by administering the drug to himself and three other volunteers. Alarmed by symptoms of poisoning, the men took strong vinegar to induce vomiting, but it took several days for the symptoms to completely disappear.[8]

Sertürner recognized that morphine was alkaline in nature, but it was the French chemist Joseph Gay-Lussac and pharmacist Pierre Robiquet who most clearly saw the significance of this discovery. They predicted that morphine was just the first of a whole new class of organic bases. By 1820, at least eight alkaloids had been discovered, with the French pharmacists Pierre-Joseph Pelletier and Joseph Caventou leading the way by isolating strychnine, quinine, and several other plant bases. The generic term "alkaloid" was introduced for these plant bases in 1818, although it did not come into general use until much later.[9]

The French physiologist François Magendie, mentioned earlier as one of the founders of the science of experimental pharmacology, clearly understood the significance of the alkaloids for therapeutics. He himself collaborated with Pelletier in investigating the properties of emetine, an alkaloid isolated from ipecacuanha root by Pelletier and Caventou. Magendie postulated that one could develop a more rational therapeutics through the experimental investigation of the physiological effects of chemically pure substances. He even published a formulary based on these pure chemicals, which largely consisted of the few alkaloids known at the time and several other substances such as the inorganic iodine salts. The first edition of the work, in fact, contained only twelve substances, but it was well received and went through nine editions between 1821 and 1836.[10]

The Study of Structure-Activity Relationships

Once scientists were able to isolate pure chemicals such as the alkaloids from crude drug sources, such as plant leaves, it was natural for them to begin to investigate the composition and structure of these chemical substances. Questions also arose as to the way in which the chemical composition and structure of a substance affected its action on the living organism. At least since the seventeenth century, there had been speculation about the relationship between the medicinal or toxic properties of a substance and its chemical nature. The so-called iatrochemists, for example, tried to associate the remedial action of medicines with their acidic and basic properties. Adherents of the corpuscular philosophy, such as Robert Boyle and John Locke, attempted to explain the action of drugs and poisons in terms of the size, shape and motion of their corpuscles or atoms.[11]

By the nineteenth century, however, advances in chemistry and pharmacology made it possible to go beyond speculation in investigating the subject. Most drugs were organic compounds, however, and the understanding of the structure of organic molecules was still in its infancy in the first half of the nineteenth century. It is understandable, therefore, that early investigators into the relationship between chemical structure and pharmacological activity concentrated on linking specific physiological effects to the presence of certain elements or functional groups in a compound, rather than considering more complicated questions involving the general structure of the molecule.[12]

The first scientist to make a serious beginning in the study of structure-activity relationships was James Blake, an English physician who later emigrated to America. Blake's studies, begun in the late 1830s, initially involved an investigation of the effects of a wide array of compounds, both organic and inorganic, but this sweeping approach proved too complex. He was able only to group his substances in very broad general classes, one of which was for those substances that did not fit into the other groups. He then decided to focus his efforts on a series of inorganic salts, and was struck by the relationship that he found between chemical composition and physiological action. The different salts of a given metal, such as sodium, produced essentially identical pharmacological effects.

Blake continued his experiments and was soon able to divide the elements into various groups according to the physiological effects produced by their salts. In 1841, he announced that elements that were isomorphic (i.e.,

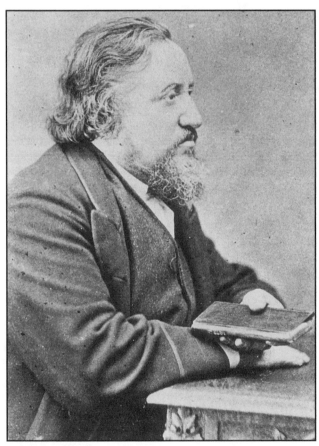

Benjamin Ward Richardson was one of the pioneers in the study of structure-activity relationships in drugs. (Courtesy of the National Library of Medicine.)

had the same crystalline form) generally had very similar pharmacological properties. Some of Blake's groupings of elements, incidentally, were very similar to those used by Mendeleev almost two decades later in constructing his periodic table, but Blake was unaware of any periodic relationship of the elements. His work was important because it demonstrated that a relationship could be established between the pharmacological action and the chemical nature of a substance. He himself noted:

> I think that the facts above are sufficient to show that there exists some intimate connection between the chemical properties of substances, and their physiological action, the investigation of which promises to furnish a rich field for physiological researches.[13]

The subject did indeed provide a rich field for investigation. Given the fact that the composition and properties of organic compounds were still imperfectly understood at the time, it is understandable that Blake limited his studies to inorganic substances. As previously noted, however, the most interesting drugs were organic compounds. While structural organic chemistry was still in its infancy, the British physician Benjamin Ward Richardson made perhaps the earliest systematic effort to investigate structure-activity relationships in organic compounds.

Between 1864 and 1870, Richardson published a series of papers in which he described his experiments with hydrocarbon compounds, involving a comparison of the effects of different functional groups on the pharmacological action of these substances. He was able to associate certain functional groups with specific physiological properties. For example, the nitrite group was shown to be associated with vasodilation and quickening of the heart, and the hydroxy or alcohol group with depression of the active functions of the cerebrospinal system. Richardson was thus at least able to show a crude relationship between structure and activity.[14]

The study that really called attention to the field of structure-activity relationships, however, was that of the chemist Alexander Crum Brown and the pharmacologist Thomas Fraser, both at Edinburgh University. They began their first paper on the subject, in 1869, with a declaration of faith:

> There can be no reasonable doubt that a relation exists between the physiological action of a substance and its chemical constitution, understanding by the latter term the mutual relations of the atoms in the substance.[15]

Although Brown and Fraser recognized the need to relate activity to the structure of a molecule, and not just its chemical composition, the structure of most organic compounds was not known at the time. They refused to allow such considerations to deter them, however, reasoning that one should still be

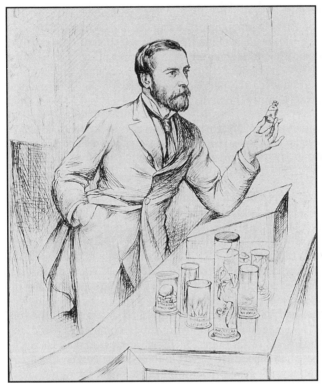

Thomas Fraser, shown lecturing on materia medica about 1884, collaborted with Alexander Crum Brown on ground-breaking research in the field of structure-activity relation-ships. (Courtesy of the National Library of Medicine.)

able to discover the nature of the relationship between structure and activity at least in an approximate manner. Their approach was to produce a known change in structure that would be the same in a number of different compounds, and then observe the effect on physiological activity. Their examination of the literature had convinced them that physiological activity was often associated with an unsaturated valence, i.e., with the presence of an atom that could undergo further addition. Chemical addition often seemed to remove or diminish physiological activity. For example, carbon monoxide is highly toxic, but addition of another oxygen results in a much less toxic substance, carbon dioxide.

Brown and Fraser decided to work with alkaloids, because, as we have seen, many important drugs fall into this class. In addition, there was some evidence that the addition of methyl iodide to these compounds, the process of methylation, destroyed or diminished their physiological activity. This fact supported their theory about the relationship of addition and saturation to activity.

Working with a number of alkaloids, they found that upon methylation, the ability of these alkaloids to produce convulsions disappeared. The narcotic properties of morphine and codeine were also diminished. At the same time, the methylated compounds were not inactive, but exhibited a very different toxic effect. The methylated derivatives all exhibited a paralyzing effect similar to that of the arrow poison curare. A relatively small change in structure had thus produced a dramatic change in the pharmacological properties of the alkaloids.

The two Scottish scientists expanded their experiments to other substances, and soon found that in general compounds known as quaternary ammonium salts (which included the methylated alkaloids) were associated with a paralyzing action. They had been extremely fortunate in their choice of compounds to study, because such clear-cut relationships between structure and activity are not common. Their success encouraged others to undertake investigations in this field.[16]

At first there was considerable optimism that a general law, or a few generalizations, describing the relationship between structure and activity would be discovered. There were also high hopes for the therapeutic applications of structure-activity research. In 1869, Benjamin Ward Richardson, whose work was discussed earlier, wrote:

> I am certain that the time must soon come when the books we call 'Pharmacopoeias'
> will be everywhere constructed on this basis of thought and the chemist and the
> physician will become one and one.[17]

The British physician Thomas Lauder Brunton echoed these sentiments a decade later, suggesting that the time was not far off when the physician would be able to predict the pharmacological action of any compound from its chemical constitution.[18] And the previously cited quotation from Huxley about the cunningly contrived torpedo was also uttered in response to these developments in pharmacology.

Chemists in the German dye industry also developed an interest in the relationship between chemical structure and the properties of molecules, such as color and the ability to hold fast to a cloth. In the late nineteenth century, encouraged by their own success in manipulating dye molecules to produce desired properties and by the pharmacological studies of Brown and Fraser and their colleagues, the research laboratories in these firms began altering the structure of substances to see if they could produce useful, marketable drugs from the by-products of dye production.[19]

Some synthetic drugs were developed in the last decades of the nineteenth century as a result of structural considerations. For example, the Bayer Company was able to modify the structure of para-nitrophenol, a by-product of the dye industry, to produce a useful antipyretic, phenacetin. In this case, there was a conscious effort to create a substance with a structure similar to that of a known antipyretic. Often, however, success in producing new synthetic drugs owed as much to luck as to correct structural reasoning. For example, Ludwig Knorr attempted to synthesize a quinine-type structure in 1883, although the structure of quinine was not completely known at the time. He did succeed in producing a new antipyretic, antipyrine, but its structure was not what he had expected and did not resemble that of quinine.[20] By the end of the century, it was becoming obvious that determining the relationship between structure and activity was going to be much more difficult than originally anticipated. The practical results of this approach for therapeutics had not been as great as expected. In 1901, British biochemist F. Gowland Hopkins summed up the situation when he wrote:

> It is a matter for some disappointment, and perhaps for surprise, that we should, today, after thirty years, be able to point to very few general relations bearing the stamp of such definiteness and simplicity as are found in the case brought to light by Crum Brown and Fraser; and that even now the results of those investigators may be quoted as the most satisfactory instance to hand, of obvious relation between chemical constitution and physiological action.[21]

Ehrlich and Magic Bullets against Microbes

In spite of the disappointment expressed by Hopkins, chemists had had some success in elucidating the chemical composition and sometimes even the structural formulas of drugs, and a number of new synthetic drugs had entered the market. The establishment of the germ theory of disease in the late nineteenth century also provided an understanding of the cause of infectious disease, and some hope that drugs could be found to combat the pathogenic microbes responsible for these diseases. Joseph Lister had shown that microbes could be destroyed in the operating room by disinfectants, thus reducing infections during surgery, and there were hopes that "internal disinfectants" could be found to combat microorganisms inside the body. Caustic substances such as carbolic acid could be used as effective disinfectants in the operating room, but the damage that they could cause to body tissues limited their scope for internal use. What was needed were substances that would specifically destroy microorganisms within the body without unduly harming the human host. Thomas Lauder Brunton recognized, for example, that many drugs might be injurious to both microorganisms and to the host tissues, but one could hope to find substances that were not equally harmful to both.[22]

As historian John Crellin has shown, there was a significant effort in the late nineteenth century to find internal antiseptics or disinfectants, and compounds such as the sulfocarbolates, the phenols, and the salicylates were tried internally (by oral, hypodermic, and inhalation routes) for diseases such as tuberculosis, diphtheria, and urinary tract infections. These trials, however, produced little or no results of substantive value for therapeutics.[23]

We now come full circle and return to Paul Ehrlich, who wove together the various strands of structure-activity studies, dye chemistry, and the search for internal disinfectants in producing his own theory of chemotherapy.[24] Ehrlich developed an interest in the selective action of drugs and chemicals while he was still a medical student in Germany in the early 1870s. He read a work on lead poisoning that intrigued him because the author had found re-

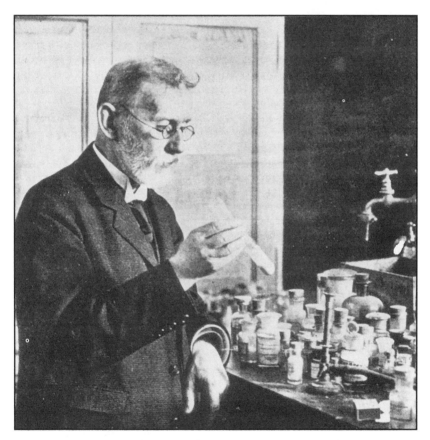

Paul Ehrlich, the founder of modern chemotherapy, introduced the concept of "magic bullets" against infectious disease. (Courtesy of the National Library of Medicine.)

markable differences in the amounts of lead absorbed by the different organs. Ehrlich became fascinated with the question of the selective distribution of substances in the different organs and tissues. He decided to study this problem using dyes because they would allow him to easily determine distribution by color. These studies introduced him to the field of dyes and also to questions involving the relationship of the chemical structure of a substance to its distribution in the body.[25]

It was also in the course of his studies on dyes that he developed his side chain theory of cell function, which he eventually applied to his work in immunology and chemotherapy, using it to explain the selective action of immunological agents such as antibodies and antitoxins and also of drugs. In the case of drugs, Ehrlich argued that these substances had specific chemical groups that allowed them to combine with chemical side chains or receptors in the cell and thus exert their physiological effects. The substance had a chemical structure that allowed it to fit the receptor like a key fits a lock, thus explaining the specificity of action. Ehrlich's work, along with that of the English physiologist James Newport Langley at about the same time, mark the beginnings of our contemporary drug receptor theory.[26]

Ehrlich's research in immunology had so impressed him with the specificity of the antibodies produced by the organism, which specifically target an invading microorganism without harming the host, that he referred to these immunological agents as "magic bullets." Shortly after the turn of the twentieth century, he began in earnest a program to try to synthesize chemical magic bullets to combat infectious diseases, substances that would specifically combine with and poison pathogenic microorganisms while leaving the host cell largely unaffected.

He began by studying dyes as potential drugs against the microorganism known as trypanosomes, which cause diseases such as sleeping sickness. Later he extended his studies to include arsenic compounds, and also to test his compounds against the newly discovered cause of syphilis, an organism known as the spirochete. It was not enough to test the properties of these substances in the test tube, or even in healthy animals. Ehrlich emphasized the need to study the effects of these compounds in animals that had been infected with the disease in question.[27]

Many of the substances tested had activity against the microorganisms, but they proved to be too toxic to the animal host for therapeutic use. In 1905, for example, British researchers discovered that atoxyl, an organic arsenic compound, had significant activity against trypanosomes, but it damaged the optic nerve and caused blindness in higher animals. Ehrlich and his coworkers elucidated the structure of atoxyl and reasoned that it should be possible to modify the structure of the chemical in such a way as to retain its activity against trypanosomes but to reduce or eliminate its toxic effect on the optic nerve. Hundreds of compounds were synthesized and tested in Ehrlich's institute in a systematic effort to find the compound that met the requirements to serve as a "magic bullet." The work was carefully directed by Ehrlich. Every morning he would provide his team of investigators with detailed instructions for their day's work, and he expected these instructions to be obeyed exactly.[28]

Finally in 1909 it was discovered that compound number 606 was effective against syphilis, as well as certain trypanosome infections, in experimental animals. Ehrlich arranged for clinical tests of the drug, and in April of 1910 he was able to report very encouraging results at the Congress of Internal Medicine in Wiesbaden. The announcement of the discovery of a specific for syphilis was greeted with great enthusiasm, and the demand for the drug soon outgrew the ability of Ehrlich's laboratory to produce it. He then arranged for the Höchst Chemical Works to manufacture 606 under the tradename Salvarsan.[29]

For much of the rest of Ehrlich's life (he died in 1915), he was absorbed by questions concerning the production and distribution of Salvarsan and problems involving its use. He devoted a substantial amount of time to educating physicians in the proper use of the drug and in trying to improve methods of administration. Reports of its toxic side effects deeply concerned him.[30]

Although Salvarsan seems to us in retrospect less than an ideal drug, and has since been replaced by more effective and less toxic medicines such as penicillin, in its day it did indeed seem like a miracle drug for a much feared disease. Ehrlich had developed the first chemical synthetic drug that had significant success against an infectious disease, and his triumph gave new hope to scientists, physicians, and the public. His theories of chemotherapy and receptors also provided working hypothesizes that stimulated further research. There was hope that perhaps scientists could indeed systematically design "magic bullets" against a variety of diseases.

Conclusion

We have come a long way in the twentieth century in our quest for magic bullets, and the list of effective drugs developed in the laboratory is impressive indeed. We have also learned, however, that it is difficult to find true "magic bullets," which cure the disease while doing no harm to the host. Often there are undesirable side effects that we must accept as part of the package. And the process of developing drugs for specific purposes still has more guesswork in it than we would like. In spite of our remarkable progress, we still have not fulfilled the hopes of some of the early investigators in the field of structure-activity relationships. We still cannot completely predict the pharmacological action of any compound by merely inspecting its structural formula, not can we design drugs at will for specific diseases.

Notes and References

1. For examples of the use of the "magic bullet" metaphor in relation to social problems, see Eunice Kennedy Shriver, "Rx for Teen Pregnancy," *Washington Post*, March 19, 1987, A23 and J.P. Newhouse, "Economists, Policy Entrepreneurs, and Health Care Reform," *Health Aff.* 14 (1995): 182-98.

2. See, e.g., Paul Ehrlich, "Address Delivered at the Dedication of the Georg-Speyer Haus" [1906], English translation, in *The Collected Papers of Paul Ehrlich*, ed. F. Himmelweit, vol. 3 (London: Pergamon Press, 1960), pp. 53-63 (the specific reference to "magic bullets" is on p. 59).

3. Melvin Earles, "Early Theories of the Mode of Action of Drugs and Poisons," *Ann. Sci.* 17 (1961; publ. 1963): 97-110.

4. John K. Crellin, "Internal Antisepsis or the Dawn of Chemotherapy?" *J. Hist. Med.* 36 (1981): 9-18.

5. Thomas Huxley, "The Connection of the Biological Sciences with Medicine," *Nature* 24 (1881): 346.

6. Paul de Kruif, *Microbe Hunters* (New York: Harcourt, Brace and Company, 1926).

7. Glenn Sonnedecker, revisor, *Kremers and Urdang's History of Pharmacy*, 4th ed. (Philadelphia: J. B. Lippincott, 1976), pp. 353-61.

8. John Lesch, "Conceptual Change in an Empirical Science: The Discovery of the First Alkaloids," *Hist. Stud. Phys. Sci.* 11 (1981): 305-328 and Rudolf Schmitz, "Friedrich Wilhelm Sertürner and the Discovery of Morphine," *Pharm. Hist.* 27 (1985): 61-74.

9. Lesch, "Conceptual Change" (n. 8), p. 324.

10. On Magendie's work in pharmacology, see John Lesch, *Science and Medicine in France: The Emergence of Experimental Physiology, 1790-1855* (Cambridge, MA: Harvard University Press, 1984), pp. 99-165 and J.M.D. Olmsted, *François Magendie* (New York: Schuman's, 1944), pp. 35-44.

11. See, e.g., Robert Boyle, *On the Reconcileableness of Specific Medicines to the Corpuscular Philosophy* (London: Samuel Smith, 1685).

12. For more detailed discussions of the early history of structure-activity studies than can be presented here, see John Parascandola, "Structure-Activity Relationships: The Early Mirage," *Pharm. Hist.* 13 (1971): 3-10 and William Bynum, "Chemical Structure and Pharmacological Action: A Chapter in the History of 19th Century Molecular Pharmacology," *Bull. Hist. Med.* 44 (1970): 518-38.

13. James Blake, "On the Action of Certain Inorganic Compounds When Introduced Directly into the Blood," *Edinburgh Med. Surg. J.* 56 (1841): 124. For further details on Blake's work, see the references cited in n. 12.

14. On Richardson's work, see the references cited in n. 12.

15. A. Crum Brown and Thomas Fraser, "On the Connection between Chemical Constitution and Physiological Action. Part I. - On the Physiological Action of the Salts of the Ammonium Bases, Derived from Strychnia, Brucia, Thebaia, Codeia, Morphia, and Nicotia," *Trans. Roy. Soc. Edinburgh* 25 (1869): 151.

16. For further details on the work of Crum Brown and Fraser, see the references cited in n. 12.

17. Benjamin Ward Richardson, "Report on the Physiological Action of the Methyl and Allied Series," *Brit. Assoc. Rep.* 39 (1869): 421.

18. T. Lauder Brunton, *An Introduction to Modern Therapeutics* [Croonian Lectures for 1889]

(London: Macmillan, 1892), p. 4.

19. On the development of the German dye industry and its relationship to the development of pharmaceuticals, see John J. Beer, *The Emergence of the German Dye Industry* (Urbana: University of Illinois Press, 1959) and Anthony S. Travis, "Science as Receptor of Technology: Paul Ehrlich and the Synthetic Dyestuffs Industry," *Science in Context* 3 (1989): 383-408.

20. Hans-Joachim Flechtner, *Carl Duisberg* (Dusseldorf: Econ Verlag, 1959), pp. 108-110; Carl Duisberg, "Zur Geschichte der Entdeckung des Phenacetins," *Z. angew. Chem.* 26[I] (1913): 240; anon., "Discoverer of Antipyrin. A Note on Ludwig Knorr (1859-1912)," *Chem. Drugg.* 172 (1959): 508; Milton Silverman, *Magic in a Bottle* (New York: Macmillan, 1941), pp. 180-182.

21. F. G. Hopkins, "on the Relation between Chemical Constitution and Physiological Action," in *Textbook of Pharmacology and Therapeutics*, ed. W. Hale-White (Edinburgh: Young J. Pentland, 1901), p. 3.

22. T. Lauder Brunton, *A Text-book of Pharmacology, Therapeutics, and Materia Medica* (Philadelphia: Lea Brothers, 1885), p. 104.

23. Crellin, "Internal Antisepsis" (n. 4).

24. For a detailed discussion of Ehrlich's work in chemotherapy, see John Parascandola, "The Theoretical Basis of Paul Ehrlich's Chemotherapy," *J. Hist. Med.* 36 (1981): 19-43.

25. Parascandola, "Chemotherapy" (n. 24), 22-24.

26. On the development of the receptor theory, see John Parascandola and Ronald Jasensky, "Origins of the Receptor Theory of Drug Action," *Bull. Hist. Med.* 48 (1974): 199-220 and John Parascandola, "The Development of Receptor Theory," in *Discoveries in Pharmacology*, ed. M. J. Parnham and J. Bruinvels, vol. 3 (Amsterdam: Elsevier, 1985), pp. 129-156.

27. Parascandola, "Chemotherapy" (n. 24), pp. 20-21, 26-30.

28. Parascandola, "Chemotherapy" (n. 24), pp. 31-32. For more information on Ehrlich's personality and work habits, see Martha Marquardt, *Paul Ehrlich* (New York: Henry Schuman, 1951) and Ernst Bäumler, *Paul Ehrlich: Scientist for Life*, translated by Grant Edwards (New York: Holmes and Meier, 1984).

29. Parascandola, "Chemotherapy" (n. 24), pp. 33-34.

30. Marquardt, *Ehrlich* (n. 28), pp. 188-206.

The Discovery of Insulin: The Inside Story

by *Michael Bliss*

T HE isolation of insulin and its immediate application as a therapy for diabetes in 1921-22 was one of the most remarkable and dramatic events in the history of medicine. The story of insulin's emergence is a splendid verification of the maxim that chance favors the prepared mind. It also underlines the notion of a seamless connection between bench and bedside in the development of therapeutic agents; demonstrates the value of well-funded, collaborative research both within the university and between the university and the private sector; shows the folly that can result from personal ambition and paranoia in science; and is a spectacular, immensely moving example of medicine's ability to conquer disease.

In 1889 Oskar Minkowski in Germany formulated the hypothesis that a substance in the pancreas must regulate metabolism, somehow preventing the formation of diabetes mellitus[1]. A massive search immediately began for the substance, but no one could find it. In the meantime, type I or juvenile diabetes was a fatal disease, whose victims could only be treated by severe starvation diets, leaving them faced with a choice between death from starvation or death from diabetes, plus perhaps the dashed hopes that would come from trying one of the many quack remedies on the market. Despite researchers' gradual revelation of the existence of an endocrine system in the body, a concrete demonstration a pancreatic "internal secretion" continued to defy investigation. By definition the substance would not be proven to exist until administration of it as a replacement therapy inhibited or reversed the development of diabetes mellitus. In other words you would have to be able to treat diabetics with it.[2]

In 1920 a Canadian physician and surgeon with an interest in research, Frederick Banting, jotted down an idea involving ligating the ducts of the

93

pancreas in a living animal. He hoped that the resulting degenerated pancreas would contain the internal secretion in a relatively uncontaminated state:

Diabetus

> Ligate pancreatic ducts of dog. Keep dogs alive till acini degenerate leaving Islets.
> Try to isolate the internal secretion of these to relieve glycosurea.

Banting proposed to demonstrate the relief of "glycosurea" by transplanting parts of that pancreas into a depancreatized animal.[3]

Banting took his idea to his alma mater, the University of Toronto, where the Professor of Physiology, J. J. R. Macleod agreed to supply him with laboratory space, experimental animals, and a skilled student assistant. Macleod, who knew a lot about carbohydrate metabolism, but appears to have pretty well given up belief in an internal secretion, thought the antici-pated negative result of Banting's work would be useful. In any case, he had unused facilities and underemployed students on his hands in a university whose willingness to support research was outpacing the energies of its staff.[4]

In the summer of 1921, Banting and his helper, Charles Best, carried out a series of experiments depancreatizing dogs, ligating ducts, and adminis-tering extracts of a degenerated pancreas. They relied on blood sugar mea-surements as a monitor of the dogs' diabetic condition and were excited when their extract appeared to drive down the blood sugar of depancreatized ani-mals. Everyone knew, however, that a little bit of blood sugar reduction was only a start and much more would have to be done in the way of repeating and expanding the work. The research went forward under Macleod's direc-tion, despite serious personal friction between himself and Banting, mainly concerning the resources and priority the work should receive.[5]

Michael Bliss (M.A., Ph.D., F.R.S.C.) is a professor of History at the University of Toronto, Resident Scholar in the History of Medicine programme, and a Fellow of the Royal Society of Canada. He is the author of ten books and numerous articles in several areas of Canadian history, and has received the highest prizes for history given by the Canadian Historical Association and the Royal Society of Canada. His book, *The Dis-covery of Insulin*, published in 1983, was honored by the Hannah Medal of the Royal Society of Canada and the Welch Medal of the American Association for the History of Medicine. In 1984 a sequel, *Banting: A Biography*, was published. These books were adapted for television by Gemstone Productions of Toronto as the award-winning four-hour miniseries, "Glory Enough for All" (shown on PBS's "Masterpiece Theatre").

Professor Bliss has lectured widely about insulin and related topics through-out Europe as well as the United States and Canada. In addition to his scholarly work, he writes extensively in Canadian magazines and newspapers and has won two Canadian National Magazine Awards; he often comments on Canadian public affairs in the broad-cast media. He is now writing a biography of Sir William Osler.

Banting was a rough-and-ready surgeon with no training in research; Best was a recently graduated student. Their laboratory work was flawed by errors, sloppiness, and conceptual confusion.[6] Banting's main interest that autumn seems to have been getting back to pancreas transplants. He and Best did discover that they could use fresh whole pancreas with the same results on diabetic animals, thus completely bypassing the whole ligation procedure (that had been the rationale for the research in the first place). Even then they found they could not regularly repeat their results and when they tentatively, and secretively, tried their extract on a human diabetic, a classmate of Banting's named Joe Gilchrist, that did not work either.[7]

Nonetheless, Banting and Best's extracts had lowered blood sugar often enough in diabetic animals that Macleod became convinced that they probably contained the elusive pancreatic secretion. As formal director of the research he agreed to push on with it, and agreed with Banting's suggestion in December 1921 that they strengthen their team by adding a trained biochemist, J. B. Collip (who happened to be in Toronto on sabbatical from the University of Alberta that year working with Macleod on a quite different problem). Collip's advent, and his work on problems suggested by Macleod, marked the beginning of rapid advances in the research, including the discovery that the extract made possible glycogen formation in the liver, that it combated ketoacidosis in diabetic animals, and that it would lower the blood sugar of normal animals.[8]

When the Toronto team moved to formal clinical testing of their extract on a fourteen-year-old human diabetic, Leonard Thompson, in January 1922, Collip's role became crucial. The first extract used on Thompson on January 11th was made by Banting and Best, and it failed to improve his condition. On January 19th, however, J. B. Collip discovered a method by which he could precipitate out most of the toxic contaminants from the crude extract, thus producing a substance that contained the active principle in a pure enough form that when it was tested on Thompson on January 23rd it produced unequivocally positive results.[9] At that point the research team began to know they had isolated the internal secretion that physiologists had long dreamed of—they knew it because their extract worked so beautifully clinically as a replacement therapy.

A number of earlier researchers, such as Georg L. Zuelzer in Germany, N. C. Paulesco in Roumania, and E. L. Scott and Israel Kleiner in the United States, had almost reached this same goal, but all of them had stopped their research for want of financial support, research animals, or collaborative assistance in surmounting roadblocks.[10] Although Banting and to a degree Best were very energetic in spreading myths about having been underfunded and underappreciated, the dominant fact about the Toronto research was that it had evolved into a very high-powered collaboration among the two enthusiasts, Banting and Best, a world-class physiologist and expert in carbohydrate metabolism in Macleod, and an intuitive wizard of biochemistry, Collip. They were using first-rate facilities, and had access to all the dogs and other apparatus they needed. Their success rested particularly clearly on advances others had been making in recent years in blood sugar estimation; indeed the ability to do reasonably quick serial blood sugars, which had not existed before 1910, was a *sine qua non* to the insulin research.

The whole research endeavor had begun with the chance appearance of Banting in Macleod's lab, had been kept going when Macleod, cautious as he was, thought Banting and Best's results were worth developing, and came to triumphant completion when the prepared professional Collip, got to work on the extract. If Collip had not joined the insulin team in December, 1921, I suspect that the clinical triumphs would have taken place somewhere in the United States within about six months.

It was a great personal and institutional tragedy that the Toronto insulin team proved impossibly volatile even as the work continued. Banting had never liked Macleod; he soon became intensely suspicious of Collip. By the time of Collip's breakthrough, Banting had become positively paranoiac in his belief that the two senior members of the team were conspiring to appropriate the credit and the glory of being the discoverers of insulin. On the night of Collip's breakthrough he and Banting came to blows in the lab, which commenced a struggle for glory that lasted, in evolving form, for the rest of the discoverers' lifetimes and beyond. "In insulin there is glory enough for all" Lewellys Barker said at Toronto's 1923 dinner to honor its newly-minted Nobel laureates, but to Banting and Best's great discredit they did not heed him.[11]

The more important problem the Toronto group experienced in the spring of 1922 was its inability to capitalize on the discovery of insulin without outside help. The attempt in Toronto to move from discovery to clinical and commercial development of insulin floundered almost immediately when Collip, working in the university's fledgling Connaught Anti-Toxin Laboratory, found he could not produce insulin in larger batches. Indeed, after his first few batches he could not make potent insulin at all. The group were like explorers who had found the promised land and then lost it in a fog. There was a desperate insulin "famine" in Toronto in the spring of 1922 that only finally ended when the research team began collaboration with Eli Lilly and Company of Indianapolis. Lilly, in those days a medium-sized ethical drug company, had expressed interest early on in the work (its research director, G. H. A. Clowes had heard about the research and attended the New Haven presentation). Lilly had been held at bay by the Toronto team, and was finally brought on board in what proved a very fruitful collaboration for them and the University only after Toronto realized it just could not make insulin with its own resources. The Lilly-University of Toronto relationship worked well and became an important model for other collaborative efforts in the 1920s and 1930s.[12]

The human impact of the discovery of insulin was implicit in its very discovery—you knew you had it when you saw the sensational impact it had on diabetics. We do not know much about Leonard Thompson, the first patient: he was a charity case who survived fourteen years on insulin but we have a large roster of other patients whose stories are the stuff of high drama. These include the first American patient, James Havens, whose father had given up hope for his life in the spring of 1921 and who lived for 38 years on insulin; the first child to come out of coma by the use of insulin, Elsie Needham; and Banting's prize case, Elizabeth Hughes, the daughter of the United States Secretary of State and future Chief Justice, Charles Evans Hughes. Elizabeth was fifteen years old, five feet tall, and thanks to her starvation diet, weighed only forty-five pounds when she first began receiving insulin in August 1922. The ability of insulin to pull these children back from the edge of the grave was spectacular. The greatest thrills of my professional life as an historian came, first when I discovered in 1980 that Elizabeth Hughes was still alive; and, second, when in 1990 for our opening of an historical display on the discovery of insulin in Toronto we were able to have present one of the original patients, Mr. Theodore Ryder, who in 1992 became the first human to survive seventy years on insulin. Ted died in 1993. On the day in 1996 that I wrote the version of this essay to be published, I

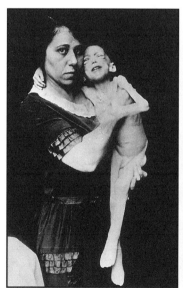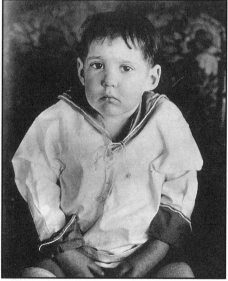

The use of insulin in diabetes produced many "before and after" images like those shown here. (Courtesy Eli Lilly and Company Archives.)

learned of the continuing survival of Mr. William Rounds of Granbury, Texas. He has been receiving insulin since 5 April 1923, in the first year of his life.[13]

The discovery of insulin had an enormous and as yet largely unexamined impact on biomedical sciences, clinical practice, and the mythology and symbolism of modern medicine. But for those contemporaries who were touched by the insulin research, and for many people involved with insulin and diabetes today, the best description of the transcendent meaning of this therapeutic breakthrough was given by Elliott Joslin of Boston. "By Christmas of 1922," Joslin wrote:

> I had witnessed so many near resurrections that I realized I was seeing enacted before my very eyes Ezekial's vision of the valley of dry bones:
>
> ...and behold, there were very many in the open valley; and lo, they were very dry. And he said unto me, Son of Man, can these bones live?
>
> And...lo, the sinews and the flesh came upon them and the skin covered them above: but there was no breath in them.
>
> Then said He unto me, "Prophesy unto the wind, prophesy, Son of Man, and say to the wind, Thus saith the Lord God: "Come from the four winds, O breath, and breathe upon these slain, that they may live."
>
> So I prophesied as he commanded me, and the breath came into them, and they lived, and stood up upon their feet, an exceeding great army.[14]

Notes and References

1. For a detailed account of these events see Michael Bliss, *The Discovery of Insulin* (Toronto, 1982; Chicago, 1983; 2nd ed. , Toronto, 1996); for Minkowski's work, see J. Von Mering, and O. Minkowski "Diabetes mellitus nach Pankreasextirpation," *Arch. Exp. Pathol. Pharmacol., Leipzig* 26(1890): 371-87; S. Zeller, and M. Bliss, "Minkowski," *Dictionary of Scientific Biography*, Sup II (New York: Scribner's, 1990), 626-633.

2. F. G. Young, "The Evolution of Ideas About Animal Hormones," in J. Needham, ed., *The Chemistry of Life* (Cambridge, 1970), 125-155.

3. F. G. Banting Initial Notebook, Thomas Fisher Rare Book Library, University of Toronto.

4. See M. Bliss, "JJR Macleod and the discovery of insulin," *Quarterly Journal of Experimental Physiology* (1989), 74, pp. 87-96; also Macleod, "History of the researches leading to the discovery of insulin," *Bull. Hist. Med.* 52,3,(Fall 1978), 295-312.

5. Banting and Best Notebooks, Banting Papers, Fisher Library; Macleod, "History" (n. 4); M. Bliss, ed., "Banting's, Best's, and Collip's accounts of the discovery of insulin," *Bull. Hist Med.* 56 (Winter 1982-83): 554-68.

6. Banting and Best Notebooks; F. G. Banting and C. H. Best, "The internal secretion of the pancreas," *J. Lab. Clin. Med.* 9(1954): 281-289.

7. Banting and Best Notebooks; Banting index cards, Banting Papers, Box 22.

8. Bliss, "Banting's, Best's, and Collip's accounts," (n. 5).

9. F. G. Banting, C. H. Best, J. B. Collip, W. R. Campbell, A. A. Fletcher, "Pancreatic extracts in the treatment of diabetes mellitus. preliminary report," *CMAJ* 2, 141(March 1922): 141-146; Bliss, "Banting's, Best's, and Collip's accounts" (n. 5); Macleod, "History" (n. 4).

10. Bliss, *Discovery of Insulin* (n. 1), 28-42, 209-210; see esp. E. S. Kleiner, "The action of

intravenous injections of pancreas emulsions in experimental diabetes," *J. Biol. Chem.* 40(1919):153-170.

11. Bliss, "Banting's, Best's, and Collip's accounts" (n. 5); F. G. Banting, "The story of insulin," unpublished ms, 1940, Banting Papers; M. Bliss, *Banting: A Biography* (Toronto, 1984; 2nd ed., Toronto, 1992); M. Bliss, "Rewriting medical history: Charles Best and the Banting and Best myth," *J. Hist. Med.* 48(July 1993): 253-274.

12. See John P. Swann, *Academic Scientists and the Pharmaceutical Industry* (Baltimore, 1988).

13. Personal communication, Dr. David B. Wilson to Dr. Bernard Zinman, Mount Sinai Hospital, Toronto, February 29, 1996; the records of Ryder, Hughes, Havens, and the other early patients are in the Banting Papers.

14. Eli Lilly & Company Archives, Joslin address at the opening of the Lilly research Laboratories, 1934.

The Discovery of M & B 693 (Sulfapyridine)

by John E. Lesch

Late in 1943, at the height of the Second World War, Winston Churchill visited the Middle East for conferences with Britain's allies. He met Chiang Kai-shek in Cairo, then flew to Teheran to talk with Stalin, and finally returned to Cairo for a meeting with President Roosevelt. Exhausted from work and travel, he boarded an airplane at 1 a.m. on 11 December for a flight to Tunisia, where he was to stay at Dwight Eisenhower's villa near Carthage. Off course, the plane made an unscheduled stop forty miles from its destination. Churchill sat on his luggage on the runway in a cold wind for an hour before completing his journey. Later that day Churchill had a pain in his throat and a bad headache. The next day he had a fever of 101 . Lord Moran, Churchill's personal physician, called in nurses and a pathologist from Cairo. A portable x-ray machine was brought from Tunis. X-rays showed a shadow on Churchill's lung, which the doctors diagnosed as pneumonia. Moran immediately put Churchill on one of the recently developed sulfa drugs manufactured by the British company May & Baker, and familiarly known as M & B. Churchill began to have heart trouble.[1]

Alarmed and fearing the worst for his 69-year-old-patient, Moran called in leading specialists from the Mediterranean theater. From Cairo came Brigadier D. Evan Bedford, a prominent heart specialist, and from Italy Lt.-Colonel G. A. H. Buttle, who as a civilian researcher before the war had conducted some of the earliest animal trials of sulfonamides in Britain and who was now regarded as an expert on the administration of M & B. Churchill's condition continued to deteriorate. His lungs became congested. He had heart fibrillations. A planned side trip to Italy to visit the troops was canceled, and Churchill's stay at Carthage was extended indefinitely. Then, much to the relief of everyone around him, he began to improve. By Christmas Day he was

101

feeling better and working. On December 27 he flew to Marrakesh to continue his convalescence, during which he worked on plans for the Anzio invasion, the Normandy invasion, and other, lesser, operations. From Marrakesh he flew to Gibraltar in mid-January, and from there sailed for England, arriving on 17 January 1944.[2]

No one, not Churchill himself, not his doctors, not the press or the public who anxiously followed the Prime Minister's illness and recovery, doubted that he had been brought back from the brink of death by the new medicine, that is by "M & B." After arriving in Marrakesh, Churchill issued a bulletin that was immediately printed in the British newspapers, and that said in part

> This admirable M & B, from which I did not suffer any inconvenience, was used at the earliest moment; and after a week's fever the intruders were repulsed. I hope all our battles will be equally well conducted. . . .The M & B, which I may also call Moran and Bedford [Churchill could not resist the joke on his physicians' names], did the work most effectively. There is no doubt that pneumonia is a very different illness from what it was before this marvelous drug was discovered.[3]

All very good. But what was "M & B?" Martin Gilbert's otherwise exhaustive biography of Churchill is not more specific, nor is Richard Lovell's biography of Lord Moran. A compound called M & B 760 (chemical name: sulfathiazole) may have been used. One of the specialists attending Churchill, a Lt.-Colonel R.J.V. Pulvertaft, had participated in research on penicillin with the British Middle East forces. But the presumption of most doctors, the press, and the public was that the drug that had saved Churchill's life was M & B 693, or sulfapyridine.[4]

Thanks to Churchill's recovery, M & B 693 enjoyed its most brilliant moment in the public eye. M & B was a "miracle drug" that had not existed six years earlier. And even as it was reported that Churchill had taken it, M & B 693 was being displaced by newer, more effective or less toxic medicines, first other sulfas such as M & B 760, later by penicillin. M & B 693, in fact,

John E. Lesch, Ph.D., teaches the history of science at the University of California, Berkeley, where he is Associate Professor of History. He is the author of a number of publications on the history of biology and medical sciences from the eighteenth to the twentieth century, most notably a book, *Science and Medicine in France: The Emergence of Experimental Physiology 1790-1855* (Cambridge, Mass. and London: Harvard University Press, 1984). He is writing a book on the history of the sulfa drugs, for which he has received research grants from the National Science Foundation, the National Institutes of Health, and the John Simon Guggenheim Memorial Foundation.

was one of a flood of sulfonamide derivatives that appeared from the late 1930s to the late 1940s. It was but one instance of a spreading revolution in the therapeutics of bacterial infections set in motion by the introduction of the first sulfa drugs, Prontosil and sulfanilamide, in 1935. With the way shown by Prontosil and sulfanilamide, pharmaceutical companies in several countries had joined an intensive search for new derivatives to treat a widening spectrum of bacterial diseases with lower risks to the patient.[5]

By 1945, a decade after the entry of Prontosil into medical practice, over 5,000 compounds had been synthesized, and some small fraction of these had gone on the market. Chemotherapies were available for many infections previously untreatable, or treated only with great difficulty, including puerperal fever, erysipelas, septicemia, urinary tract infections, gonorrhea, bacillary dysentery, and bacterial pneumonia. At the end of the war penicillin was beginning to displace the sulfas as the drug of choice in bacterial infections, but for most of World War II it was the sulfas that carried the main therapeutic burden.[6]

The first sulfas, Prontosil and sulfanilamide, were effective mainly against streptococcal infections. M & B 693 burst on the medical scene in 1938 as the first effective chemotherapy for bacterial pneumonia, a major scourge counted by William Osler among the "captains of the men of death." A study of case fatalities in pneumonia published in the *American Journal of Public Health* in 1943 showed a drop in mortality from over 20% in the period 1935-1937 to less than 4% between 1939 and June 1942. The same study estimated that by 1943 M & B 693 and other sulfa drugs were saving at least 25,000 lives a year in the working population of the United States alone. Churchill was only the most celebrated beneficiary of the new medicines.[7]

M & B 693 enjoyed about five years in the limelight as a miracle drug. In the brevity of its career it exemplified the fate of other medicines in the fast-changing domain of bacterial chemotherapy, where patents were often rendered superfluous by the pace of obsolescence. It may be representative of the new generation of sulfa drugs in other respects, and not least in the way it was "discovered."

M & B 693 emerged from an industrial research effort in which a deliberately constructed system of methodical trial and error was complemented by serendipity. It was greeted by the medical community with measured but genuine enthusiasm, and was appropriated by the popular press in ways that frequently exaggerated, misrepresented, or distorted its significance. Viewed in retrospect by participants and observers, the discovery of M & B 693 became subject to competing interpretations, most of which, nevertheless, presupposed that the discovery could be isolated to a single point in time, and that credit could be assigned to one or two individuals.

Assessing the meaning of "discovery" in the case of M & B 693 turns out to be more complicated than one might expect. Here I will give a short narrative of the brief but heroic life of this medicine, with emphasis on what I take to be the key events relevant to its discovery. With this story as a basis, I will offer a few reflections on what "discovery" can mean for this kind of drug.

Structure of Prontosil, from H. J. Barber, "Antibacterial dawn and antiprotozoal noon," in Historical Aspects of Chemotherapy: Six Essays *(Dagenham: May & Baker Ltd., 1976), pp. 24-32.*

The first of the sulfa drugs, Prontosil, was the product of the pharmaceutical research laboratories of I. G. Farbenindustrie at Elberfeld, Germany. The principal medical researcher involved in the development of Prontosil, Gerhard Domagk—who later received a Nobel Prize in Physiology or Medi-

Structure of sulfanilamide, from H. J. Barber, "Antibacterial dawn and antiprotozoal noon," in Historical Aspects of Chemotherapy: Six Essays *(Dagenham: May & Baker Ltd., 1976), pp. 24-32.*

cine—first published his findings in 1935. Prontosil was an azo dye, and so had the characteristic aromatic groups joined by a double bond between two nitrogens. The I. G. Farben researchers thought that Prontosil's biological activity was connected to its nature as a dye. But later in 1935 a team at the Pasteur Institute in Paris showed that Prontosil could be broken in two at the azo bond, and that one of the parts, a colorless compound later named sulfanilamide, was alone responsible for the therapeutic action.[8]

In principle, the Pasteur Institute discovery opened the way for a new program of chemotherapeutic research based on substitution for the hydrogen atoms in the sulfanilamide molecule. In practice, it seems that it was not immediately obvious to industrial researchers which direction to take, and response was slower than one might think in retrospect. One complication was that it took a while for researchers and doctors to be convinced that Prontosil itself worked, and still longer for them to recognize that sulfanilamide was Prontosil's equal. This was especially true in Britain and the United States.[9]

At the laboratories of May & Baker, at Dagenham outside London, interest in the sulfa drugs did not surface until January 1936 when George Newbery, one of the company's small staff of research chemists, synthesized Prontosil. Even then, a crash program of sulfonamides research was not in the works, still less one that took as starting point the Pasteur Institute finding published two months earlier. Company chemists made a few azo compounds, evidently with the thought of extending the Prontosil model. At research director A. J. Ewins's instigation they also synthesized a number of stilbene compounds. Stilbene derivatives, with their aromatic groups linked by a double bond between two carbon atoms, were important in the dye industry, and their structural analogy to azo dyes may have prompted Ewins's interest in their possible therapeutic activity. At the same time, however, company chemists were working on compounds without direct relation to the sulfonamides, including cyano compounds and oil-soluble arsenicals.[10]

It was only in May 1936 that Newbery turned to making derivatives of sulfanilamide. Two explanations may be suggested for this shift. One is that Newbery was asked to do so by his superior, Ewins, who was in turn asked to initiate research on sulfanilamide derivatives by his superior, Nicholas Grillet. Grillet was general manager of the French chemical firm, Rhône-Poulenc. In 1927 one of the parent companies of Rhône-Poulenc, Poulenc Frères, had bought a controlling interest in May & Baker, and this was retained after the merger that gave rise to Rhône-Poulenc in 1928. Grillet, a manager who understood research problems, therefore presumably had the

Possible substitutions in the sulfanilamide molecule. From H. J. Barber, "Antibacterial dawn and antiprotozoal noon," in Historical Aspects of Chemotherapy: Six Essays *(Dagenham: May & Baker Ltd.), pp. 24-32.*

authority to direct Ewins to initiate a new line of research. That he did so was later asserted by Jacques Billon, another manager at Rhône-Poulenc. Billon wrote that Grillet ordered A. J. Ewins at May & Baker, and Edmond Blaise, the scientific director of Rhône-Poulenc, to divide up the work in the search for derivatives of sulfanilamide. Rhône-Poulenc was to concentrate on derivatives substituted in the N^4 position, that is the amino group. May & Baker was to concentrate on derivatives substituted in the N^1 position, that is the sulfonamide group.[11]

A second explanation for the May & Baker research staff's shift of attention to sulfanilamide derivatives points to sources closer to home. In the Spring of 1936 G. A. H. Buttle, a researcher at Wellcome Laboratories in

London, was following up on the Pasteur Institute discovery by testing the therapeutic efficacy of sulfanilamide and its derivatives in animal trials. Word of his success with sulfanilamide itself and with one derivative may have reached May & Baker staff even before Buttle published his first results in June 1936.[12]

Either or both explanations may be correct, although the Billon story is placed in some doubt by the circumstance that May & Baker chemists did not confine themselves to preparation of N^1-substituted derivatives, but also made N^4-substituted ones. In any case, one day in the Spring of 1936 Ewins met with two of his chemists, George Newbery and Montague Phillips, and agreed on a program for synthesis of various derivatives of sulfanilamide. No written record of the plan survives, but according to recollections of at least one chemist who was working in the laboratory at the time, the idea was to look for water-soluble compounds. This would make sense, because one drawback of sulfanilamide as a medicine was that it was relatively insoluble. Part of the aim was apparently to increase the basic quality of the molecule so that it would form neutral salts with an inorganic acid.[13]

The first sulfanilamide derivative was entered in the laboratory test book in May 1936. Thereafter the program was pursued, sporadically, through the rest of 1936 and the first ten months of 1937. By June, 1936, the May & Baker chemists had entered into a collaboration with Lionel Whitby, a pathologist at Middlesex Hospital in London, to conduct trials of the new compounds on experimental infections in mice. Some fifty sulfonamide compounds were made, many of them by Newbery, who was simultaneously engaged in other projects.[14]

One day in October 1937, someone in the laboratory, possibly Newbery himself, noticed an old bottle sitting on the shelf. It turned out to be a sample of the base aminopyridine, prepared by a chemist named Eric Baines back in 1930 for another chemist who had since left the company. The sample had been moved from Wandsworth to Dagenham when the company relocated in 1934, and had stood on the shelf collecting dust ever since. Looking back two and a half decades later, company chemists, including Baines, agreed that it would have been very unlikely that this compound would have been prepared for use in the sulfanilamide derivatives program. But since it was there, "at the front of the third shelf on the left hand side of the cupboard," as another chemist, L. E. Hart, recalled, it was used. "Well, you know what would happen very much in those days," Baines remarked to company colleagues in 1961, "you would set out to try and make something, and you would find something on the shelf, and you would try it."[15]

On 29 October 1937, a laboratory assistant named Alexander, probably on the direction of Newbery, condensed the aminopyridine with acetanilide sulfonyl chloride. The result was a compound called acetyl sulfapyridine. Ordinarily in preparing sulfanilamide derivatives the acetyl group would be re-

Treatment of acetyl sufapyridine with acid or alkali: products. From H. J. Barber, "Antibacterial dawn and antiprotozoal noon," *in* Historical Aspects of Chemotherapy: Six Essays *(Dagenham: May & Baker Ltd.), pp. 24-32.*

moved with hydrochloric acid. Memories of laboratory workers differ on whether this was actually attempted. If it was, it failed, yielding merely sulfanilic acid. What is certain is that four days later, on November 2, Montague Phillips successfully removed the acetyl using the unconventional sodium hy-

Page taken from May & Baker's Test Register, *showing the entry for T693.*

droxide, yielding sulfapyridine. The new compound was duly entered in the test book as T693.[16]

At this stage, it must be emphasized, T693 was nothing special, just another compound to be sent on to Whitby for animal trials. Chemists who were present in the May & Baker laboratories at the time or shortly thereafter recalled that when the first sample of T693 was sent to Whitby he was away from his laboratory, perhaps on holiday. Moreover his laboratory was temporarily out of streptococcus-infected mice, the standard subjects for tests with sulfonamide compounds. In this situation Whitby's assistant, acting on a hunch, decided to try T693 on mice with pneumococcal infections. Contrary to expectation, the first results were positive. So too were trials in mice with streptococcal, meningococcal, staphylococcal, and gonococcal infections.[17]

At some time in November or early December 1937, A. J. Ewins sent a sample of T693 to Richard Wien, a researcher at the Pharmacological Society in London, for toxicity tests. The report came back on December 23. It must have been favorable, for Ewins wrote to Wien a few days later thanking him and remarking that "this product becomes more and more interesting." "Interesting" was also the word used by Whitby to describe his first impressions of T693 to Ewins. In the meantime one or more healthy members of the company research staff had swallowed T693 without ill effect.[18]

It is clear that by late December the May & Baker research team was beginning to focus its attention on T693, and that hopes were on the rise for the new stuff. Still, it was by no means clear to them yet exactly what they were dealing with, either biologically or chemically. One incident is revealing. A sample of sulfapyridine prepared after the first one supplied by Phillips was found to have a melting point 7-8 higher than Phillips's sample. L.E. Hart recalled that there was a big flap, and "we were virtually told that we hadn't made the right material." But then they found that Phillips, "in his inimitable way," had not done a thorough job in determining the melting point. The chemists were also concerned that later samples of sulfapyridine, not prepared with what one chemist called the "scruffy," impure sample of aminopyridine used by Phillips, although less toxic, would turn out to be therapeutically inactive. Fortunately Whitby found that this was not the case.[19]

In January 1938 May & Baker production chemists, under technical manager R. W. E. Stickings, began working on the first larger batch of T693. Ron Welford, who was delegated much of the work, recalled that the first production equipment was improvised from whatever things were available around the works. For example, since the chemists lacked a vacuum still for distillation of aminopyridine, Welford carried out the distillation in one- or two-liter flasks in the semi-technical laboratory next to the research lab. "After much struggling," Welford remembered, "just over a kilogram of T693 emerged sometime in February." It came out "a glorious pink color." Unfortunately, it was supposed to be white. Stickings intervened, and further operations produced a liquid closer to the proper color and largely free of acetic acid. The chemists called this kilogram or so of T693 "Batch 1."[20]

By mid-February 1938 Ewins was convinced of the low toxicity of the compound, and was talking of clinical trials. Sometime in March a decision was made to give T693 to a human patient. The man selected was a Norfolk farm laborer thought to be near death from lobar pneumonia. When treated with T693 from Batch 1, his condition improved, and he went on to a full recovery.[21]

If there was any more doubt in the minds of Ewins and his staff, this cure must have ended it. The production chemists were asked to raise their output to the maximum that was feasible. From January to October 1938 they struggled with inadequate equipment, intermediates of low quality or insufficient quantity, and kinks in the production processes. In smoothing out the latter they were helped by Rhône-Poulenc, which now entered the program to develop T693. In March, May & Baker also made arrangements with physicians at Dudley Road Hospital in Birmingham to treat patients admitted for pneumonia with T693 over several months.[22]

Meanwhile Whitby continued his animal trials of T693, publishing his first results in *The Lancet* at the end of May. His conclusions were forthright and unequivocal: "These experiments represent the one striking success in the chemotherapy of pneumococcal infections in an assessment of no less than 64 related sulfanilamide compounds [all obtained from May & Baker]," he wrote. Not only did M & B 693 (as Whitby now referred to it) possess "great chemotherapeutic activity against pneumococci of several types," but it was also as effective as sulfanilamide against hemolytic streptococcal and meningococcal infections, and apparently of low toxicity.[23]

Publication of the first clinical trial followed five weeks later in *The Lancet*. Between March and June 1938, G. M. Evans and Wilfrid F. Gaisford, physicians at Dudley Road Hospital in Birmingham, treated about 100 patients suffering from lobar pneumonia with M & B 693. One hundred other patients admitted with lobar pneumonia during the same period were given the conventional non-specific treatment by other physicians. In the control group the mortality was twenty-seven percent, a figure very close to the case mortality rate for lobar pneumonia in the same hospital in the preceding year and a half. In the treated group the rate was eight percent. Gaisford and Evans called this "a striking fall in mortality" and hoped that others would confirm their findings.[24]

Whitby continued his animal tests, and the company made arrangements for further clinical trials. In the eyes of May & Baker executives, however, enough was already known to justify making the new compound generally available to doctors. In September 1938, M & B 693 went on the British market under the trade name Dagenan. Great pressure was placed on the company's production team, which put its first plant in operation in October. By the end of the year, May & Baker had licensed Merck to make and distribute sulfapyridine in the United States, which it did in time for the pneumonia outbreak that winter.[25]

M & B 693 was enthusiastically embraced by many physicians, and increasingly also by the public, which began to hear of "miracle cures" by the wonderful new drug. But as awareness of the medicine spread, a gap began to open up between the intensive and sometimes unrestrained use by practicing doctors and the more deliberate pace of research. Researchers worried about side effects and dosage, and discussed the continuing value of serum therapy in pneumonia. Doctors went ahead and treated their patients with M & B 693. In March 1939 the Medical Research Council's Therapeutic Trials Committee concluded that more clinical study was needed. Lionel Whitby also believed that use had outrun knowledge, and complained about the same time that "pounds if not tons of the drug . . . have been used and abused in the past six months."[26]

In the United States, the divergence between cautious researchers and enthusiastic practitioners and patients was, if anything, more pronounced. In February 1939 the AMA's Council on Pharmacy and Chemistry received a report on sulfapyridine—the generic name they had approved in January—from Johns Hopkins researchers Perrin H. Long and Eleanor Bliss. Long and Bliss had largely confirmed Whitby's experimental findings on mice, published nine months earlier, and recommended careful clinical trials. The Council approved the report and at the same time published a recommendation that sulfapyridine *not* be approved for sale in interstate commerce "at the present time."[27]

Under the recently passed Food, Drug, and Cosmetic Act, the U.S. Food and Drug Administration had to pass judgment on sulfapyridine. Asked by the FDA for advice, the AMA's Council on Pharmacy and Chemistry in turn consulted 100 physicians who had used sulfapyridine in treatment of 1800 cases of pneumonia in adults, and 650 cases in children. Although it still expressed reservations, the Council interpreted the physicians' experience as showing that sulfapyridine was a "useful remedy." In March 1939, the FDA approved sulfapyridine for sale in interstate commerce. Simultaneously the Council voted to include sulfapyridine in its list of New and Nonofficial Remedies, and to review brands of the drug submitted by various manufacturers. Despite the Council's hesitations, the floodgates had been opened. By May 1939 the AMA's *Journal* was "overwhelmed" with papers submitted by physicians wanting to report their experiences with sulfapyridine.[28]

By November 1939, eighteen months after Whitby's first publication, sulfapyridine had been used to treat thousands of cases of pneumonia in many countries. An article in the *British Medical Journal* reviewing the literature concluded that "it is now established that sulfapyridine is a most ef-

fective agent against infections by pneumococci of all types," and "an outstanding medical advance." The article stated that the relative value of
sulfapyridine in most other bacterial infections compared to other sulfonamides remained to be determined, but noted that it was already shown to be
the most effective of the sulfas against gonorrhea.[29]

From the time that Whitby did his first mouse trials of T693 in 1938 to
Churchill's cure in 1943, sulfapyridine was tried in the treatment of many
kinds of human bacterial infections. The *British Medical Journal* reported trials in meningitis of several varieties (pneumococccal, staphylococcal, meningococcal, Pfeiffer's bacillus), in pneumococcal peritonitis, in human anthrax,
in bacterial endocarditis, in gas gangrene, in cerebrospinal fever, in acute bacillary dysentery, in suppurative otitis media, and in corneal ulcers. Tests of
M & B 693 in gonorrhea had begun by the summer of 1938, and by June

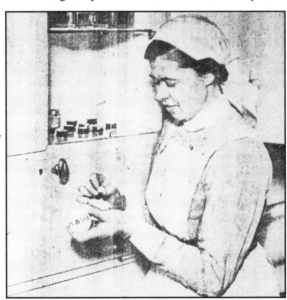

A nurse taking a tablet of
M & B 693. From
Glasgow Evening Times.

1941 sulfapyridine treatment of gonorrhea was routine in the British army. As
one harried production chemist who had rushed to meet the early demand recalled, "there seemed to be no end to its uses."[30]

Churchill's cure, not once but twice in 1943 at the height of the war,
made M & B a household word in Britain. The caption of a photograph that
appeared in the *Glasgow Evening Times* was representative: "A nurse taking
a tablet of M & B 693, the famous sulphonamide drug that has twice saved
the life of Mr. Churchill. The drug is the one powerful specific against pneumonia, and has literally saved thousands of lives." M & B seemed to be ev-

erywhere, even at the circus where the medicine was reported to have "pulled Nero, Royal circus lion, through pneumonia," and at the London Zoo where Winnie the lioness was also treated with M & B 693 for pneumonia. For some reason the initials invited humor, as Churchill's Moran and Bedford joke was joined by others. A cartoon in the *Yorkshire Evening Post* showed a man with a visibly shiny nose in bed, attended by his wife and doctor. The wife remarked to the doctor "M & B? If that means mild and bitter he's been taking it for years." Another cartoon, in *The Wall Planet*, showed two German civilians rushing for a bomb shelter as one said to the other "Ja, that man Churchill uses the code M & B—and that means More on Berlin."[31]

In its most emphatic version, the story went: M & B had saved Churchill, Churchill led the nation, therefore M & B had saved the nation. And how appropriate that M & B was a British invention, made by a British company. National pride did not yet have to contend with the complication that May & Baker was French-owned, a fact that was not available even to most of the company's employees. But what was M & B? As noted above, press reports often failed to distinguish between M & B 693 (sulfapyridine) and a related compound also developed by May & Baker, M & B 760 (sulfathiazole). In this they seem to have followed the lead of the doctors and nurses, who often spoke loosely of "M & B." What was certain, in the messages that reached the public, was that M & B was a cure for pneumonia. Other diseases were sometimes mentioned in the press, but tended to be eclipsed by the great killer.[32]

The British popular press tended to assimilate the story of M & B 693 to a simplified model of discovery that included several elements. Struggling to convey the stunning impact of the new medicine, writers alternated between, or mixed, religious and military metaphors. Lives were saved by the new "miracle drug," or "the intruders were repulsed" (Churchill's phrase) and the foe conquered. Credit could be assigned to a single heroic discoverer. He might be aided by others, but would have to overcome difficulties. He was modest, perseverant, and dedicated to the welfare of humanity. In the case of M & B 693 this role sometimes fell to Lionel Whitby, especially in the earlier reports, but increasingly the mantle was shifted to A. J. Ewins, research director of May & Baker. As one newspaper put it, "The number 693 means that shy, 61-year-old Dr. Ewins perfected the drug at the 693rd attempt. If he had said 'I am sick of this' and given up at number 692 there would have been thousands more deaths last year—and one of them almost certainly would have been Mr. Winston Churchill." Often in popular press accounts the discovery could be located at a precise moment in time. One day there was no M & B 693, the next day there was. In these versions of the story the discovery extended at most from the moment of synthesis to Whitby's first animal experiments. Finally, the medicine cured a single disease. In the case of M & B, of course, this was pneumonia, although the drug's cure of other diseases was

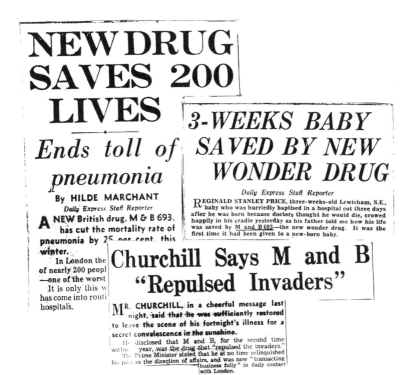

Headlines from the British press extol virtues of M & B 693.

occasionally reported with dramatic effect.[33]

In one respect at least the popular press accounts could not be faulted. Against the backdrop of the heavy mortality from pneumonia, M & B 693 did indeed appear to many as a kind of miracle, a wonder drug, a powerful weapon against an enemy of mankind. Only such strong language could adequately convey the impact of a medicine that meant the difference between life and death for hundreds of thousands of people.

In other ways, however, the prevailing popular presentation of the discovery was wrong. M & B 693 was not discovered by a single person. It was not discovered at a precise moment. It was not a cure for one disease only.

Take just one fragment of the story, the initial synthesis of the compound. Where is credit to be assigned? To Grillet, who may have initiated the program to make sulfanilamide derivatives and divided the labor between Ewins and Blaise? To Ewins, who led his part of the program at May & Baker? To Newbery, who (probably) asked Alexander to carry out the condensation reaction? To Alexander, who actually carried it out? To Phillips, who came up with a way to deacetylate the product of the condensation reaction? To all of the above? Even if we could answer this in a satisfying way, we have to remember that at this stage, November 2, 1937, T693 was just one more in a long list of compounds entered in the laboratory test book. No one knew that it had any biological activity, much less therapeutic efficacy.

So, was "M & B 693" discovered yet? No. Beyond this lay Whitby's animal studies, Evans and Gaisford's first series of clinical trials, and years of efforts by many doctors in many countries to probe the potentials of sulfapyridine as a medicine and the nature and extent of its hazards. The questions of who discovered sulfapyridine and when are difficult ones to answer not only because many people were involved over a matter of months or years, but also, and more importantly, because the nature of the "discovery" was plural, not singular, and changed shape over time. What sulfapyridine was conceived to be in November 1937 was different from what it was conceived to be in December 1937 or March 1938 or July 1938 or November 1939. In fact its medical identity continued to be in flux right up to the time that Churchill took it, when it was already beginning to be displaced by other sulfa drugs and by penicillin.

To some degree there was a convergence between popular versions of the discovery and the ways in which it was rewarded by academic science and medicine. No Nobel Prize followed, although the magnitude of M & B 693's impact on medicine might have justified one. But A. J. Ewins was elected a Fellow of the Royal Society. Lionel Whitby was knighted, and as Sir Lionel Whitby went on to serve as Vice Chancellor of Cambridge University. The company gained financial rewards and an enhanced reputation. For the most part, however, the other characters in the story here told disappeared from the official account of the discovery and from public view.

One who tried not to disappear was Montague Phillips, who had effected an important step in the synthesis of T693, and whose name appeared with that of Ewins on the original patent. In 1964 the Science Museum in London opened an exhibit on medicinal drugs. The exhibit showcased M & B 693, and curators sought May & Baker's advice on the history of the discovery. The display included a photograph of A. J. Ewins, but none of Montague Phillips, although Phillips was mentioned in the accompanying text. Phillips, outraged at what he took to be a slight to his own role, went to the press, bringing with him a bottle purportedly containing a sample of the first batch of M & B 693.[34]

It was not the first time that Phillips had gone public in an effort to assert his role, which was rarely mentioned in early press reports on M & B 693. After leaving May & Baker and setting up his own chemical consultant business, Phillips had given an account to a newspaper in 1944 that made him co-responsible with Ewins for the discovery, and that also brought out the element of luck in the form of the presence of the old sample of the compound on the laboratory shelf. Now, in 1964, he was described as angry and bitter as a result of "27 years of frustration and disappointment over his success with M & B 693," and prepared to give "the inside story of how M & B 693 was discovered." The inside story consisted, first, of a debunking of the notion that M & B 693 was the result of 693 experiments, a version that had sometimes appeared in early press reports but that was never put forward by May & Baker or by other participants in the research. Second, Phillips asserted that M & B 693 was the result of "three astonishing accidents": the use of an old chemical from the shelf; Phillips's own "gamble" in using an alkali rather than an acid in one step of the synthesis; and the availability of pneumococcus-infected mice in Whitby's laboratory when the first sample of T693 arrived. Why had credit been withheld? Phillips recalled that "Dr. Ewins was never friendly to me," and speculated that Ewins had looked down on him as a man of working class background who had worked his way up within the company, obtained his degrees by attending evening classes, and held unorthodox ideas in politics. "The result," complained the writer for *The People*, "is this present scandalous insult to a distinguished scientist in the exhibition at the Science Museum."[35]

Phillips had a combative personality. When he died in 1972 he was portrayed as a self-made man who, in his widow's words, "liked to champion the small person against the establishment," was "eccentric and bad tempered," and "always tended to be extreme and was non-conformist in every way." He was a severe critic of the pharmaceutical industry who for many years sought compensation for thalidomide children. No doubt he saw himself as yet another victim of an unjust establishment, and this generalized resentment was part of what drove him to a public attack on the official history of M & B 693.[36]

Also driving Phillips's attack was a particular view of the discovery. Insofar as this view called for more explicit recognition of Phillips's contribution and brought forward the role played by chance, it is consistent with the present study. In making his case, however, Phillips fell into the same error as many of the accounts that drew his ire by equating the discovery with the chemical synthesis of the compound, and indeed even more narrowly with the last step in the original synthesis, the step that he had effected. Only on this view could the reporter for the *Recorder Review* state flatly that "the historic discovery was made on November 2, 1937." And only on this view could credit for the discovery be assigned to one or two individuals.[37]

For better or worse the reward system of science has been long preoccupied with questions of individual achievement and priority. However appropriate this method of assigning credit may be for academic science, it leaves much to be desired as a way of understanding the development of medicinal drugs. A model of innovation that begins with the presupposition that the appearance of a new medicine may be located at a discrete moment and in the mind of an individual investigator will often obscure or efface essential features of the events it seeks to illuminate. The leadership roles of research managers, the collaborative nature of research, the multiple stages of the development process—from definition of goals through chemical synthesis, laboratory and clinical testing, patenting, manufacture, and large-scale use by physicians—may all be lost from view, or at best may be viewed through a distorted lens.

"Discovery" may not be the best way to characterize the emergence of a new medicine like M & B 693. If the term is to be retained it must be on the understanding that it frequently covers a chain of events that have extension in time and that involve numbers of individuals of diverse expertise as well as, usually, an industrial research organization. For this process the phrase "industrialized invention" is more appropriate, since it connotes a corporate institutional setting and a collaborative, multi-step process of research and development.[38]

M & B 693, like other sulfa drugs, was a product of an industrial system of invention in which individuals played crucial but partial roles. Recognition of this fact does no dishonor to those who participated in the process, but does allow us to begin to recover in its full complexity the path by which a new medicine came into the world.

Notes and References

1 . Martin Gilbert, *Road to Victory: Winston S. Churchill 1941-1945* (London: Heinemann, 1986), pp. 603-604; Richard Lovell, *Churchill's Doctor: A Biography of Lord Moran* (London: Royal Society of Medicine, 1992), pp. 228-35.

2 . Gilbert, *Road to Victory*(n.1), pp. 603-54; Lovell, *Churchill's Doctor* (n.1), pp. 228-35.

3 . See e.g., "Mr Churchill's own bulletin," *Yorkshire Post*, December 30, 1943; "Premier off to convalesce," *East Anglian Times*, December 30, 1943; and "Premier goes to convalescence: 'Destination unknown'," *Newcastle Journal*, December 30, 1943.

4 . Montague A. Phillips, a chemist who had contributed to the development of M & B 693 (about whom more below), guessed that Churchill had been treated with M & B 760. *Northern Daily Telegraph*, December 30, 1943. So did the writer of an unsigned article in the *Wolverhampton Express & Star* for December 30, 1943. On Pulvertaft and penicillin see *News Chronicle*, December 17, 1943. Examples of the more representative focus on M & B 693 are "New drugs can defeat pneumonia," *News Chronicle*, December 17, 1943; and "M & B—Churchill version," *Norwich Eastern Daily Press*, December 30, 1943.

5 . For surveys of the history of the sulfonamides see Daniel Bovet, *Une chimie qui guérit: histoire de la découverte des sulfamides* (Paris: Payot, 1988); and Marcel H. Bickel, "The development of sulfonamides (1932-1938) as a focal point in the history of chemotherapy," *Gesnerus* 45 (1988): 67-86.

6 . Ronald D. Mann, *Modern Drug Use: An Enquiry on Historical Principles* (Lancaster, Boston, The Hague, Dordrecht: MTP Press Limited, 1984), pp. 556-57; Bickel, "The develop-

ment of sulfonamides (n.5)," pp. 75-76; Elmore H. Northey, *The Sulfonamides and Allied Compounds* (New York: Reinhold Publishing Corporation, 1948), p. v.

7 . H. E. Ungerleider, H. W. Steinhaus, and R. S. Gubner, "Public health and economic aspects of pneumonia: A comparison with pre-sulfonamide years," *American Journal of Public Health* 33 (1943): 1093-1102.

8 . On the development of Prontosil see John E. Lesch, "Chemistry and biomedicine in an industrial setting: The invention of the sulfa drugs," in *Chemical Sciences in the Modern World*, ed. Seymour H. Mauskopf (Philadelphia: University of Pennsylvania Press, 1993), pp. 158-215. On the Pasteur Institute work see Bovet, *Une chimie qui guérit* (n.5), pp. 37-53.

9 . Bovet, *Une chimie qui guérit* (n.5), pp. 167-201.

10 . M & B Test Register, Compound Nos. 1-606, and M & B Test Register, Compound Nos. 607-1358, May & Baker archives. Prontosil was entered as compound 576 on January 17, 1936. See also H. J. Barber, "Antibacterial dawn and antiprotozoal noon," in idem., *Historical Aspects of Chemotherapy: Six Essays* (Dagenham: May & Baker Ltd., 1976), pp. 24-32. On the research establishment at May & Baker see Judy Slinn, *A History of May & Baker 1834-1984* (Cambridge: Hobsons Limited, 1984), esp. pp. 95-126.

11 . On Rhône-Poulenc's ownership of May & Baker, see Slinn, *A History of May & Baker* (n.10), pp. 95-99; and Fred Aftalion, *A History of the International Chemical Industry*, trans. by Otto Theodor Benfey (Philadelphia: University of Pennsylvania Press, 1991), p. 196. The argument for a division of labor is made by Jean-Pierre Billon, "La découverte des sulfamides: implication et contribution de l'industrie," (Paris-La Défense: Rhône-Poulenc Santé, n.d.), 11 pages and 4 tables, May & Baker archives. On the chemical possibilities as perceived at the time see Barber, "Antibacterial dawn" (n.10), p. 27.

12 . G. A. H. Buttle, W. H. Gary, and Dora Stephenson, "Protection of mice against streptococcal and other infections by p-aminobenzenesulphonamide and related substances," *Lancet* 1 (1936): 1286-90; A. J. Ewins, "British achievements in sulphonamide research and production," *The Pharmaceutical Journal*, April 28, 1951, 312-314.

13 . "Transcription of a tape recording made at a meeting on the discovery of M & B 693 Held 2.6.61," File 270, May & Baker archives, pages 5-6, 8. Present at this meeting were H. J. Barber, L. E. Hart, E. J. Baines, and a Mrs. Wragg. Barber, Hart, and Baines, all of whom had worked in May & Baker's pharmaceutical research division, were attempting to reconstruct the discovery of M & B 693 for an exhibition then being planned at the Science Museum in London. In one of the cited passages Hart was drawing upon memories of another colleague, F. W. Bampton.

14 . M & B Test Register, Compound Nos. 1-606, and M & B Test Register, Compound Nos. 607-1358; "Transcription" (n.13), pp. 8-11.

15 . "Transcription" (n.13), pp. 4-13 (quotes on pp. 4, 5).

16 . "Transcription" (n.13), 11-13; and M & B Test Register, Compound Nos. 607-1358.

17 . R. F. B. Welford, personal communication, February 21, 1994; J. F. Hodgson, personal communication, February 11, 1994; M & B Test Register, Compound Nos. 607-1358; Lionel E. H. Whitby, "Chemotherapy of pneumococcal and other infections with 2-(p-aminobenzenesulphonamido) pyridine," *Lancet* 9(May 28, 1938): 1210-1212.

18 . R. Wien to A. J. Ewins, December 3, 1937, and A. J. Ewins to R. Wien, December 28, 1937, both in File 269, May & Baker archives; "Transcription" (n.13), 14; M. A. F. Lake, "25 years of sulfapyridine," nonpaginated reprint from *The Chemist and Druggist*, October 26, 1963.

19 . "Transcription" (n.13), p. 14.

20 . R. F. B. Welford, personal communication, February 21, 1994.

21 . R. F. B. Welford, personal communication, February 21, 1994; M. A. F. Lake, "25 years of sulfapyridine" (n.18).

22 . R. F. B. Welford, personal communication, February 21, 1994; G. M. Evans and Wilfrid F. Gaisford, "Treatment of pneumonia with 2-(p-aminobenzenesulphonamido) pyridine," *Lancet* (July 2, 1938): 14-19.

23 . Whitby, "Chemotherapy of pneumococcal and other infections" (n.17), p. 1212.

24 . Evans and Gaisford, "Treatment of pneumonia" (n.22).

25 . A. J. Ewins to R. Wien, January 5, 1939 [Letter is dated 5th January 1938 but internal evidence clearly indicates that the year is 1939], File 269, May & Baker archives; Merck & Co. Inc., Report to Stockholders, 1939; Slinn, *A History of May & Baker* (n.10), p. 124; R. F. B. Welford, personal communication, February 21, 1994.

26 . Two samples of press reports are "Pneumonia robbed of its terror—Experiments with a wonderful new drug," *News of the World*, June 19, 1938; and "New drug cures dread disease—Wolverhampton girl's recovery-'dramatic response'," *Morning Advertiser*, September 9, 1938. For physicians' and medical researchers' cautions, see A. J. Ewins to R. Wien, January 5, 1939, File 269, May & Baker archives; "Sulfapyridine," *British Medical Journal* (March 25, 1939): 623-624; Therapeutic Trials Committee, meeting of March 28, 1939, Medical Research Council Minute Book, MB 55; and "Recent advances in treatment of pneumonia," *British Medical Journal* (April 8, 1939): 741-743 (quote on 743).

27 . Council on Pharmacy and Chemistry, "Preliminary report of the council," and Perrin H. Long, "Sulfapyridine," *Journal of the American Medical Association* 112 (1939): 538-539.

28 . Council on Pharmacy and Chemistry, "Special report of the council: sulfapyridine," *Journal of the American Medical Association* 112 (1939): 1830; "New and nonofficial remedies," *Journal of the American Medical Association* 112 (1939): 1831; and editorial, "Sulfapyridine," *Journal of the American Medical Association* 112 (1939): 1833.

29 . H. L. Marriott, "Sulphapyridine (M & B 693) and pneumococcal infections," *British Medical Journal* (November 11, 1939): 944-947. The article concluded with 122 citations to the British and overseas medical literature.

30 . M. H. Hughes, "Otogenic cellular meningitis treated with M & B 693," *British Medical Journal* (February 4, 1939): 214-215; A. Morton Gill, "Staphylococcal meningitis treated with sulphapyridine: Recovery," *British Medical Journal* (May 18, 1940): 810; D. F. Johnstone and P. Forgacs, "Cerebral symptoms occurring during sulphapyridine treatment of meningococcal meningitis," *British Medical Journal* (May 24, 1941): 772-774; G. Marsden Roberts, "Sulphapyridine and soluseptasine in meningitis due to Pfeiffer bacillus: Recovery," *British Medical Journal* (November 25, 1939): 1041; John M. Teasdale, "Pneumococcal peritonitis with bilateral pneumococcal empyemata—Treatment with M & B 693: Recovery," *British Medical Journal* (June 10, 1939): 1179; Wm. Bonnar, "Sulphapyridine in human anthrax," *British Medical Journal* (March 9, 1940): 389; G. A. Richards, "Sulphapyridine in bacterial endocarditis," *British Medical Journal* (April 13, 1940): 637; R. J. McNeill Love, "Treatment of gas gangrene with sulphapyridine," *British Medical Journal* (June 1, 1940): 908; J. H. Jordan, J. H. Blakelock, and W. R. Johnston, "Treatment of cerebrospinal fever with sulphapyridine," *British Medical Journal* (June 22, 1940): 1005-1008; Rudolf Reitler and Kurt Marberg, "Note on the treatment of acute bacillary dysentery with sulphapyridine," *British Medical Journal* (February 22, 1941): 277-278; V. Ruth Sharp, "Sulphapyridine in suppurative otitis media," *British Medical Journal* (August 9, 1941): 211; Sydney Tibbles, "Corneal ulcers cured by sulphapyridine," *British Medical Journal* (August 23, 1941): 292; F. J. T. Bowie, "Chemotherapy in gonorrhea: A preliminary report on the use of 2-(p-

aminobenzenesulphonamido) Pyridine, M & B 693," *British Medical Journal* (August 6, 1938): 283-284; R. M. B. MacKenna, "Recent experiences in the treatment of gonorrhea in the male," *British Medical Journal* (June 28, 1941): 958-961; R. F. B. Welford, personal communication, February 11, 1994.

31 . Photo in *Glasgow Evening Times*, December 31, 1943; "Churchill drug saves lion too," *Glasgow Evening News*, January 7, 1944; "M & B lioness is improving," *Sunday Chronicle*, January 30, 1944; Cartoon, *Yorkshire Evening Post*, January 21, 1944; Cartoon, *The Wall Planet*, reproduced in Slinn, *A History of May & Baker (n.10)*, 135.

32 . On the conflation of different May & Baker products, see "The development of sulphonamides," two-page typescript, n. d., File 131, May & Baker archives. On M & B as a source of national pride, see e. g., "Pneumonia robbed of its terror: Experiments with a wonderful new drug," *News of the World*, June 19, 1938. The article reported that "British doctors and British chemists are rejoicing in the knowledge that the drug is a product of one of our own research laboratories. The new drug is the answer to criticisms so often made that research in chemistry in this country is a long way behind that in Germany and America."

33 . See e. g., "'Miracle' drug saves life of W'ton girl," *Express and Star* (Wolverhampton), September 9, 1938; "Pneumonia discovery," *Evening Standard*, July 2, 1938; "Pneumonia discovery," *Lancashire Daily Post*, January 4, 1938; "Brilliant young scientist," *Hastings Evening Argus*, July 11, 1938; "Disease you need no longer dread—New drug conquers deadly germ," *Everybody's*, July 25, 1938; James Harpole, "'This marvelous drug'," *Sunday Graphic*, January 2, 1944; and "Miss 1944 gets a gift from science—10 years of extra life," *Sunday Pictorial*, January 2, 1944 (quote).

34 . Peter Bishop, "Why leave this genius out in the cold?" *The People*, June 21, 1964.

35 . "Luck led to this great discovery," *Sunday Pictorial*, February 2, 1944. One exception to Phillips's lack of notice was "Birthplace of a new drug," *Romford Times*, September 7, 1938. Romford was Phillips's place of residence. The "inside story" is in Bishop, "Why leave this genius out in the cold?" Phillips's later career as a chemical consultant is reported in Jo Weedon, "Fighting doctor who discovered a miracle," *Recorder Review*, October 20, 1972.

36 . Jo Weedon, "Fighting doctor" (n.35).

37 . Jo Weedon, "Fighting doctor" (n.35).

38 . Lesch, "Chemistry and biomedicine in an industrial setting" (n.8).

The Introduction of the Thiazides: A Case Study in Twentieth-Century Therapeutics

by Robert M. Kaiser

First synthesized and marketed by Merck, Sharp, and Dohme in the late 1950s,[1] the thiazide diuretics are now four decades old. Proclaimed as "wonder drugs" for high blood pressure and congestive heart failure on their introduction, they are still in widespread use in the 1990s. Although their place in the history of medical practice is well known to clinicians,[2] their story is less familiar to historians. Compared to penicillin, the century's most famous pill, the thiazides may seem a mere footnote, but their relative obscurity in the annals of therapeutics is undeserved. The following paper will recount the advent of this class of drugs and recall their considerable impact on American therapeutic behavior and practice at mid-century.

Certainly no accident of history, the thiazide diuretics were the product of highly specialized, technically sophisticated research in a burgeoning post-World War II pharmaceutical industry, one that effectively harnessed science for economic gain. The adoption of these drugs is an illuminating example of the rapidly changing therapeutic landscape of the 1950s. Their ultimate success depended upon carefully cultivated connections between pharmaceutical companies and physicians outside of industry, who tested the drugs in clinical trials and who served as some of its most fervent advocates. The quick acceptance of the thiazides in practice was driven by medical need, utility, professional interest, and corporate salesmanship. Chronic disease had displaced infectious disease as the leading cause of death in mid-century America and

121

physicians were enjoined to battle this newly-perceived scourge by the government, by their professional organizations, and by their peers. In patients with congestive heart failure or hypertension, the thiazides provided a novel, practical, and relatively benign tool to treat these common, deadly diseases. The abundance of positive reports about the thiazides in the medical literature were reinforced by a well-financed marketing effort to accelerate their acceptance, which came quickly resulting in tens of millions of dollars in profits. The success of the thiazides, propelled by science and by the profit-making imperatives, was also shaped by the small-scale contingencies of the doctor-patient relationship, contingencies that gave physicians great latitude and discretion in the management of chronic diseases.

The Epidemic of Chronic Disease

By the 1950s, heart disease had surpassed infectious disease as the leading cause of death in the United States. A consensus emerged in the medical community: the challenge of infectious disease had been supplanted by a more daunting epidemic. The problem was well documented and publicly proclaimed. In 1948, with the formation of the National Heart Institute of the National Institutes of Health, the U.S. government launched an ambitious program of research in cardiovascular disease. This multimillion-dollar effort encompassed basic laboratory science and large-scale population studies. The initiative was announced in the first national conference on cardiovascular diseases held in 1950 in Washington, D.C., a jointly sponsored effort of the National Heart Institute and the American Heart Association.[3]

The conference report identified cardiovascular disease as a major public health problem that deserved serious attention:

> Cardiovascular diseases killed 637,679 persons—equal to the population of San Francisco—in 1948. . . .

> As the expectation of life increases, cardiovascular diseases take a heavier toll. In 1935 they accounted for only 33 percent of mortality, compared to 44 percent in 1948. . . .

Dr. Kaiser received an A. B. in History from Duke University and an M. A. in History of Medicine from The Johns Hopkins University. After completeing the M. D. at The Medical College of Pennsylvania, he trained in Internal Medicine at the University of Minnesota Hospital in Minneapolis. He was subsequently Robert Wood Johnson Clinical Scholar and Fellow in General Internal Medicine at the University of Pennsylvania. He is currently Assistant Professor of Medicine at the University of Pennsylvania, where he practices and teaches general internal medicine and conducts research in the history of medicine.

Two things are essential for further progress. First, there must be broader knowledge of cardiovascular diseases. . . . Research will take time, but no time need be
lost in acting on the second requisite for progress: fuller application of existing
knowledge. The Washington conferees recommended that all professions related
to the prevention and treatment of heart disease make greater use of the facts that
are known today.[4]

Essential hypertension, or high blood pressure of unknown cause, was
identified by the conferees as one of the most pressing cardiovascular problems. The conference called for a multi-disciplinary approach to the disorder,
emphasizing "those studies which elucidate the physiological and chemical
aspects of the circulation."[5] They acknowledged that "few methods of treatment have become established on the basis of adequate evidence,"[6] and concluded that there was, at that time, "no sure way to prevent hypertension."[7]

The focus of the federal research effort also encompassed epidemiology. In 1949, under the direction of William Kannel, and others, a long-term
prospective study of coronary heart disease began in Framingham, Massachusetts. Chosen randomly, 4469 patients were examined twice a year and observed for evidence of coronary heart disease; the data was supplemented by
information obtained from the patients' families and individual physicians, as
well as from hospital records and death certificates. Blood pressure was one
of many parameters that was measured. The first Framingham reports were
published in 1957 and 1958. The reports confirmed what some had suspected—that coronary artery disease was associated with certain risk factors—among them, hypertension.[8]

**An Industry Come of Age: The Growth of American Pharmaceutical
Research**

Federal governmental efforts in the post World War II period did not
occur in isolation. They were complemented by research in the pharmaceutical industry. A fledgling enterprise in 1900, it had grown considerably in size
and sophistication by 1950. As historian John Swann has shown in his work,
American pharmaceutical firms lagged somewhat behind Europe in their
funding and promotion of research. By the turn of the century, the need to
produce standardized drugs led firms like Parke-Davis, Lilly, and Searle to
engage scientists on their staffs. With the discovery of diphtheria antitoxin in
the 1890s, pharmaceutical firms were eager to move quickly to initiate large-
scale manufacture of the antitoxin. They therefore developed links with academic institutions to accomplish that goal.[9]

The commitment of pharmaceutical companies to research was a reflection of the emergence of industrial research generally not only in drug manufacturing but also in the chemical, electrical, and petroleum industries. The

advent of World War I accelerated the development of industrial research. The war created tremendous demand for sophisticated electronic, chemical, and pharmaceutical products. This trend continued during the 1920s and 1930s. In 1927, there were 1000 industrial laboratories with research staffs totaling 19,000; thirteen years later, in 1940, 2264 labs existed employing a staff of 58,000, three times the previous level.[10]

In the period between the world wars, the drug industry began to attract talented young scientists to work for them. By the 1930s, several leading American pharmaceutical companies had set up research divisions, among these the Merck Institute for Therapeutic Research (1933), the Lilly Research Laboratories (1934), the Squibb Institute for Medical Research (1938), and the Abbott Research Laboratories (1938). Their opening was heralded not only by industry but also by foundations, universities, and government officials. Once reviled for their mercenary tendencies, shameless commercialism, and unscrupulous promotion of suspect remedies, pharmaceutical firms had, by the 1930s, earned a modicum of respect for their dedication to science and for their support of basic research.[11]

The Merck Institute, which opened in 1933, exemplified this search for recognition and respectability. Chief Executive George Merck aspired to create a first-class research laboratory. At the recommendation of his distinguished consultant, Alfred N. Richards of the University of Pennsylvania, Merck hired a well-known Viennese pharmacologist, Hans Molitor, to head the new institute. Richards considered Molitor to be a scientist of the highest caliber.[12] Under his direction, the Institute became a leader in pharmacology research. The published output of the Institute was steady and impressive: thirty papers in the first five years and nearly fifty papers from 1939 to 1941.[13] The company provided generous research support: annual expenditures for research at the Institute increased six-fold over a nine-year period, from $146,000 in 1931 to $906,000 in 1940.[14] In the next two decades, Merck funded multimillion dollar annual budgets for research and development.[15]

Serendipity and Scientific Acumen: The Invention of the Thiazide Diuretics

The invention of the thiazides was both systematic and serendipitous. The details of this story have been described in several articles and books by experimental scientists who participated in their discovery and have been best summarized in the classic account by Thomas Maren.[16] The lack of access to archival materials and laboratory notebooks from pharmaceutical firms has hindered this author from the construction of a more precise historical narrative of these events. The account that follows draws upon Maren's history, other personal histories, the abundant medical literature of the period, and drug industry trade journals.[17]

In post-World War I Vienna, a medical student named Alfred Vogl accidentally stumbled upon one of the twentieth century's first effective diuretics, the organomercurials, when he injected the antisyphilitic Novasurol into one of his edematous patients, causing a profound increase in urine production.[18] Although the clinical effects of the organomercurials were dramatic, their need to be injected was inconvenient and their prolonged use resulted in toxic side effects. These disadvantages impelled pharmaceutical firms to search for a less toxic medical alternative, one that could be administered orally rather than parenterally, and one with fewer side effects. This led first to the development of carbonic anhydrase inhibitors and eventually to the synthesis of thiazide diuretics.[19]

Cornell University Professor Robert Pitts, in the mid-1940s, linked sulfanilamide—a sulfonamide drug originally synthesized as an antibacterial agent—with the inhibition of the enzyme carbonic anhydrase in the kidney, an enzyme that had been characterized earlier in the decade. He showed experimentally that sulfanilamide interfered with the normal process of urinary acidification. William Schwartz, a physician and fellow in training at Boston's Peter Bent Brigham Hospital soon capitalized clinically on this published fact. He administered ten grams of sulfanilamide to a woman patient with rheumatic heart disease and congestive heart failure. She was no longer responding to mercurial diuretics, but in response to the large dose of sulfanilamide, the patient produced urine, excreting large amounts of sodium and potassium. Richard Roblin, a scientist with the pharmaceutical company American Cyanamid immediately recognized the potential promise of sulfonamides after contact with Schwartz, and new derivatives of sulfanilamide were quickly developed. This resulted in the synthesis of the carbonic anhydrase inhibitor known as compound 6063, later named acetazolamide, or Diamox. This drug, although nontoxic, was only variably effective as a diuretic, but was nonetheless used widely for the treatment of patients with congestive heart failure in the 1950s.[20]

It was a group of scientists at Sharp and Dohme in the early 1940s (and later Merck, Sharp, and Dohme after a merger in the early 1950s) that succeeded by 1955 in synthesizing the carbonic anhydrase inhibitor, 6-chloro-7-sulfamyl-1,2,4-benzothiadiazine-1,1-dioxide, also known as chlorothiazide or Diuril, the first thiazide diuretic to be marketed by an American pharmaceutical company. This group of researchers, working together in Sharp and Dohme's Renal Research Program, included among them Karl Beyer, a talented physiologist recruited from the University of Wisconsin in 1943, chemists James Sprague and Frederick Novello, and biologist John Baer. Under the leadership of Beyer, these scientists looked systematically for an agent that would inhibit the reabsorption of sodium and chloride ions in the tubules of the kidney and result in increased urine production, without disturbing the body's balance of electrolytes. Fully aware of the work of Robert Pitts and William Schwartz with sulfanilamide, they sought to avoid the serious disadvantages of that carbonic anhydrase inhibitor: namely, the loss of bicarbonate leading to metabolic acidosis, an unacceptable side effect of the medication, one that could spell trouble clinically for any patient over the long term. As the man who discovered probenecid, a drug that inhibited renal tubular secretion of penicillin, Beyer was pursuing a scientific strategy along the same lines in his search for an effective diuretic medication. Scientists at Sharp and Dohme prepared a dealkylated form of probenecid, yielding a simple, unsubstituted sulfonamide known as p-carboxylbenzenesulfonamide. Beyer's team tested this substance in dogs, finding it to cause a diuresis of both sodium and chloride; it was also given to three physicians to test in three hypertensive patients, and the effect was confirmed clinically. The compound tested was about five times as active as sulfanilamide, but Merck scientists needed a drug with even greater activity. They initially sought to substitute additional sulfamoyl groups on the sulfonamide. They eventually developed a more potent compound in which the sulfamoyl and amino groups were bonded together on the benzene ring, yielding a benzothiadiazine heterocyclic nucleus, or, in short, a thiazide.[21]

Merck gave chlorothiazide to physician William Wilkinson to test in several of his hypertensive patients with edema and he found it to be effective.[22] Its clinical efficacy was confirmed and first reported by several groups of clinical investigators at American universities, including Freis, Wanko, and Wilson,[23] Hollander and Wilkins,[24] and Moyer, Ford, and Spur.[25] The drug was tested in clinical trials by a total of 1000 physicians beginning in October 1956. Fourteen months later, the drug was approved for release.[26]

A parallel research effort on the thiazides was conducted by scientists George DeStevens and his group at CIBA. This eventually produced a second generation thiazide, hydrochlorothiazide, simultaneously synthesized by Merck researchers. Both companies shared the patent for this second generation drug, although the drug carried different brand names and was marketed separately by each firm.[27] Hydrochlorothiazide, named Hydrodiuril and Esidrix respectively by Merck and CIBA, began to be sold commercially in January 1959.[28]

Enthusiasm and Economic Success: The Clinical Reception of Thiazides

The introduction of chlorothiazide was announced by Merck on 30 January 1958. The press release was simple and straightforward, stating that the new drug, Diuril, "is expected to be of special benefit to cardiac patients through more effective treatment of congestive heart failure and high blood pressure."[29] The subsequent repercussions in the pharmaceutical industry were dramatic. As Beyer himself attested: "The effect of . . . pilot chlorothiazide studies . . . was explosive. An avalanche of publications attesting to the efficacy and safety of chlorothiazide evoked a chemical effort in the worldwide pharmaceutical industry that could not be kept up with. Every company seemed to want its own very patentable thiazide"[30]

In 1957, the initial clinical reports on chlorothiazide appeared in the *Medical Annals of the District of Colombia,*[31] the *Boston Medical Quarterly,*[32] *Proceedings of the Society of Experimental Biology and Medicine,*[33] and the *Annals of the New York Academy of Medicine.*[34] In November of 1957, its utility in hypertension and congestive heart failure was propounded by Robert Wilkins[35] and Robert Schreiner[36] in articles in *The New England Journal of Medicine.* Wilkins' report was particularly laudatory. He stated: "it is my hope that the general physician who reads this report will find it of assistance in making his way among the maze of new preparations available commercially for the treatment of hypertension. Some of these, particularly chlorothiazide, promise to increase greatly the effectiveness of drugs in management of this disease."[37] Two months later, at the time of chlorothiazide's release, the *Journal of the American Medical Association* featured four favorable reports on the new drug.[38] Over the next two years, reports on the utility of the thiazides were published in *The Annals of Internal Medicine*[39] and *The Mayo Clinic Proceedings,*[40] in state and local medical journals throughout the

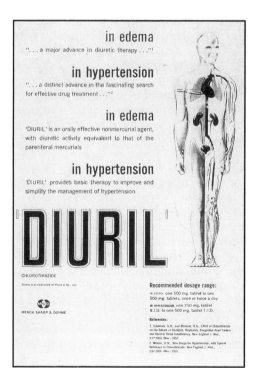

Merck advertised Diuril to physicians in their company publication, Seminar Report, *in 1959.*

country, including Delaware,[41] Minnesota,[42] Mississippi,[43] Nebraska,[44] New Jersey,[45] Ohio,[46] and Seattle[47]; in clinical journals such as *GP*,[48] *Postgraduate Medicine*,[49] *International Record of Medicine*,[50] and *Medical Times*[51]; in the *Journal of the National Medical Association*,[52] and in the subspecialty journals *Circulation*[53] and the *American Journal of Cardiology*.[54] Reports on chlorothiazide were also featured in lay publications such as *Science Digest*,[55] *Today's Health*,[56] and *U.S. News and World Report*.[57] The newly inaugurated *Medical Letter*, more objective and less prone to hyperbole than almost any other medical publication, regarded chlorothiazide as a valuable drug, eminently superior to the organomercurials and to oral diuretics like the carbonic anhydrase inhibitors.[58] The permeation of the medical literature was broad and deep, and the reaction was unmistakably positive.

Here is a sampling of these reports. *Minnesota Medicine* praised the medical utility and underscored the clinical importance of chlorothiazide: "The advent of potent oral diuretics such as chlorothiazide . . . promises to revolutionize the treatment of hypertension. These agents have a modest hypotensive action when administered alone, and they are even more effective in enhancing the hypotensive response of ganglionic blocking agents."[59] The *Delaware State Medical Journal* praised Diuril as innovative and effective: "The use of this agent may stand the test of time as the most vital and specific weapon in the treatment of a relatively non-specific disease . . . . Chlorothiazide now appears to be the drug of choice when initiating therapy in the average hypertensive patient."[60] The *Nebraska State Medical Journal* was also laudatory: "Chlorothiazide, a potent nonmercurial diuretic, as effective orally as parenteral mercurial diuretics, and well tolerated chronically . . . is now employed with other hypotensive drugs in the treatment of hypertension. . . . In general, chronic administration of oral chlorothiazide is well tolerated."[61]

These reports in the medical literature were echoed by generous amounts of advertising. Editor Milton Moskowitz of *Advertising Age* magazine reported in *The Nation* in 1957 that one in every five dollars in drug sales was allocated toward marketing of medications.[62] Half of those promotional expenses paid for detailing (personal visits by drug company representatives to physician offices and hospitals). Physicians also received a barrage of promotional material by mail. Moskowitz reported that, on average, a general practitioner in New York received 5000 pieces of direct mail per year. The *Journal of the American Medical Association*, in 1956, ran 5200 pages of advertising, worth $5.2 million.[63] The actual promotional expenses allocated for Diuril are unpublished; employing Moskowitz's formula, the promotional expenditures for Diuril would have been, at a minimum, several million dollars.

In its first year of release, chlorothiazide was tremendously popular and extremely lucrative. Thirteen million prescriptions were issued for Diuril, the trade name for the Merck drug. One million diuretic patients and half a million hypertensive patients were taking it, according to the trade journal, *Drug and Cosmetic Industry*.[64] In 1958, Merck, Sharp, and Dohme recorded $20 million in sales for Diuril, representing 75% of the total market for diuretics.[65] The company retained a comparable share of an expanding market in 1959, even in the face of competition from other pharmaceutical firms, and nearly the same share in 1960.[66] By any conservative estimate, chlorothiazide quickly found a niche in the therapeutic armamentarium.

This niche was secured because chlorothiazide satisfied an existing demand for the treatment of edema and congestive heart failure, which at that time had been dominated by the comparatively toxic organomercurials. It was also introduced during a decade when high blood pressure treatment was changing. Chlorothiazide benefited from this dynamic therapeutic environment in which a less nihilistic approach to a very prevalent condition was taking hold; according to the U.S. National Health Survey conducted from 1957-1959, 5.3 million Americans were classified as hypertensive.[67] Diuril was also introduced at a time when physicians recoiled from the more harmful side effects of available medicines, particularly the ganglionic blockers, which could cause severe orthostatic hypotension; the initial studies on chlorothiazide showed it could be used effectively in combination with these medications, thereby reducing the doses required, and minimizing the anticipated side effects.

By 1950, a surgical innovation of the 1940s, the thoraco-lumbar sympathectomy, had begun to influence how physicians perceived the treatment of essential hypertension. Adson and Peet, and then Smithwick, developed an operation in which the splanchnic roots of the sympathetic nervous system were cut, thereby producing a fall in blood pressure in certain patients. Smithwick reported his extensive series of over a thousand patients at a national symposium on hypertension held at the University of Minnesota in September 1950. Smithwick operated on a group of hypertensive patients and compared them to a group that did not receive surgery, and found that the first group survived longer.[68]

As drugs for the treatment of hypertension became available in the 1950s—including reserpine, hydralazine, and the ganglionic blockers—physicians began using them to treat certain types of patients, particularly those in the more threatening malignant phase of hypertensive disease. Reports appearing by the late 1950s confirmed prolongation of survival in patients with malignant hypertension who were treated with medication. Fewer of those patients had complications such as renal damage and retinal deterioration.[69]

The unsettled question by the late 1950s was whether or not treating hypertension in an earlier stage, before patients developed renal and vascular complications, might be beneficial. Some physicians believed that treatment should be postponed until evidence from long-term clinical trials became available, while others felt that prophylactic treatment should begin in light of evidence that had already been reported. This issue was the subject of discussion by a panel of experts at the first national symposium on hypertension held at Philadelphia's Hahnemann University in 1958. Here is an excerpt of that exchange:

> **Dr. Schmidt**: Should antihypertensive drug therapy be limited to the more severe cases of hypertension which already show organic damage?

> **Dr. Finnerty**: I am sure that the average patient who comes to the doctor's office shows very little vascular disease. . . . What does the doctor do with this patient?

> **Dr. Beyer**: I have been interested in this question from the standpoint of pharmacologic approach to preventive medicine. . . . If therapy is started early, you can arrest the progression of the disease at an early stage rather than trying to reverse a disease process which has already progressed to the point that you know you can't do anything about it.

> **Dr. Heider**: If we were to subscribe to the idea that hypertension ultimately ends up in producing damage to one organ or another, we are forced into having to treat it. This disease starts somewhere and it progresses—it's not here today and gone tomorrow. I believe that the sooner you treat it the better.

> **Dr. Beyer**: This is in large measure contingent on a safe mode of therapy.

> **Dr. Schroeder:** I think that is right, Dr. Beyer, but we haven't got a completely safe form of therapy yet. So, I think we have to progress in stages. Obviously, when we evaluate the status of a patient we take our chances with the severe or fatal side effects of any regimen. . . . And when the chances of the drug doing harm are less than the disease, then we take the chance and treat the disease.[70]

Those who looked at the epidemiologic evidence also found convincing reasons to treat hypertension before complications developed. For example, Jeremiah Stamler, an epidemiologist from Chicago, was among the most vocal advocates of preventive treatment. In the 1958 Proceedings of the Council of High Blood Pressure Research of the American Heart Association, he declared that risk factors for cardiac disease identified in the Framingham reports—obesity, smoking, hypercholesterolemia, diabetes, and hypertension—should be minimized before they did damage, even in advance of definitive, long-term studies.[71] Stamler's enthusiasm notwithstanding, the Council could make no such endorsement at that point, stating, "There is a wide divergence of opinion as to whether uncomplicated essential or primary hypertension should be treated at any age."[72]

One can reasonably conclude, based on multiple statements in the medical literature, that the control of elevated blood pressure was left to each doctor's individual judgment. Hypertension was compared by practitioners of the time to diabetes, an illness that demanded individualized care, with therapy tailored to each patient's circumstances. J. Earle Estes described this particular therapeutic imperative in his review of hypertensive treatment for the *Medical Clinics of North America* in 1958:

> There are no generally accepted statistics on the prognosis of untreated hypertensive
> patients. Also the wide variation in severity of hypertension and the variable re-
> sponse of afflicted persons add to the problem of evaluating treatment.
> Antihypertensive therapy is not standardized and patients vary greatly in their
> adherence to a therapeutic program. Each of us must establish goals of
> antihypertensive therapy and then measure as accurately as possible how these
> goals are achieved.[73]

In the context of such uncertainty, the characteristics of chlorothiazide
as a relatively benign medication held attractions for those who had fewer
reservations about treating their hypertensive patients. Based on the available—and arguably imperfect—evidence in the medical literature and trade
journals, one can deduce that a substantial number of patients with mild disease were treated with the new drug, given the number of prescriptions written, even though the raw data do not permit a definitive conclusion. Even in
advance of completion of the VA Cooperative Trial, the first randomized
clinical trial of antihypertensive medications initiated in the late 1950s (but
not finished until the next decade), and the Framingham study, a long-term
prospective study of cardiac risk factors—physicians were willing to treat patients for hypertension as long as suggestive evidence pointed to probable potential benefits.

Dr. Edward Freis, a prominent physician at the Veterans Administration
Hospital in Washington, D.C., and an acknowledged expert on hypertension,
describes this likely early transition toward treating hypertension more ag-
gressively:

> Therapeutic philosophy in many diseases carries with it a therapeutic tradition
> from the past. In the case of hypertension this tradition from older times is one of
> therapeutic nihilism. The administration of the unsatisfactory therapeutic agents
> available twenty years ago was rightly looked upon as bordering upon charlatansim.
> Our elders' attitude can be sensed in the very name "essential" hypertension sug-
> gesting that the elevated blood pressure was a compensation and was necessary
> in some way for the patient's welfare.
>
>
> Rightly or wrongly, a negativistic attitude persists in many quarters today. These
> critics point out that a controlled study over a period of sufficient time to deter-
> mine the value of blood pressure reduction has not been carried out. But, such a
> study would involve a collaborative effort of several hospitals and a time period
> of five to ten years or more. . . . Are we justified in doing nothing about early
> hypertension while awaiting for final proof? Let us examine the argument from
> another aspect.

Antihypertensive therapy is based on a rationale here described. It is granted that we do not know, and hence, cannot remove the ultimate cause of essential hypertension. Therefore, we cannot cure. But to an increasing degree from year to year as more effective agents are developed we can control the hypertension. If the level of blood pressure can be controlled at normotensive or nearly normotensive levels, then the organic progression, such as cardiac hypertrophy and vascular degenerative changes, will not occur."[74]

These remarks, written several years prior to the publication of results of long-term randomized clinical studies of hypertension in the literature, suggest that clinical judgment superseded science, at least in many cases, in the use of new antihypertensive medications. As one of the widely heralded treatments for hypertension, the thiazides certainly played a role in this therapeutic change.

Conclusion

The thiazides represent both an evolutionary, and revolutionary, development in the history of American medical practice. The synthesis, testing, promotion, and adoption of these drugs demonstrate the maturity and economic power of the pharmaceutical industry to influence therapeutic practice in a systematic and influential way. The evolution of the industry into a sophisticated research and marketing enterprise is evident in the quick success and immediate acceptance the thiazides enjoyed. These drugs were also revolutionary in their therapeutic application: as oral, noninvasive treatment alternatives for diseases such as congestive heart failure and hypertension, new treatments that had a measurable impact on morbidity and mortality. In 1959, the American Heart Association and the National Institutes of Health reported declining death rates from cardiovascular disease over the preceding ten years, which were partly attributed to the use of new anti-hypertensive medications.[75]

This paper has left certain questions about the thiazides incompletely answered. The organizational arrangements for research and the way in which they influenced events are largely hidden from view and worthy of further characterization. The rich and complicated relationships between pharmaceutical companies and physicians in academic institutions, hospitals, and private practice is one that can be inferred but not described in detail. The future availability of archival materials may offer further insight into those important and salient connections.

Ultimately, the use of the thiazides was shaped not only by corporate power and skillful entrepreneurship but also dictated by the individual biases and priorities of doctors and patients in the treatment of chronic disease. These very specific, and necessarily idiosyncratic, details are the most difficult to discern in writing an accurate therapeutic history of this new class of medications. In all probability, these novel drugs were seen generally as a welcome innovation that favorably altered the clinical outcome of patients with hypertension and congestive heart failure, an advance that could be adopted even in advance of definitive scientific evidence proving their clinical effectiveness. It is also safe to assume that the frequency with which the thiazides were prescribed may have varied widely, according to race, economic or social class, or locality, especially in an American medical culture in which treatments were not standardized and physicians exercised large amounts of individual discretion. The undiscovered intricacies of this therapeutic tale certainly deserve further exploration.

As an enduring staple of the therapeutic armamentarium, the thiazides today remain remarkable for their resilience. Once a symbol of corporate innovation and state-of-the-art science during a crucial decade in the history of therapeutics, they now represent reliable, sensible, inexpensive remedies for edema and hypertension. Far from anachronistic, they have retained a place in medical practice, even though their past symbolism has now been forever altered in the present. They remain comfortable old warhorses in an age of cost-effective care.

Notes and References

Acknowledgments: The author would like to acknowledge the generous research support of the Robert Wood Johnson Foundation Clinical Scholars Program.

1. F.C. Novello and J.M. Sprague, "Benzothiadizine dioxides as novel diuretics," *Journal of the American Chemical Society* 79(1957): 2028-2029; K.H. Beyer, et. al., "Chlorothiazide (6-chloro-7 sulfamyl-1,2,4-benzothiadiazine-1,1-dioxide): The enhancement of sodium chloride excretion," *Federal Proceedings* 16 (1957): 282.

2. Thomas H. Maren, "Diuretics and renal drug development," in *Renal Physiology: People and Ideas* (Bethesda: American Physiological Society, 1987), pp. 407-436;Karl Beyer, "Chlorothiazide: How the thiazides evolved as antihypertensive therapy," *Hypertension* 22 (1993): 388-391; Julius H. Comroe, Jr., M.D., *Exploring the Heart: Discoveries in Heart Disease and Blood Pressure* (New York: Norton, 1983), pp. 295-304; F.O. Simpson and J.V. Hodge, "The evolution of antihypertensive therapy," *New Zealand Medical Journal* 67 (1968): 271.

3. William H. Stewart, "Research progress report: High blood pressure," *Public Health Reports,* 70 (1955): 64-66; *Proceedings of the First National Conference on Cardiovascular Diseases* (New York: American Heart Association, 1950).

4. *Report of the National Conference on Cardiovascular Diseases* (New York: American Heart Association, 1950), pp. 5-6.

5. *Proceedings of the First National Conference on Cardiovascular Diseases* (n. 3), p. 126.

6. *Proceedings of the First National Conference on Cardiovascular Diseases* (n. 3), p. 125.

7. *Proceedings of the First National Conference on Cardiovascular Diseases* (n. 3), p. 126.

8. Thomas R. Dawber, F.E. Moore, and G.V. Mann, "II. Coronary heart disease in the Framingham study," *American Journal of Public Health* 47 (1957): 4; Abraham Kagan, Tavia Gordon, William Kannel, and Thomas Dawber, "Blood pressure and its relation to coronary heart disease in the Framingham study," in *Hypertension Vol. VII, Proceedings of the Council for High Blood Pressure Research, American Heart Association, November, 1958* (New York: American Heart Association, 1959), pp. 53-81; see also William B. Kannel, "Factors of risk in the development of coronary heart disease— Six-year follow-up experience: The Framingham study," *Annals of Internal Medicine* 55 (1961): 33-50.

9. John Swann, *Academic Scientists and the Pharmaceutical Industry: Cooperative Research in Twentieth Century America* (Baltimore: Johns Hopkins University Press, 1988), pp. 1-23.

10. Swann, *Academic Scientists* (n. 9), pp. 15-16.

11. Swann, *Academic Scientists* (n. 9,) pp. 41-49.

12. Swann, *Academic Scientists* (n. 9), p. 71.

13. Swann, *Academic Scientists* (n. 9), p. 47.

14. Swann, *Academic Scientists* (n. 9), p. 36

15. Louis Galambos and Michael S. Brown, *Values and Visions: A Merck Century* (Merck and Company, 1991), p. 185. Research and development expenditures for the company actually topped one million dollars beginning in 1941.

16. Maren, "Diuretics and renal drug development" (n. 2), pp. 407-436; Beyer, "Chlorothiazide: How the thiazides evolved as antihypertensive therapy" (n. 2), pp. 388-91; Comroe, *Exploring the Heart* (n. 2), pp. 295-304; and Simpson and Hodge, "The Evolution of Antihypertensive Therapy" (n. 2), p. 271.

17. See in particular Bernard Idson, "Diuretics and edema," *Drug and Cosmetic Industry* 85 (1959): 466-67, 548-53.

18. Maren, "Diuretics and renal drug development" (n. 2), pp. 411-13.

19. Maren, "Diuretics and renal drug development" (n. 2), pp. 416-22, 423-27.

20. Maren, "Diuretics and renal drug development" (n. 2), pp. 416-22.

21. Maren, "Diuretics and renal drug development" (n. 2), pp. 423-27. See also Karl Beyer's own recent account in Karl Beyer, "Chlorothiazide: How the Thiazides Evolved as Antihypertensive Therapy" (n. 2), pp. 388-91.

22. Beyer, "Chlorothiazide: How the thiazides evolved as antihypertensive therapy" (n. 2), p. 390.

23. E.D. Freis, A. Wanko, and I.M. Wilson, "Potentiating effect of chlorothiazide (Diuril) in combination with other antihypertensive agents: Preliminary report," *Medical Annals of the District of Colombia* 26 (1957): 468, 516.

24. W. Hollander and R.W. Wilkins, "Chlorothiazide: A new type of drug for treatment of arterial hypertension," *Boston Medical Quarterly* 8(1957): 69-75.

25 J.H. Moyer, R.V. Ford, and C.L. Spurr, "Pharmacodynamics of chlorothiazide (Diuril), an orally effective non-mercurial diuretic agent," *Proceedings of the Society of Experimental Medicine and Biology* 95 (1957): 529-31.

26. Milton Moskowitz, "Diuril creates a new market," *Drug and Cosmetic Industry* 87 (1960): 843.

27. Maren, "Diuretics and renal drug development" (n. 2), p. 426.

28. Moskowitz, "Diuril creates a new market" (n. 26), p. 843.

29. Press Release, Merck, Sharp, and Dohme, January 30, 1958, Merck Archives, White House Station, New Jersey.

30. Beyer, "Chlorothiazide: How the thiazides evolved as antihypertensive therapy" (n. 2), p.

390.

31. Freis, Wanko, and Wilson, "Potentiating effect of chlorothiazide (Diuril)" (n. 23), pp. 468, 516.

32. R. W. Wilkins, "New drugs for the treatment of hypertension, with special reference to chlorothiazide," *New England Journal of Medicine* 257 (1957): 1029-30.

33. Moyer, Ford, and Spurr, "Pharmacodynamics of chlorothiazide (Diuril)" (n. 25), pp. 529-31.

34. Edward D. Freis, et. al., "Chlorothiazide in hypertension," *Annals of the New York Academy of Medicine* 71 (1957): 450.

35. Wilkins, "New drugs for the treatment of hypertension" (n. 32), pp. 1026-30.

36. George E. Schreiner and H. Allan Bloomer, "Effect of chlorothiazide on the edema of cirrhosis, nephrosis, congestive heart failure, and chronic renal insufficiency," *New England Journal of Medicine* 257 (1957): 1016-22. Schreiner stated: "Most therapeutic enthusiasts, aware of the generally safe record of mercurial diuretics in uncomplicated congestive heart failure, do not heed the warnings concerning their use in active renal disease. They are likely to reply, 'What else do we use?'

Acetazolamide has provided only a partial answer to that question. It has not proved to be a striking diuretic agent clinically and becomes less effective on repetition as the serum bicarbonate is depleted. . . .

We believe that the experience with chlorothiazide described above provides a significantly more effective answer to the question."

37. Wilkins, "New drugs for the treatment of hypertension" (n. 32),p. 1026.

38. Ralph V. Ford, et. al., "Choice of a Diuretic Agent Based on Pharmacologic Principles," *JAMA* 166 (1958): 129-136; Edward D. Freis, et. al., "Treatment of essential hypertension with chlorothiazide," *JAMA* 166 (1958): 137-40; Frank A. Finnerty, Joachim H. Buchholz, and John Tuchman, "Evaluation of chlorothiazide (Diuril) in the toxemias of pregnancy, " *JAMA* 166 (1958): 141-44; John H. Laragh, Henry O. Heinemann, and Felix E. Demartini, "Effect of chlorothiazide on electrolyte transport in man: Its use in the treatment of edema of congestive heart failure, nephrosis, and cirrhosis," *JAMA* 166 (1958): 145-52.

39. Wilkins, "New Drugs for the Treatment of Hypertension" (n. 32), pp. 1-10.

40. J.A. Spittel, R.W. Gifford, and R.W.P. Anchor, "Treatment of hypertension with hydrochlorothiazide as the sole antihypertensive agent," *Mayo Clinic Proceedings* 34 (1959): 256-62.

41. David J. Reinhardt, "The impact of chlorothiazide (Diuril) on therapy in arterial hypertension," *Delaware State Medical Journal* 30 (1958): 1-3; David J. Reinhardt, "Experience with chlorothiazide (Diuril) in hypertensive patients," *Delaware State Medical Journal* 31 (1959): 44-52.

42. John F. Briggs, Arthur H. Wells, and Henry G. Moehring, "Antihypertensive agents: The role of diuretics," *Minnesota Medicine* 42 (1959): 939-40.

43. Joseph C. Edwards, " Management of hypertension," *Mississippi Valley Medical Journal* 81 (1959): 149-50.

44. Walter E. Judson, "Combination of new drugs in treatment of hypertension," *Nebraska State Medical Journal* 44 (1959): 305-11.

45. Marvin C. Becker, et. al, "Chlorothiazide as a diuretic and hypotensive agent," *Journal of the Medical Society of New Jersey* 55 (1958): 427-34.

46. John Messina, "Diuril in hypertension," *Ohio State Medical Journal* 55 (1959): 344-46.

47. Fred T. Darvill, "A controlled (placebo) study of the antihypertensive effects of chlorothiazide," *Northwest Medicine* 58 (1959): 707-709.

48. Richard B. Freeman, Brooks W. Gilmore, and Robert J. Gill, "Chlorothiazide in the Treatment of Arterial Hypertension," *GP* 20 (1959): pp. 99-104.

49. Harriet P. Dustan, "Diuretics in the treatment of hypertension," *Postgraduate Medicine* 25 (1959): 446-449; John H. Laragh, "Diuretics in the treatment of congestive heart failure," *Postgraduate Medicine* 25 (1959): 528-34; Ray W. Gifford, "Chlorothiazide in the treatment of hypertension," *Postgraduate Medicine* 25 (1959): 559-71.

50. Karl H. Beyer and John E. Baer, "The pharmacology of chlorothiazide and its analogues," *International Record of Medicine* 172 (1959): 413-59; Nemat O. Borbani, "The use of chlorothiazide and other thiazide derivatives in the treatment of hypertension," *International Record of Medicine* 172 (1959): 509-50.

51. Caroline Bedell Thomas, "Current views on diagnosis and management of hypertension," *Medical Times* 87 (1959): 1085-91.

52. Edward D. Freis, "Rationale and methods for the treatment of early essential hypertension," *Journal of the National Medical Association* 50 (1958):405-12.

53. Frank A. Finnerty, et. al., "Evaluation of chlorothiazide alone in the treatment of moderately severe and severe hypertension," *Circulation* 20 (1959): 1037-42.

54. John H. Moyer and John Beem, "Treatment of hypertension in the ambulatory patient," *American Journal of Cardiology* 3 (1959): 199-213; Marvin Moser and Alice Macaulay, "Chlorothiazide as an adjunct in the treatment of essential hypertension," *American Journal of Cardiology* 3 (1959): 214-19.

55. Robert W. Wilkins, "How to live with hypertension," *Science Digest* (April 1959): 37-41.

56. Robert W. Wilkins, "Drugs to aid hypertension," *U.S. News and World Report* (February 27, 1959): 75; "New drugs for overweight, pain, high blood pressure," *U.S. News and World Report* (November 16, 1959): 73

57. "High blood pressure: How dangerous is it," *Today's Health* (June 1960): 61, 65-67.

58. "Diuril," *The Medical Letter on Drugs and Therapeutics* , Pre-publication issue (1959): 3-4; "Diuril, Hydrodiuril, and Esidrix," *The Medical Letter on Drugs and Therapeutics* 1 (1959): 33-34.

59. Briggs, et. al. ,"Antihypertensive agents" (n. 42), p. 939.

60. Reinhardt, "The impact of chlorothiazide" (n. 41), p. 3.

61. Judson, "New drugs in hypertension" (n. 44), p. 309.

62. Milton Moskowitz, "Wonder profits in wonder drugs," *The Nation* 184 (1957): 357-60.

63. Moskowitz, "Wonder profits" (n. 62), pp. 357-359.

64. Moskowitz, "Diuril creates a new market" (n. 26), p. 843.

65. Moskowitz, "Diuril creates a new market" (n. 26).

66. Moskowitz, "Diuril creates a new market" (n. 26), p. 845.

67. *Health Statistics from the U.S. National Health Survey: Heart Conditions and High Blood Pressure Reported in Interviews, July 1957-June 1958.* Series B, Number 13, February 1960. (Washington, D.C.: U.S. Department of Health, Education, and Welfare, Public Health Service, 1960), p. 3.

68. A.W. Adson, W.M. Craig, and G.E. Brown, "Surgery in its relation to hypertension," *Surgery, Gynecology, and Obstetrics*, 62 (1936): 314; M.M. Peet, "Splanchnic section for hypertension: a preliminary report," *University Hospital Bulletin, Ann Arbor*, 1 (1935): 17; R.H. Smithwick, "A technique for splanchnic resection for hypertension," *Surgery*, 7 (1940):1; Reginald H. Smithwick, "The effect of sympathectomy upon the mortality and survival rates of patients with hypertensive cardiovacular disease," in E.T. Bell, ed., *Hypertension: A Symposium* (Minneapolis, University of Minnesota Press, 1951), pp. 429-448; Reginald H.

Smithwick, "Splanchniectomy in the treatment of essential hypertension," in John H. Moyer, ed., *Hypertension: The First Hahnemann Symposium on Hypertensive Disease*, (Philadelphia: W.B. Saunders, 1959), pp. 681-690.

69. H.M. Perry, Jr. and H.A. Schroeder, "Studies on control of hypertension. vi. some evidence for reversal of the process during hexamethonium and hydralazine therapy," *Circulation* 13 (1956): 528; H. M. Perry, Jr. and H.A. Schroeder, "The effect of treatment on mortality rates in severe hypertension," *Archives of Internal Medicine* 102 (1958): 418; J.H. Moyer, C.H. Heider, J.K. Pevey, and R.V. Ford, "The vascular status of a heterogeneous group of patients with hypertension, with particular emphasis on renal function," *American Journal of Medicine* 24 (1958): 164; John H. Moyer, "The Effect of blood pressure control on renal vascular damage associated with hypertension," in John H. Moyer, ed., *The First Hahnemann Symposium on Hypertension*, pp. 484-96.

70. Discussion," in Moyer, *The First Hahnemann Symposium on Hypertensive Disease*, (n. 69), pp. 598-599.

71. J. Stamler, et. al, "Epidemiological analysis of hypertension and hypertensive disease in the labor force of a Chicago utility company," *Hypertension* VII (1958): 48-49. Stamler declared: ". . . it is all too evident what will happen to high risk men if they are left alone. Moreover, it is quite clear that the measure available for correcting abnormalities are simple, practicable, reasonable, and devoid of danger. It therefore seems entirely in order to propose that the medical profession apply the knowledge from recent studies to identify the susceptibles to coronary heart disease and attempt to help them prophylactically."

72. M. Mendlowitz, et. al., "Report of the committee on chemotherapy in hypertension," *Hypertension* VI (1958): 91.

73. J. Earle Estes, "Hypertension in 1958: A tale of pills, philosophy, and perplexity," *Medical Clinics of North America* 42 (1958): 913-14.

74. Freis, "Rationale for treatment of early hypertension," (n. 52), p. 411-12.

75. Congress, House of Representatives, A Report to the Nation Presented by the American Heart Association and National Heart Institute on "A decade of progress against cardiovascular disease," Extension of Remarks by John E. Fogarty, *Congressional Record, Appendix* (19 February 1959), p. A1804.

Planning and Serendipity in the Search for a Nonaddicting Opiate Analgesic

by Caroline Jean Acker

I̶ₙ their reflective moments, pharmacologists and medicinal chemists often tell two kinds of stories. One is about the compound a chemist had made that was left sitting on the shelf because it appeared uninteresting, until, years or decades later, someone took a new look at it and found it had some fascinating properties. Another recounts how testing of a compound uncovered effects entirely unexpected—effects that may even have contradicted what was thought to be known about the compound. Unexpected or anomalous findings become serendipitous when the questions they pose open new avenues for research or suggest new explanatory models.[1]

Scientists seeking to develop new medicines must make decisions at every point regarding what kinds of compounds to strive for, what kinds of effects to test for, and whether to continue investing research and development resources in a given compound. Whether as researchers or as pharmaceutical entrepreneurs, decision makers in drug development must assess whether a compound will not just prove useful as a medicine, but useful enough to warrant the substantial engineering and marketing investments necessary to shift from making small quantities for laboratory testing to making and selling adequate supplies to fill a market need and produce profits. Pharmacologists have developed drug testing methods with these goals in mind. Individual tests of a drug's effects, however, can function in two ways—answering the question embedded in the testing method, but also failing to reveal important answers to questions not explicitly posed. Thus, testing methods can reveal, but sometimes conceal, important information.

The decades-long search for a nonaddicting analgesic that could replace morphine in the treatment of pain illustrates the interactions among planned testing sequences for new drugs, unexpected findings, and the serendipitous power of apparently anomalous findings to reveal the limitations of previous testing methods. Although German pharmaceutical manufacturers had been working toward improved opiate analgesics since the late nineteenth century, I will discuss Americans' work in this area from 1930 to the mid-1970s, with a focus on the activities of the National Research Council's Committee on Drug Addiction and its successor bodies.

The basic method of drug testing in the 1930s was the bioassay, i.e., the administration of a measured dose of a compound to a test animal and the subsequent observation of the presence and intensity, or absence, of a specific effect.[2] The mechanism whereby the compound produced this effect was not sought. In the complex matrix of mammalian physiology, with its interacting sets of control mechanisms, drugs may act in puzzling ways, as three episodes in the search for a nonaddicting opiate analgesic illustrate: the study of morphine agonists, or drugs that produce some or all of the effects associated with morphine; the discovery of the opiate antagonists, drugs that could reverse the effects of morphine; and the development of compounds that combined morphine-like effects and antagonistic effects, a class called mixed agonist-antagonists.

In the early 1970s, opioid[3] pharmacology became linked to studies of neurotransmission in the brain, as compounds produced in the search for analgesics functioned as useful probes of brain function. At this time, the older, narrower goal of identifying a nonaddicting analgesic broadened, as chemists produced compounds, and pharmacologists studied them, not just in the search for new medicines, but in the hopes of better understanding brain function.

The Quest for a Nonaddicting Opiate Analgesic

By the late nineteenth century, the phenomenon of addiction to opium and morphine, its chief active ingredient, was well recognized. Some Ameri-

---

Caroline Jean Acker is an Assistant Professor of History at Carnegie Mellon University in Pittsburgh, Pennsylvania. During 1993-1994, she was the DeWitt Stetten, Jr., Memorial Fellow in the History of Twentieth-Century Biomedical Research and/or Technology at the National Institutes of Health. She received her Ph.D. in History of Health Sciences from the University of California, San Francisco, in 1993. Her publications include "Addiction and the Laboratory: The Work of the National Research Council's Committee on Drug Addition, 1928-1939," which appeared in *Isis* in 1995, and "Stigma or Legitimation? A Historical Examination of the Social Potentials of Addiction Disease Models," which appeared in *The Journal of Psychoactive Drugs* in 1993.

can physicians, especially those active in the reform of medical education and the transformation of the American Medical Association (AMA) into a powerful advocate for the practicing physician urged caution in the prescribing of opiates, and by 1910, physicians were prescribing opiates less often than before.[4] But morphine, because of its analgesic, cough relieving, and antidiarrheal properties, remained an essential tool for the physician. Most importantly, morphine relieved serious pain better than any other known drug. Despite the serious liability posed by morphine's addictiveness, physicians found it essential to their practice. At the same time, the motives for relying less on morphine were becoming stronger. Physicians were blamed, both within and without the profession, for causing much unnecessary addiction through overprescribing of morphine.[5] And in the early decades of the twentieth century, as morphine and heroin were used recreationally among new social groups in American cities, the idea that addiction to opiates represented a serious social problem gained urgency. A drug that could relieve pain as powerfully as morphine did, but would not lead to addiction, would be highly desirable.

Heroin

Diaceticacidester of morphin.

To be kept in a dry and cool place and well-corked.

THE SAFE SUBSTITUTE FOR THE OPIATES.

Asthma coughs, especially in phthisis, bronchitis and laryngitis.

White crystalline powder, having a melting point of 171 to 172°, dissolving with difficulty in water, but readily soluble in alcohol and in water to which a little acetic acid has been added; incompatible with alkalies, such as sodium bicarbonate, ammonium carbonate.

The dose of Heroin varies from 1-24 to 1-12 grain in adults, three or four times daily, and taken preferably after ingestion of food. Children require proportionately *much smaller* doses. It is best given in powder, pills or tablets, avoiding combinations with alkalies such as sodium bicarbonate, etc. A solution in water can be readily prepared by adding a few drops of acetic acid.

If administered properly, beginning with minimum doses, Heroin is the safest and most efficient remedy for the relief of cough and dyspnea in phthisis, bronchial and laryngeal affections, emphysema, pneumonia, etc. It has also been employed with much success in hay-fever.

The description of heroin in the wholesale price list for Bayer Pharmaceutical Products (April 1, 1907) focuses on the product's usefulness as a cough remedy and a safe substitute for opiates. (Kremers Reference Files, University of Wisconsin School of Pharmacy.)

In 1929, the National Research Council (NRC) established a Committee on Drug Addiction whose goal was to identify just such a drug. A nonaddicting opiate analgesic had been sought at least since the late nineteenth century; the introduction of heroin in 1898 was just one—but certainly the most notorious—example of premature claims that a newly developed opiate was not addicting. Confusion over addictiveness reflected the lack of any reliable method for testing new compounds for addictive potential.

The NRC's involvement in drug development began when the Bureau of Social Hygiene, a Rockefeller-funded New York philanthropy, offered a three-year grant of $286,000 if the NRC would agree to assume leadership in the scientific study of opiate addiction. Although the Bureau's concerns regarding addiction were primarily social, the Bureau's director, Lawrence B. Dunham, shared the hope, widespread among reformers in the 1920s, that scientific research would provide solutions to vexing social problems.

Before deciding to pass its scientific program to the NRC, the Bureau of Social Hygiene had funded a variety of kinds of research, including physiological studies of morphine effects in animals and humans and surveys of medical and nonmedical use of opiates in several American cities.[6] At the NRC, however, largely at the urging of Harvard pharmacologist Reid Hunt, the newly formed Committee on Drug Addiction chose to devote the funds to a single project: the search for a nonaddicting substitute for morphine.[7] Hunt's recommendation reflected the aspirations of American pharmacologists who sought to build a drug development infrastructure in this country to rival that of the world's leading producer of new pharmaceuticals, Germany. The recent war with Germany had both revealed American dependence on German pharmaceuticals and provided an impetus for American firms (and academic scientists) to begin investing in research and development to produce new drugs.[8] The scientists on the Committee on Drug Addiction believed that mounting a search for a nonaddicting opiate would produce two benefits. First, a nonaddicting opiate analgesic would replace morphine in medical use and once morphine was no longer medically necessary, both scientists and policymakers believed, it would be possible to prevent importation of morphine and substantially eradicate the problem of opiate addiction—clearly an overly optimistic projection. Second, setting up such a project would result in drug development facilities modeled after those that characterized German pharmaceutical development in academic and industrial settings. Pharmaceutical research was based on the idea that a molecule's effects in the body were a direct function of its molecular structure, and that therefore modification of molecular structures was the best source of new medications. This conceptual foundation was embodied in the structure of Paul Ehrlich's Institute for Experimental Therapy in Frankfurt, where organic chemists who produced new compounds and pharmacologists who tested them in animals worked closely together. Ehrlich's metaphor of the "magic bullet" captured what for pharmacologists would be the ideal medicine: a compound with a single, therapeutically desirable action of desired intensity at a particular site in the human body (or acting only on an infectious pathogen in that body).[9] By contrast, morphine possesses several therapeutically desirable actions (including analgesia and cough relief) as well as undesirable actions (addictiveness and respiratory depression). Researchers seeking to improve on morphine would try to pare away or diminish undesired effects, and to separate desirable effects from each other, so that one compound might be used for pain relief, another to treat cough, and so forth.

Although the Committee on Drug Addiction did not gather its researchers at a single site, committee members envisioned a closely coordinated team of chemists and pharmacologists. To produce new compounds to be studied, the Committee hired Lyndon F. Small, an organic chemist who had spent two years in Heinrich Wieland's laboratory in Munich studying alkaloids found in the opium poppy. The Committee arranged with the University of Virginia, where Small was a member of the chemistry department, to set up a laboratory there. Small brought the German chemist Erich Mosettig to join him; while Small focused on breaking down the morphine molecule and adding structural components to it, Mosettig would seek a synthetic route to the desired drug, working with the phenanthrene structure, which could be derived from coal tar byproducts and which duplicated important structural elements of the morphine molecule. In the Drug Addiction Laboratory at the University of Virginia, Small built a program for training graduate students and postdoctoral fellows. Thus, a product of the laboratory would also be skilled chemists, many of whom moved from Small's laboratory to research jobs in the American pharmaceutical industry and at other universities.

The pharmacological studies would be conducted at the University of Michigan, where pharmacologist Nathan B. Eddy set up a laboratory to test the various compounds emerging from Small's laboratory in animals for therapeutic effect and for toxicity, including the potential to produce addiction. For compounds deemed promising enough, the Public Health Service would oversee clinical studies. An important site for these studies would be the Public Health Service Narcotic Hospital at Lexington, Kentucky. The legislation authorizing the establishment of this institution (and a companion narcotic hospital in Fort Worth, Texas) passed through Congress in 1929, the same year that the NRC created its Committee on Drug Addiction.

From the outset, the Committee researchers planned to move systematically through whole sets of structural variants on the morphine molecule and the phenanthrene structure and, equally systematically, to determine the whole range of physiological effects these compounds produced in animals. The keystone for measurement was the bioassay with special attention to dose. Researchers sought to determine the minimum dose at which a given effect appeared, how that effect intensified as the dose was increased, and at what dose toxic effects set in. The resulting data, in the form of dose-response curves, was the foundation for assessing a compound's utility: for example, was the therapeutic dose range sufficiently lower than the toxic dose to insure relative safety? These research methods comprise what pharmacologists today refer to as "classical pharmacology." The procedures grew directly from the aim of the work: the production of compounds with specific therapeutic effects. As it was not necessary to know how the drug produced these effects, the test animal functioned like a black box, receiving the input of dose and exhibiting a measurable response like respiration rate.

While the wide-ranging testing of opiate effects was intended to add to general knowledge about the effects of these drugs, a more targeted approach was necessary to identify those compounds that were serious candidates for testing in humans. In the earliest months of its operation, the Committee hired Cornell pharmacologist Robert Hatcher to survey the pharmacological literature on opiates and advise the Committee on how to set up its testing systems. Hatcher's advice reflected both the Committee's specific objective and the current state of the art in the testing of opiates. Since the Committee was seeking a nonaddicting analgesic, and since methods existed for testing analgesic potency but not for assaying addictiveness, Hatcher suggested that all compounds first be tested for pain relieving effects. Any compound showing analgesic effectiveness comparable to morphine's (and acceptable toxicity and side effect profiles) should then be examined to determine addictive potential. As for how to detect addictiveness, Hatcher noted that earlier drugs like heroin had been thought of first as cures for morphine addiction because they completely relieved the distresses of the withdrawal syndrome; but continued experience showed the drug to be addicting in the same manner as morphine. Hatcher hypothesized that any drug that suppressed the withdrawal syndrome associated with cessation of chronic morphine use would in fact be addictive in the same manner as morphine.[10]

Eddy followed Hatcher's suggested sequence, first testing compounds for analgesia before confronting the problem of addictiveness. He refined the mouse tail flick test as a measure of a compound's pain-relieving power. Baseline data were produced by observing how long it took the rodent to lift its tail from a warming hot plate; if a drug lengthened the time the animal allowed the tail to lie on the plate, it was assumed to be blunting the animal's sensation of pain. The standard to be matched or surpassed was the analgesic power of morphine. The first compound from Small's laboratory to show analgesic potency greater than that of morphine was dihydrodesoxymorphine-D, later named desomorphine.

Eddy then faced the problem of determining whether desomorphine was addictive in animal studies. He administered the drug continuously to dogs, cats, and monkeys, watching carefully for the development of tolerance (needing increased doses to maintain effects); then he stopped administration and watched for withdrawal symptoms. Although cats developed tolerance to certain of desomorphine's effects, in general, signs of tolerance or withdrawal were faint enough to leave Eddy optimistic that desomorphine represented the sought-after nonaddicting analgesic. The next step was to test the drug in humans.

Pending construction and opening of the Lexington Narcotic Hospital in 1935, addicted federal prisoners were being housed at the Fort Leavenworth Prison Annex in Kansas. The Public Health Service assigned physician Clifton K. Himmelsbach to undertake clinical studies with promising compounds emerging from Small's and Eddy's laboratories. At the Leavenworth Prison Annex (and later at Lexington), Himmelsbach had an experimental resource that proved crucial in developing an effective method for determining a compound's addictiveness: adult males who were addicted to morphine or heroin but were otherwise healthy. Drawing on what he had learned about tolerance and cross tolerance[11] during a training visit to Eddy's and other laboratories of pharmacology, Himmelsbach reasoned that a drug addictive in the same manner as morphine would likely substitute for morphine in preventing withdrawal symptoms.[12] He first developed a method for measuring the intensity of morphine withdrawal syndromes. He grouped the symptoms into categories of mild, moderate, marked, and severe. Using incoming prisoners who were still addicted to morphine as subjects, he observed them carefully as they went through withdrawal and plotted the onset of symptoms over time. The resulting curve indicated that mild symptoms like watery eyes appeared within the first day after cessation of drug use; the withdrawal syndrome peaked at about the third day with severe symptoms like vomiting, and all symptoms faded by about the seventh day. The severity of symptoms experienced by a given individual reflected the dose of morphine or heroin he regularly took.

To test desomorphine, Himmelsbach first stabilized a group of subjects on doses of morphine sufficient to prevent withdrawal symptoms. Then he substituted desomorphine for the morphine they were receiving, and continued giving them desomorphine at regular intervals. No withdrawal symptoms appeared. After about ten days, he abruptly ended the doses of desomorphine, and the well-recognized signs of withdrawal began to appear right on schedule. Himmelsbach concluded that desomorphine had prevented withdrawal because it was addicting in the same manner as morphine, and that the appearance of withdrawal symptoms after cessation of desomorphine further indicated the drug was addicting. Moreover, he was convinced he had developed a reliable method for testing any opiate compound for addictiveness. By ranking the symptoms of withdrawal according to their severity, Himmelsbach created a quantitative measure of the intensity of the withdrawal syndrome as a function of the dose of a drug. The more intense the withdrawal syndrome a compound produced (at comparable dose levels), the more addictive that compound was judged to be.

Nathan Eddy and the NRC committee members were initially reluctant to accept Himmelsbach's findings, since they meant that desomorphine represented no improvement over morphine, but subsequent tests bore out

Himmelsbach's ideas. He was able to demonstrate in terminal cancer patients who had never received morphine that prolonged administration of desomorphine produced definite addiction. Meanwhile, Eddy tried the morphine-substitution procedure with animals and found that desomorphine's addictiveness clearly emerged. By developing and standardizing the morphine substitution test in animals, Eddy also brought animal and human testing methods into closer correspondence with each other, to the end of gaining more reliable predictability from animal tests as to how compounds would behave in humans.[13]

The morphine substitution test meant that addictiveness could be understood as a measurable side effect like any other. It was the final step in the development of the standard sequence of tests that compounds moved through as they emerged from Small's laboratory. With the general toxicity and side effects tests, as well as the crucial analgesia and addictiveness assays, the researchers believed they could successfully screen out undesirable drugs and identify a nonaddicting analgesic. Of course, the vast majority of compounds were screened out early in the process (several hundred compounds had been developed and tested by 1939), and the desomorphine experience cautioned against excessive optimism and braced the investigators for a potentially long quest. But the testing procedures, and the project more generally, received some vindication in metopon, a compound Small developed in 1936.

Metopon, like desomorphine, showed significant analgesic potency. More importantly, the morphine substitution test showed it produced a much milder withdrawal syndrome than morphine when given at clinically useful doses for analgesia. Although metopon was not the nonaddicting analgesic researchers were seeking, it was used in hospitals as an analgesic until the early 1950s.[14] Despite its limited clinical utility, the committee and its researchers saw in metopon a theoretical vindication for their methods. The demonstrably lower addictive liability of metopon as compared to morphine suggested that addictiveness and analgesia varied independently of each other, and that further chemical modifications were therefore likely to produce an analgesic that lacked any addiction liability.

In 1932, when the Bureau of Social Hygiene's initial grant ran out, the Rockefeller Foundation funded the work of the Committee on Drug Addiction. In 1939, the Rockefeller Foundation ended its relationship with the committee. However, the Public Health Service connection provided the means for a transition to a new home for the researchers. At the recommendation of Surgeon General Thomas Parran, Nathan Eddy, Lyndon Small, and several of their colleagues came to the National Institute of Health (NIH) to form a chemotherapeutic unit. This move brought together into the same building the chemists and pharmacologists who had been collaborating at long distance. At Parran's request, the NRC continued its involvement by providing advice and coordination. In 1947, the NRC again appointed a formal committee to perform these functions, now named the Committee on Drug Addiction and Narcotics.[15]

The move to NIH reflected the importance of the opiate research to the federal government in two policy domains. The opening of the Public Health Service Narcotic Hospitals marked a strong federal investment in the problem of treating opiate addicts, and Parran favored the addition of a relevant research unit at the NIH, also a part of the Public Health Service. Keeping the work in the Public Health Service also insured links to the critical resource represented by Lexington inmates. The Addiction Research Center at Lexington became the place for testing new opiates for addictiveness, and not just for compounds emerging from Small and Eddy's work. The availability of incoming addicted prisoners as research subjects made it the only place where the morphine substitution test could be carried out on humans, and the existence of the test meant it was no longer acceptable to introduce new opiates with unsupported claims that they were not addicting.

In 1939, the German researchers O. Eisleb and O. Schaumann introduced meperidine, the first analgesic with morphine-like actions to be developed from a purely synthetic route. Himmelsbach subjected it to the morphine substitution test and demonstrated that its similarities to morphine included addictiveness.[16] The Addiction Research Center became the standard testing site to check new opioid compounds for addictiveness, and the Committee on Drug Addiction and Narcotics gradually assumed the role of coordinating the testing of opiates from any source at the ARC.[17]

A second concern prompting federal interest in opiate research was the looming war in Europe. Since opium poppies could not, by law, be grown in the United States, the country was dependent on imports from abroad for the most valuable analgesic in treating the pain resulting from wounds and surgery. To identify an improved, synthetic substitute that could be manufactured from materials readily available in the United States would lessen American dependence on foreign sources for morphine.

By about 1940, the committee had accomplished much, despite the failure to achieve its stated goal of producing a therapeutic replacement for morphine: A set of methods to test new candidates for such a drug were in place; the technical challenge of how to test new drugs for addictiveness had been overcome; and the Addiction Research Center was becoming the recognized center for determining addictiveness in new opiates, whether produced under the committee's auspices or by other research groups. Moreover, the committee's work represented an important investment in the building of a drug development infrastructure in the United States. Two events reflected the stature achieved by the committee's work and those who carried it out. In 1939, the American Pharmaceutical Manufacturers Association gave its first Annual Scientific Award to Lyndon Small and Nathan Eddy. In 1941, the first edition of Goodman and Gilman's now-classic textbook, *The Pharmacological Basis of Therapeutics*, devoted much of its chapter on opiates to the work of the committee's researchers.[18]

The most important tests in the established procedures, given acceptable toxicity and side effect profiles, were the tests for analgesia and addictiveness. Just as Hatcher had suggested in 1930, compounds showing good analgesic potency, by means of the tail flick test, were then tested for addictiveness. This testing sequence remained in place for many years, but before long, new compounds forced new questions about the meanings of these results.

The Discovery of Opiate Antagonists

Ironically, not long after the committee's testing procedures had been established, standardized, and apparently vindicated, the testing methods themselves functioned as a barrier to recognizing the analgesic properties of a new opiate derivative, nalorphine.

Among the sites where researchers were engaged in the search for improved opiate analgesics was the laboratory of Chauncey Leake at the University of California, where graduate student Elton McCawley was testing morphine derivatives in 1940.[19] A fellow graduate student, E. Ross Hart, had found that an allyl substitution on some compounds stimulated respiration. The two decided to explore whether an allyl-substituted morphine derivative would produce an analgesic that would not depress respiration and thus would lack morphine's most dangerous toxic effect. On surveying the relevant pharmacological literature, they found that the German chemist Pohl had reported in 1915 that an allyl substituted codeine would reverse the respiratory depression produced by morphine or heroin in animals—a finding that lay dormant for 25 years.[20] Hart and McCawley set about to develop the allyl of morphine; in 1941, they announced the development of N-allylnormorphine (nalorphine) and its ability to antagonize some morphine effects.[21] Leake then approached his friend Randolph Major at the pharmaceutical firm Merck and Company to learn if the company would make larger amounts of the new compound so that more testing could be done. Further work by McCawley and independent work by Weijlard and Erickson at Merck made it clear that the original substance developed by Hart and McCawley had not actually been nalorphine (it was either a close relative to the structure they had described, or a mixture of two similar compounds). The two groups of researchers then independently produced the correct compound. That it was negative in the tail-flick test for pain relief eliminated it from consideration as an analgesic. Although both Hart at the University of California and Unna at Merck demonstrated nalorphine's capacity to reverse the effects of morphine, the therapeutic potential represented by this finding remained unexplored for almost another decade.

In 1951, Eckenhoff, Elder, and King demonstrated that nalorphine could be used to treat opiate overdoses.[22] Shortly thereafter, Abraham Wikler at the Addiction Research Center showed that when nalorphine was given to a subject addicted to morphine, the individual would go into immediate withdrawal.[23] Also at the Addiction Research Center, Harris Isbell hypothesized that adding a small amount of nalorphine to morphine might prevent the latter drug from inducing addiction when administered for pain over a long period, and this idea prompted new interest in examining nalorphine in the context of testing analgesics.

The standard methods for testing pain-relieving potency came under challenge as Harvard anesthesiologist Henry K. Beecher, based on his experience treating soldiers during World War II, rejected the utility of laboratory pain tests in assessing a drug's ability to relieve pain in the clinical situation.[24] The tail flick test exemplified animal tests for a drug's pain relieving potential. In the late 1930s, James Hardy, Harold Wolff, and Helen Goodell of Cornell developed a laboratory method for measuring pain in humans. The painful stimulus they used was heat radiating from a high-wattage lamp. Subjects noted when they first perceived the warmth as pain, and each time the pain increased perceptibly in intensity. With repeated studies, Hardy, Wolff, and Goodell developed an intensity scale of pain that enabled quantitative comparisons of pain from different causes and in different subjects. They then measured the potency of analgesics by comparing the time to first perception of pain, the total intensity of pain reached, and so forth, with the subject's reaction to the painful stimulus in the absence of drugs.

Although this method produced consistent results in the laboratory setting with healthy volunteers (including the researchers themselves) as subjects, achieving similarly reliable measures of pain relief in patients proved difficult. Following his wartime observations of the different reactions to pain by soldiers recovering from surgical repair of wounds from what he was used to seeing in civilian patients, Beecher argued that the subjective component of pain—the individual's reaction to the painful situation—powerfully affected the individual's perception of pain's intensity. Beecher had observed that soldiers recovering from wounds reported significantly less pain, and required less medication for it, than civilian patients who had undergone similar operations. He concluded that the difference could be accounted for by the very different reactions of the soldier relieved to be off the battlefield and the civilian whose normal life had been interrupted by the need for surgery. Beecher and his colleagues, fellow anesthesiologist Arthur D. Keats, pharmacologist Louis Lasagna,[25] internist Jane Denton, and statistician Frederick Mosteller, conducted a systematic series of tests of known and potential new analgesics in which they relied on patients' reports of the degree of pain relief they experienced to measure the power of the analgesic. Individual patients were given more than one preparation (including placebos) so they could compare their own reactions to different drug regimens.

In 1948, Beecher had begun reporting his studies of pain and analgesia to CDAN, and shortly thereafter, the Committee began contributing funds to support his work.[26] Harris Isbell in 1953 proposed that Beecher's group assess the effectiveness of the nalorphine-morphine combination that he had suggested might deliver morphine's analgesic power without causing addiction. Beecher's group administered nalorphine alone to some patients as a control in accordance with the systematic nature of the trials. To everyone's surprise, these patients reported pain relief from nalorphine alone—despite the drug's earlier failure to produce a positive result in the tail-flick test for analgesia. Some patients also reported highly unpleasant psychological reactions, and this side effect precluded clinical use of nalorphine. Perhaps for this reason, the possibilities suggested by nalorphine's unexpected analgesic power were not further explored.

The ability of nalorphine to produce analgesia, even as it reversed some effects of morphine, meant that it was not simply a morphine antagonist, as had earlier been thought. Rather, the compound combined agonist and antagonist properties. The first pure antagonist emerged in 1961 when Blumberg and colleagues announced the development of naloxone.[27] This short-acting drug effectively blocked or reversed the effects of morphine but produced no observable effects itself. It became the standard treatment for opiate overdose. With the development of naloxone, pharmacologists had identified a range of opiate compounds that included pure agonists like morphine, pure antagonists like naloxone, and compounds that combined agonist and antagonist properties.

Exploring the Agonist-Antagonist Concept

As correlations between structure and activity in the opiate family were amassed, chemists and pharmacologists were increasingly able to make informed conjectures about the implications of specific molecular modifications. Lyndon Small had begun in 1930, systematically producing whole sets of possible modifications to the morphine molecule, and the collaboration with Eddy's group produced data on several hundred compounds by 1940. In the early 1940s, Hart and McCawley had worked from a specific hypothesis that an allyl substitution on the morphine molecule would alter morphine's effect of depressing respiration. Meperidine and methadone, two synthetics with marked differences from the morphine structure but with comparable constellations of effects, suggested new synthetic routes toward the target of improved analgesics.[28] The accidental discovery that nalorphine, the first presumed morphine antagonist, also produced analgesia, opened up a more complex conceptual framework for considering the range of possibilities with opiate and opioid drugs. The possibilities posed by compounds that combined agonist and antagonist properties attracted the interest of various research groups, including that of chemist Everette May who, at the National Institutes of Health, collaborated closely with Nathan Eddy.

Everette L. May came to Lyndon Small's laboratory at the University of Virginia as a graduate student in 1935. He worked most closely there with Erich Mosettig, whose synthetic approach (with the phenanthrene ring as the starting point) differed from Small's approach, which began with the morphine molecule itself. May received his Ph.D. in 1939, spent two years working in industry, and then joined Small, Mosettig, and Nathan Eddy at the National Institutes of Health in 1941. Here he continued to focus on synthetic, rather than derivative, approaches to developing new analgesics.[29] Meperidine had been the first compound shown to act like morphine (both as an analgesic and as an addicting drug) that seemed structurally unrelated to morphine. However, as May later noted, the two compounds did share some structural elements, and these formed the focus of exploration by a number of investigators.[30] Methadone also produced morphine-like effects despite structural dissimilarities from morphine. After methadone was introduced to American researchers following World War II, May examined a number of its chemical analogues as he continued to pursue structural elements essential to producing analgesia.

May also noted the work of Grewe and Schnider in the late 1940s on the morphinan series of molecules, which showed that the entire morphine molecule was not necessary to produce the constellation of analgesic and addictive effects associated with morphine. Drawing on these findings, May began mentally paring away parts of the morphine molecule and devising three approaches to isolating the essential structural components. From these possibilities, he selected the benzomorphan family of compounds and suggested it be explored as potential analgesics employing the antagonist principle. He proposed modifications to the morphine and morphinan molecules intended to dissociate the analgesic and addictive properties; with his colleagues, he produced a number of analogues in this family.

This work opened up new avenues of exploration for pharmacologists and other medicinal chemists also interested in exploring the agonist/antagonist concept. Among these were the group of Sydney Archer, N. F. Albertson, Louis Harris, and their colleagues at the Sterling-Winthrop Research Institute.[31] Surveying the research methods of the preceding two decades, they concluded that the reliance on the mouse tail flick test as a criterion for identifying analgetic compounds had actually obstructed the search for a nonaddicting opiate pain reliever. That nalorphine could produce analgesia, and at the same time antagonize the effects of morphine, had pointed up shortcomings in the commonly used analgesia assays, although these had not been recognized as such. Noting that every drug that had produced an analgesic effect in the tail flick test had also proved to be addicting, Archer, Harris, and their colleagues proposed turning the standard testing sequence on its head: "It became clear that, in order to achieve the desired separation of analgesic potency from addiction liability, the classical approach to the problem had to be abandoned."[32]

Instead of relying on the mouse analgesia tests to select drugs of interest, as researchers had been doing for decades, they chose to examine only drugs that proved negative in the analgesia assay. The class of compounds that merited exploration in their view were those with mixed agonist/antagonist properties. The research group at Sterling-Winthrop then built on May's work with benzomorphan analogues to develop pentazocine, a drug that combined agonist (morphine-like) and antagonist effects. It produced a clinically useful level of analgesia; its addiction liability was low enough to be considered negligible, and it lacked the psychotomimetic side effects that had made nalorphine unsuitable. They reported, "It appears that pentazocine is the first clinically acceptable, strong analgesic that is free of any significant addiction liability."[33]

This milestone was achieved only when assumptions built into the testing sequence developed in the 1930s were overturned, and when unexpected findings presented a more complex range of opiate effects than had previously been recognized. These apparent anomalies prompted new conceptual approaches not only to the quest for a nonaddicting analgesic, but also to questions of how opiates function in the brain.

Conclusion

In 1973, in a review article in the journal *Science*, Nathan Eddy and Everette May surveyed progress toward the goal of identifying a nonaddicting analgesic.[34] They opened their account with the introduction of heroin in 1898, seventy-five years earlier, and described the work sponsored by the NRC Committee on Drug Addiction and its successor bodies. They noted that changes in patterns of drug use had shown that developing an analgesic that lacked morphine's ability to cause physical dependence could no longer be considered an effective solution to problems associated with drug abuse. (For example, pentazocine, which was only mildly addictive, produced more powerful euphoric effects when administered in combination with the antihistamine tripelennamine, as street addicts had discovered.) The scientific benefits of the work had been substantial, however. They pointed with pride to the accumulated knowledge regarding structure-activity relationships.

The research group that began work under sponsorship of the Committee on Drug Addiction and then moved into the National Institutes of Health, provided an important model of collaborative research that promoted alkaloid chemistry and pharmaceutical science. Among the products of this research was a vast library of compounds with varying combinations of agonist and antagonist effects, usable as research tools. In their final paragraphs, Eddy and May noted that other investigators had recently undertaken to identify the biological receptor for opiates. Among the more promising leads in this direction, they believed, was a report, just a few months earlier in *Science*, by Candace Pert and Solomon Snyder, who reported the binding of opiate analgesics to receptors in the mammalian brain.

To Eddy and May in 1973, the search for a nonaddicting opiate analgesic represented the organizing principle of several decades of work. Snyder and Pert represented a separate research strain as they and other researchers, including Avram Goldstein at Stanford, Hugh Kosterlitz at Aberdeen, Lars Terenius in Sweden, and Eric Simon at New York University searched for the opiate receptor.[35] Just as the idea of structure-activity relationships had guided the search for improved analgesics, these scientists also worked from an assumption that the molecular structure of drugs was the key to understanding their function in the body.[36] However, instead of observing the physiological effects of drugs as in bioassay (for example, the effect of a drug on respiration rate), these researchers sought the site of chemical interaction between an opiate and a particular molecular location in the brain or other tissue. Rather than correlating effects with drug structures and doses, they wanted to elucidate the mechanism whereby a drug triggered a set of events in the nervous system that culminated in faster or slower respiration, or analgesia, or euphoria. More specifically, they looked for evidence that opiates and other psychoactive drugs acted in the synapse, the gap between neurons across which communication from one neuron to another occurs through the release of neurotransmitters. These compounds, released by one neuron, cross the synaptic gap and bind to receptors on a neighboring neuron. Here, they activate an electrical impulse which travels down the receiving neuron as part of an elaborate web of communication among the various parts of the nervous system.

To test the hypothesis that opiates acted at the nerve junctions involved in the body's own regulation of pain, respiration, and mood, researchers like Pert and Snyder injected radioactively tagged drugs into animals and then mapped where in the brain they bound to the brain's own molecules. The array of compounds that had emerged from the quest for a nonaddicting opiate analgesic became essential tools in this research.

A drug might bind in many parts of the brain, but researchers needed to isolate the few and particular sites where such binding achieved a given physiological effect. Evidence suggested that only very specific molecular configurations could produce these meaningful receptor-site interactions. For example, many compounds resolve into two mirror images of the same structure, but in most cases, only one of these mirror images, or stereoisomers, produces a physiological effect in the body. This stereospecificity reinforced the idea that a precise structural match was necessary to produce a given drug effect. The array of structures available in the form of the compounds produced by Small, May, and many other opiate chemists enabled precise probes of this structural interaction.

Etorphine, a drug with ten thousand times morphine's analgesic potency, when administered in extremely low blood concentrations, proved highly selective in binding only to specific brain sites; that it seemed to seek out only those sites argued for a highly specific match between its molecular structure and that of certain portions of a neuronal membrane. More importantly, the ability of antagonists like naloxone to reverse the effects of opiate agonists reliably and completely, and at low doses, provided an important means of distinguishing opiate effects from other kinds of drug activity.[37]

Moreover, important conceptual contributions to the understanding of neurotransmission and the nature of drug receptors in the nervous system came from scientists who had primarily been engaged in the search for a better medicine and had confronted the array of effects produced by different compounds. In 1967, William Martin, Chief of the Addiction Research Center at the Lexington Narcotic Hospital, suggested an explanation for the overlapping and contrasting constellations of effects produced by the families of opiate agonists, antagonists, and mixed agonist-antagonists: rather than operating in the same way at a sole receptor, the brain might contain a family of opiate receptors, differing from each other in both function and in their ability to recognize and bind with variations in the opioid molecular structures. He posited three receptor subtypes, which he named mu, kappa, and sigma. Subsequent receptor mapping studies bore out Martin's hypothesis.[38]

Asked in 1971 to state his philosophy of science, Everette May stressed the importance of serendipity.[39] Certainly, the history of both May's own career and the larger tradition of research directed toward the identification of improved opiate analgesics exemplify the power of unexpected findings in science. It was precisely the apparent anomalies that forced new questions and new approaches to old questions, though often only after long periods of inattention. The material result of attempts to resolve these serendipitous paradoxes included the hundreds of compounds that not only provided new medications but also became critical tools in the elucidation of neurotransmission. Moreover, these same puzzles provided the context for the drug development tradition's conceptual contributions to neurotransmission research. Speaking at a gathering of chemists, pharmacologists and neuroscientists in 1993, Louis Harris highlighted this interaction with a reference to William Martin's insight regarding multiple opiate receptors. This concept emerged, Harris said, "not because it was posited, but because chemists made compounds whose actions needed to be explained."[40]

Notes and References

The research for this paper was supported by the DeWitt Stetten, Jr., Museum of Medical Research at the National Institutes of Health.

1 . References to the importance of serendipity in opiate pharmacology include Nathan B. Eddy and Everette L. May, "Origin and History of Antagonists," in *Narcotic Antagonists*, ed. M. C. Braude, L. S. Harris, E. L. May, J. P. Smith, and J. E. Villarreal, *Advances in Biochemical Psychopharmacology*, Vol. 8 (New York: Raven Press, 1974), p. 9; and Kennon M. Garrett and E. Leong Way, "The History of Narcotic Antagonists," in *Psycho- and Neuro-Pharmacology*, ed. M. J. Parnham and J. Bruinvels, *Discoveries in Pharmacology.*, Vol. 1 (Amsterdam: Elsevier, 1983), p. 380. References to compounds or findings that lay dormant for long periods include Louis S. Harris, "Narcotic Antagonists—Structure-Activity Relationships," in *Narcotic Antagonists*, ed. M. C. Braude, L. S. Harris, E. L. May, J. P. Smith, and J. E. Villarreal, *Advances in Biochemical Psychopharmacology*, Vol. 8 (New York: Raven Press, 1974), p. 13; and S. Archer, N. F. Albertson, L. S. Harris, Anne K. Pierson, J. G. Bird, "Pentazocine. Strong Analgesics and Analgesic Antagonists in the Benzomorphan Series," *Journal of Medicinal Chemistry* 7(1964)2:123.

2 . On the development of bioassay as a testing method, see J. M. van Rossum and J. Th. A. Hurkmans, "Bioassay: A Pharmacological Endeavor," in *Pharmacological Methods, Receptors and Chemotherapy*, ed. M. J. Parnham and J. Bruinvels, *Discoveries in Pharmacology*. Vol. 3 (Amsterdam: Elsevier, 1986), pp. 63-95.

3 . While the term "opiate" refers to morphine-like drugs derived from the opium poppy, opioids include synthetic drugs and drugs chemically dissimilar from, but acting like, opiates.

4 . On the reform of American medical education, see Kenneth M. Ludmerer, *Learning to Heal: The Development of American Medical Education* (New York: Basic Books, 1985) and William G. Rothstein, *American Medical Schools and the Practice of Medicine* (New York: Oxford University Press, 1987). On the American Medical Association, see James G. Burrows, *A.M.A.: Voice of American Medicine* (Baltimore: Johns Hopkins University Press, 1963). On declining prescribing of opiates by physicians, see David T. Courtwright, *Dark Paradise: Opiate Addiction in America before 1940* (Cambridge: Harvard University Press, 1982) and Caroline Jean Acker, "From All Purpose Anodyne to Marker of Deviance: Physicians' Attitudes Towards Opiates in the U.S. from 1890 to 1940," in *Drugs and Narcotics in History*, edited by Roy Porter and Mikulas Teich (Cambridge: Cambridge University Press, 1995), pp. 114-32.

5 . Charles E. Terry and Mildred Pellens, *The Opium Problem* (New York: Bureau of Social Hygiene, 1928), ch. 3; Acker, "Anodyne" (n. 4).

6 . Caroline Jean Acker, "Social Problems and Scientific Opportunities: The Case of Opiate Addiction in the United States, 1920-1940," Ph.D. diss., University of California, San Francisco, 1993, pp. 57-74.

7 . This account of the NRC's creation of its Committee on Drug Addiction, and the work it accomplished through 1939, is based in part on Caroline Jean Acker, "Addiction and the Laboratory: The Work of the National Research Council's Committee on Drug Addiction, 1928-1939," *Isis* 86(1995):167-93. On the changing structures and affiliations of the committee, see Nathan B. Eddy, *The National Research Council Involvement in the Opiate Problem* (Washington, D.C.: National Academy of Sciences, 1973), p. 31. This work is an indispens-

able reference on the work of the NRC Committee on Drug Addiction and its successors, and on the chemical and pharmacological aspects of the search for a nonaddicting opiate analgesic. See also Everette L. May and Arthur E. Jacobson, "The Committee on Problems of Drug Dependence: A Legacy of the National Academy of Sciences. A Historical Account," *Drug and Alcohol Dependence* 23(1989)3:183-218; and Arthur E. Jacobson and Kenner C. Rice, "The Continuing Interrelationship of CPDD and NIDDK," in *Problems of Drug Dependence: 1991,* ed. L. S. Harris, National Institute on Drug Abuse Monograph (Washington, D.C.: U.S. Government Printing Office, 1992).

8 . On the movement of American pharmaceutical firms into research and development in the 1920s, including links between academia and industry, see John P. Swann, *Academic Scientists and the Pharmaceutical Industry: Cooperative Research in Twentieth-Century America* (Baltimore: Johns Hopkins University Press, 1988).

9 . See John Parascandola's essay in this volume.

10 . Robert Hatcher, "Report to the Committee on Drug Addiction of the National Research Council," 27 Dec. 1930, National Academy of Sciences-National Research Council Archives; NAS-NRC Central File; Division of Medical Sciences: Projects; Folder Committee on Drug Addiction Meetings: Minutes.

11 . A drug is said to create tolerance when increasing doses are necessary to maintain the same intensity of effects. Cross tolerance sometimes occurs among similar drugs: an individual tolerant to morphine, for example, has comparably high tolerance for heroin.

12 . Although Himmelsbach's procedure carried out the recommendation made by Hatcher, Himmelsbach did not recall Hatcher or the latter's work with the Committee on Drug Addiction. Personal interview, October 28, 1993, Washington, D.C.

13 . Eddy, *National Research Council Involvement* (n. 7), p. 31.

14 . Eddy, *National Research Council Involvement* (n. 7), pp. 37-41.

15 . Eddy, *National Research Council Involvement* (n. 7), p. 42-56. The impetus to form a new committee came in part from military concerns regarding strategic supplies of analgesics.

16 . Clifton K. Himmelsbach, "Studies of the Addiction Liability of 'Demerol' (D-140)," *Journal of Pharmacology and Experimental Therapeutics* 75(1942)1:64-68.

17 . Eddy, *National Research Council Involvement* (n. 7).

18 . Louis Goodman and Alfred Gilman, *The Pharmacological Basis of Therapeutics* (New York: Macmillan, 1941), pp. 212-23.

19 . Garrett and Way, "History of Narcotic Antagonists" (n. 1).

20 . Frank M. Robinson, "Chemistry of Narcotic Antagonists of the Nalorphine Type," in *Narcotic Antagonists,* ed. M. C. Braude, L. S. Harris, E. L. May, J. P. Smith, and J. E. Villarreal, *Advances in Biochemical Psychopharmacology,* Vol. 8. (New York: Raven Press, 1974), pp. 21-31; Louis S. Harris, "Narcotic Antagonists—Structure-Activity Relationships," also in *Advances,* pp. 13-20.

21 . E. L. McCawley, E. R. Hart, and D. F. Marsh, "Preparation of N-allylnormorphine," *Journal of the American Chemical Society* 63(1941):314.

22 . Garrett and Way, "History of Narcotic Antagonists" (n. 1), pp. 384-85.

23 . Robinson, "Chemistry of Narcotic Antagonists" (n. 20), p. 22; Eddy, *National Research Council Involvement* (n. 7), p. 67.

24 . Marcia Meldrum, "Departures from the Design: The Randomized Clinical Trial in Historical Context, 1946-1970," Ph.D. diss., State University of New York, Stony Brook, 1994, pp. 286-98.

25 . See Louis Lasagna's essay in this volume.

26 . Eddy, *National Research Council Involvement* (n. 7), p. 62-70.

27 . Harris, "Narcotic Antagonists" (n. 20), p. 14.

28 . Methadone, an analgesic developed in Germany and brought to the U.S. after World War II, was studied at the Addiction Research Center and shown to be addictive. A longer-acting drug than morphine, it quickly became the standard drug for detoxifying morphine and heroin addicts coming into the Lexington Narcotic Hospital through a regimen of gradually decreasing doses.

29 . Everette L. May, interviewed by Wyndham D. Miles, 4 November 1971, History of Medicine Collection, National Library of Medicine, Bethesda, Maryland.

30 . Nathan B. Eddy and Everette L. May, "The Search for a Better Analgesic," *Science* 181(1973):410.

31 . S. Archer, N. F. Albertson, L. S. Harris, Anne K. Pierson, J. G. Bird, "Pentazocine. Strong Analgesics and Analgesic Antagonists in the Benzomorphan Series," *Journal of Medicinal Chemistry* 7(1964)2:123-27.

32 . Archer et. al., "Pentazocine" (n. 31)., p. 123.

33 . Archer et. al., "Pentazocine" (n. 31)., p. 126.

34 . Eddy and May, "Search" (n. 30).

35 . Solomon H. Snyder, *Brainstorming: The Science and Politics of Opiate Research* (Cambridge: Harvard University Press, 1989).

36 . Although these groups of researchers for the most part worked separately, Hugh Kosterlitz began presenting his work to CDAN in about 1958, and CDAN began contributing funds to Kosterlitz in 1964. Eddy, *National Research Council Involvement* (n. 7), pp. 79, 169.

37 . Snyder, *Brainstorming*, (n. 35), p. 48-52.

38 . S. Archer, "State-of-the-Art Analgesics from the Agonist-Antagonist Concept," in Harris, ed., *Problems*, 74.

39 . Everette L. May, interviewed by Wyndham D. Miles, 4 November 1971, History of Medicine Collection, National Library of Medicine, Bethesda, Maryland.

40 . National Institute on Drug Abuse Technical Review Meeting: Discovery of Novel Opioid Medications, July 18-19, 1993, Bethesda, Maryland.

Section 3.

The Disciplines of Medicine Making

Across the globe thousands of men and women work every day to discover and develop new medicines. They do so in many different ways. Most of their efforts fall within the scope of well defined disciplines. Some of these fields are centuries old, others are creations of this present generation. All have been influenced greatly by scientific and technological advances during the last 20 years.

Varro Tyler begins this section with a look at the history of pharmacognosy, a discipline that nearly died out from disinterest only to flourish in recent years. No pharmaceutical subject has captured so much current public interest, yet almost no one knows the name of this field that studies medicines of natural origin.

While pharmacognosy studies the sources of drugs, pharmacology explores where drugs go in the body and what effects they have on living organisms. A discipline with a proud 150-year history, pharmacology is undergoing a revolution of focus and scope. According to George Condouris, the scientific advances of the last two decades have made Paul Ehrlich's vision of the "magic bullet" much closer to reality.

The drugs of the future are now being "rationally" designed by medicinal chemists. As John Montgomery explains, for decades possible drugs were screened through a time-consuming and repetitious process. Active compounds were then selected and modified to improve the utility as medicines. Now our greater understanding of molecular biology is opening new methods for constructing potential curative agents.

Getting drugs into the body in the best possible way is the mission of pharmaceutics, the field that is concerned with the design, development, and use of pharmaceutical dosage forms. Only through a complete understanding of the chemical and physical properties of drug molecules is this possible. George Zografi outlines the very practical challenges that confront those who seek to transform drugs into usable medicines.

159

Today we rely on clinical testing to verify the safety and efficacy of the medicines we consume. Mark Parascandola concludes this section by casting a critical eye on randomized controlled clinical trials, the basis upon which the consuming public, health professionals, and governmental regulators depend. He reminds us that this is a young discipline, only fifty years old, and one that is perhaps ready for some serious re-examination.

The Recent History of Pharmacognosy

by Varro E. Tyler

THE starting point for any discussion of pharmacognosy is a definition of the term. Although the word has been used continually in pharmacy since its introduction by J. A. Schmidt in Vienna in 1811,[1] it is a designation that remains practically unknown to lay persons, even to this day. Formed from the two Greek words *pharmakon* (drug) and *gnosis* (knowledge), pharmacognosy requires some historical background to appreciate its full meaning.

Originally, all drugs were considered under the heading "materia medica," which literally means medical matter. As these became more numerous and more complex, specialized disciplines were required. Materia medica was divided into pharmacology, which dealt exclusively with the action of drugs, and pharmacognosy, which considered all aspects of drugs with lesser emphasis on their action. Later in the nineteenth century, as synthetic chemical entities began to enter the drug field, pharmacognosy underwent a further subdivision. Medicinal or pharmaceutical chemistry considered only synthetic compounds, while the designation pharmacognosy was retained for the study of drugs of natural origin, specifically, those derived from plants, animals, and microorganisms.

Why the meanings of pharmacology and medicinal chemistry are so well-known to the public, while the term pharmacognosy remains so obscure, is a real mystery. After all, some twenty-five percent of the prescription drugs used today are derived from higher plants. If microbial and animal products are included, the figure increases to about fifty percent. Nearly all of the significant synthetic medicines utilized today are based on prototypes of natural origin.[2] Considering these facts, it is truly astonishing that pharmacognosy has not become a household term familiar to all. There is, of course, a reason.

During the first half of this century, pharmacognosy was almost obliterated by a group of well-intentioned but highly specialized educators and practitioners who approached the subject from an extremely limited viewpoint. As an examination of the most popular textbook of the period indicates, they considered the subject only as a botanical science and became obsessed with the taxonomy, morphology, anatomy, and histology of the plant that produced the active constituent rather than the chemistry, biochemistry, pharmacology, and therapeutics of that constituent.[3] In other words, they emphasized the nature of the container rather than its contents.

Such an intense focus on relatively unimportant matters nearly killed pharmacognosy. Fortunately, there were a few professionals who, in the years following World War II, recognized the problems created by this limited approach. They saw the lack of interest by young persons in entering the field, the difficulty in obtaining federal funding to support research projects and graduate students, and the diminished emphasis on pharmacognosy in pharmacy school curriculums. All of this decline occurred in spite of the fact that natural product drugs continued to play an important role in medicine. The only difference was that now it was the isolated constituents that were used,

A registered pharmacist in both Indiana and Nebraska, Varro (Tip) Tyler graduated from the University of Nebraska, studied at Yale, and received both the M.S. and Ph.D. degrees from the University of Connecticut. He taught at Nebraska and the University of Washington before becoming Dean of the School of Pharmacy and Pharmacal Sciences at Purdue in 1966. The two schools of Nursing and Health Sciences were added to his responsibilities in 1979. After twenty years as dean, Tyler was named Executive Vice President of Academic Affairs, serving there until 1991, when he returned to the School of Pharmacy as a professor. Purdue's Trustees subsequently designated him The Lilly Distinguished Professor of Pharmacognosy, his current title. Tyler currently teaches at Purdue and serves on the Board of the Greater Lafayette Community Foundation. He is presently Chairman of the Board of Directors of North Central Health Services, Inc., and North Central Physician Services, Inc.

Tyler served his profession as first president of the American Society of Pharmacognosy and as president of the American Association of Colleges of Pharmacy, the American Council on Pharmaceutical Education, and the American Institute of the History of Pharmacy. He is a fellow of the Academy of Pharmaceutical Research and Science, the American Association of Pharmaceutical Scientists, and the American Association for the Advancement of Science. Among his recognitions are the honorary Doctor of Science degree from the University of Nebraska and the 1995 Distinguished Economic Botanist award from the Society for Economic Botany.

Over 250 scientific and education publications have been authored by Dr. Tyler, including the standard text *Pharmacognosy*, the popular books *Hoosier Home Remedies* and *The Honest Herbal*, and most recently, *Herbs of Choice*, written for the healthcare professional. He serves on the editorial boards of many scientific journals as well as advising *Prevention* and *HerbalGram* (a publication of the Herb Research Foundation and the American Botanical Council).

often in slightly modified form, instead of galenical preparations made by extracting the crude drugs.

Having recognized the problem, these individuals decided to do something about it. Four new textbooks by Pratt and Youngken (Jr.), Ferguson, Claus, and Ramstad, based on the importance of the contents rather than the container, appeared in the 1950s.[4] The formation of the American Society of Pharmacognosy in 1959 provided a great impetus to natural product research, particularly as a result of its journal, initially titled *Lloydia*; subsequently, *Journal of Natural Products*. A few centers of pharmacognostical excellence developed in schools of pharmacy, and by the 1960s things were definitely looking up for the science.

This brief historical introduction brings us up to the post-1960 period that I consider to be the actual starting point of the modern era in pharmacognosy. This span of about one-third century is the one here considered as current; I shall refer to the twenty-first century as the future. What then have been the current trends 1960 to 1996? It is a most interesting period.

From the perspective of this writer and expressed in the current vernacular, pharmacognosy almost "blew it again" by placing all its eggs in one basket, in spite of the excellent prospects previously mentioned. Of course, it may be argued that there were relatively few eggs and far too few baskets during the years in question. The science rapidly disowned the botanical emphasis that had cost it so dearly and concentrated instead on the isolation and structure determination of organic compounds contained in plants. While a few other aspects, such as alkaloid biogenesis, the screening of plants for biological activity, and even historical studies were prominent during the early part of the period, by the 1980s American pharmacognosy had settled down to isolation and structure determination and little else.[5] The new U.S. textbooks of the 1950s were, with one exception, not continued beyond a single edition or revision, so there was little opportunity for students to learn that pharmacognosy was really a broad science composed of biology and chemistry in nearly equal parts. In the early years of the century, botany dominated; in the modern era, chemistry plays an equally domineering role.

These remarks are applicable primarily to affairs in the United States. In Europe, pharmacognosy retained a broader perspective, even though in some countries the name was abandoned because of its negative botany-only connotation. *Planta Medica* is a journal devoted to natural product and medicinal plant research published in Germany. It is the official organ of the Society for Medicinal Plant Research, one of the most active scientific associations in this area worldwide. *Planta Medica* routinely publishes original scientific papers devoted to a wide variety of medicinal-plant related topics including: pharmacology, toxicology, and medicinal (therapeutic) applications; biological activity, and natural product chemistry; phytochemical analysis; and reviews. This broad scope is probably the most representative of any present-day journal devoted to pharmacognosy.

In the 1980s, pharmacognosists began to encounter a phenomenon that, until now, has proved to be both a blessing and a curse to their area of interest. At that time, an enormous resurgence of interest in the use of herbal products began to occur in the United States. The reasons for this phenomenon were several. Part of it no doubt stemmed from the counterculture movement of the 1960s, and the belief that "natural" products had an innate superiority over synthetic chemicals. In addition to this throwback to vitalism, people had become quite disillusioned with mainstream medical practice, its high cost, the difficulty of access, impersonal treatment, and its inability to cure everything. Dissatisfaction with synthetic chemical drugs was also a significant factor. The high incidence of side effects discouraged many from utilizing them; numerous cancer patients, for example, were (and still are) choosing death as a desirable alternative to the rigors of chemotherapy.

Whatever the reason, the ancient herbal remedies, and a few new ones as well, became extremely popular. Because they had not been proven safe and effective by post-1962 standards as established by the Kefauver-Harris Amendments, they were sold without therapeutic claims and were not subject to any quality standards. In 1993, Food and Drug Administration (FDA) Commissioner David Kessler threatened to remove them from the market; Congress received more mail on the subject than on any issue since the Vietnam war. Under such relentless public pressure, Congress passed the Dietary Supplement Health and Education Act (DSHEA) in October 1994.[6]

The Act went far beyond just keeping such products on the market. Although final regulations are still being prepared by the FDA for implementation on 1 January 1997, it appears that DSHEA will have both positive and negative effects. Product labeling will be given special attention. Both the common and the scientific names of the plant will have to appear on the label along with the part used and the quantity of plant material present. This is a giant step forward because many current products fail to provide this vital information.

Claims regarding the effect of the herb on the structure or function of the human body will be permitted, but not therapeutic or health claims. If a structure-function claim is made, it must be followed by a disclaimer noting that the FDA has not evaluated the claim. Then a completely hypocritical statement must appear avowing that the product is not intended to diagnose, treat, cure, or prevent any disease. Whether this new permissive labeling will have a positive or negative effect on consumer health and safety remains to be seen. The structure-function claims could be helpful, provided they are supported by scientific and clinical evidence. On the other hand, the inclusion of such generalities without therapeutic specifics may tend to mislead. In short, the long-term effects of this kind of labeling are not entirely predictable.

On the definite down side, the DSHEA regulations make no provisions for quality assurance, good manufacturing practices, or truth in advertising. Further, in order to remove a product from the market, the FDA must prove that it is unsafe.[7] The Act has already been in force for well over a year, and during the period, no action has been taken on any of the numerous herbal dietary supplements known to be unsafe.

The herbal product field in the United States has long been dominated by nonscientific elements, and this shift in the burden of proof of safety has provided a field day for those who wished to take advantage of the public's gullibility. By 1995, the U.S. herbal market had reached a dollar volume of $1.5 billion at retail and was growing rapidly.[8] While a few companies had voluntarily assumed the responsibility of providing quality products in the form of standardized plant extracts, many others were marketing unproven herbal combinations, often prepared from herbs of uncertain quality and frequently containing only traces of the specified botanicals. Others were capitalizing on the American public's enthusiasm for physical activity and weight loss by marketing central nervous system (CNS) stimulants such as ephedra or stimulant laxatives such as senna in large doses without adequate health

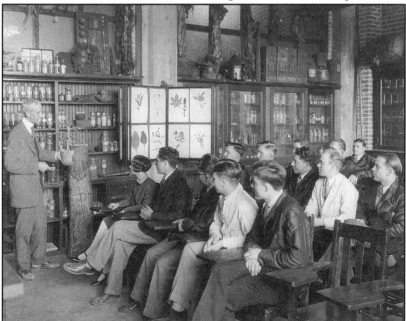

At the University of Iowa College of Pharmacy, Dean Wilber J. Teeters teaches a class in pharmacognosy in 1925. (Kremers Reference Files, University of Wisconsin School of Pharmacy Library.)

warnings. In addition, many herbs of unproven value to humans, such as ginseng and damiana, continued to be lauded and sold.[9]

Present-day pharmacognosists view these developments with ambivalence. On one hand, it is the first time during their entire lives that anyone outside their immediate circle has taken any interest in their field. And that public interest is not only intense, but intensifying. On the other hand, there is so much fraud and deception in the area of herbal medicine that some are reluctant to associate themselves with it in any way. The few who have done so have also found it an uphill battle to attempt to place this basically nonprofessional, commercially oriented industry on a sound scientific basis. A recent example will serve to illustrate the problem.

In October 1994, the FDA convened a Special Working Group to provide advice on the continued over-the-counter sale of the herb ephedra. Ephedra is one of our oldest medicines, having been found in Neanderthal tombs in Iraq dating back some 60,000 years.[10] It is a valuable bronchodilator, but it is also an active CNS stimulant, especially when consumed together with caffeine. The latter effect is responsible for its widespread presence in weight-loss and performance-enhancing herbal products. Misuse over extended periods of time has resulted in more reports of adverse reactions for ephedra than for any other herb in the United States; several deaths have also been attributed to its consumption.[11]

After extended deliberation, the Special Working Group concluded that, because of its therapeutic utility and reasonable safety when used properly, ephedra should be allowed to remain on the market as a dietary supplement, but that extensive and detailed labeling should be required.[12] Labeling should include prohibition of use by persons suffering from conditions such as hypertension or thyroid disease, as well as appropriate dosage information, time limits for unsupervised use, restrictions of sale and use by persons under age eighteen, and the like. Initially satisfied with the recommendation, pharmacognosists on the panel found, a few weeks later, that at least one herbal producer was marketing a soda pop that contained ephedra and was also planning to incorporate it in bubble gum, cookies, and breakfast cereal. All of these products are liable to be consumed and, of course, abused by children. It is difficult to help an industry in which some elements are unwilling to assume appropriate responsibility for the safety of their products and the health of those who consume them.

Another characteristic of herbal marketers in the United States is their unwillingness to devote any of their substantial profits to research. Most such companies are privately held, and their financial statements are not a matter of public record, but a conservative estimate of their annual gross profit approximates one-half billion dollars. Yet, as far as can be determined, none of this money is devoted to research, at least to studies of a publishable nature. The published investigations on garlic conducted in American medical schools recently were financed not by an American herbal company, but by a German phytomedicine producer.[13]

The American companies have even been unwilling to finance studies to determine the safety of their products. For this reason, safety of the popular botanical chaparral still remains questionable.[14] Products such as comfrey and coltsfoot remain on the American market, even though their toxicity on internal consumption is well established. Of course, it must be noted that, like all sweeping statements, this blanket condemnation of the ethics of the American herbal industry is not universally applicable. There are a sufficient number of exceptions to the rule to provide some hope that the industry as a whole can be salvaged. Still, it has placed pharmacognosists today in an ethical dilemma. The herbal renaissance has popularized their field beyond measure, yet the herbal industry as a whole has been extremely slow to respond in any way to attempts to render it professional and responsible. That challenge makes for very exciting times in pharmacognosy today.

The current worldwide search for new plant species yielding new, physiologically active constituents of patentable nature has not yet been mentioned. While neglecting the classic plant drugs because of the difficulty in obtaining a market exclusive on them, American pharmaceutical manufacturers are busily engaged in screening thousands of new chemical compounds isolated from plants obtained in obscure parts of the world ranging from the Brazilian rainforest to Samoa to China. Thus far, the search has not been an especially productive one, but that is true of all searches for new drugs from all sources, including chemical synthesis. With rare exceptions, the history of new drug development in this modern era is a story of minor molecular modifications, not outstanding breakthroughs.[15]

There is little more to be said about the present. What about future trends? The battle of science and professionalism versus hyperbole and commercialism in the herbal field could go either way. If the FDA fails to develop and to implement sensible regulations to control the unbridled development and sale of useless herbs and combinations, the public will suffer losses in both health and wealth. Eventually, under capitated health-care plans, unapproved products will probably cease to be used for the simple reason that patients will not be reimbursed for their purchase. Therefore, it is absolutely mandatory that effective botanicals and especially the phytomedicines prepared from them be recognized as approved drugs.[16] There are many of these. Ginkgo for cerebrovascular insufficiencies, garlic for hypercholesterolemia, echinacea for colds and related viral infections, feverfew for migraine prevention, saw palmetto for benign prostatic hyperplasia, and St. John's wort for depression, are just a few examples.[17]

If they are approved as drugs, standardized extracts of these and many others will be extremely popular due to their lesser side effects and greatly reduced costs. Whether this will actually come to pass is still uncertain. An extremely large number of variables, ranging from the attitude of FDA officials to whether there is a real desire to control the costs of health care in the United States, make the outcome difficult to predict.

As for future trends in the search for new drugs, it is steadfastly predictable that the empirical methods employed by human beings since the beginning of time will gradually fade away. As we learn more and more about the nature and function of receptor sites in various organs, tissues, and cells of the body, it becomes more certain that such important late twentieth-century activities as the ethnobotanical approach to new drug discovery will cease. Computers will eventually design drugs, and if chemists are unable to synthesize by conventional means the complex molecules required, biosynthetic techniques utilizing bioengineered microorganisms will carry out the task even more efficiently.[18]

However, such futuristic trends of computational chemistry need not cause us undue concern now. Future developments will occur gradually, not precipitously. For the foreseeable future, drugs old and new will continue to be derived from higher plants; and plants capable of yielding new and better drugs will be sought for in every part of the world.

A factor that may have tragic consequences, even in the near term, is the destruction of the native habitats of many plants before their potential utility can be evaluated. Population pressure and related factors such as the need for more agricultural land, coupled with logging and mining activities, are destroying natural Rainforest acreage at an unprecedented rate. Remembering that an area the size of a football field is being lost each second is an easy way to help one understand the magnitude of this loss. Knowledge that silphium, a plant widely used in the ancient world as a contraceptive, was the first plant to be rendered extinct through overharvest causes thinking persons to long for the return of it, or some readily available contraceptive like it, to help preserve our important natural resources from the scourge of overpopulation.[19]

This overview of present and future trends in pharmacognosy has pointed out the hazard and the harm that can be wrought by the excessive narrowing in perspective of what is naturally a broad field of science. This has occurred in American pharmacognosy twice this century, early on overemphasizing botany, and now, isolation and structure determination. The review has also noted the precarious relationship between the science of pharmacognosy and the, all too often, nonscience of herbal medicine in this country. Finally, it has discussed the present and future of drug development, with particular emphasis upon natural products.

When observed from afar, our survey reveals a checkerboard pattern of red and black, a phasic pattern of ups and downs, a judgmental pattern of goods and bads that characterizes not only pharmacognosy, but all aspects of human endeavor. It is a simple matter to know where one is. It is much more difficult to predict where one is going.

I have relatively little concern about the future of pharmacognosy, or the study of natural drug products, or whatever it may be called now or in the future. In my opinion, the science is now on the way up, and the immense public interest currently displayed in it will cause it to remain up for the indefinite future. There are hazards lurking along the path it follows; but they are only hazards, not major obstacles. None can deny that pharmacognosy enjoys a most interesting present and, in all probability, a truly enviable future. Fortunately, all of us will have at least some opportunity to see, and to benefit from, that future. It has been, is, and will be a better world for all, thanks to the numerous contributions of pharmacognosy.

Notes and References

1. K. Ganzinger, "Uber die Termini 'Pharmacognosis' und 'Pharmacographia', ein Beitrag zur Geschichte der pharmazeutischen Wissenschaften," *Medizinhistorisches J.* 14 (1979): 186-95.
2. J. E. Robbers, M. K. Speedie, and V. E. Tyler, *Pharmacognosy and Pharmacobiotechnology* (Baltimore: Williams & Wilkins, 1996), p. 3.
3. H. W. Youngken, *Textbook of Pharmacognosy*, six editions (Philadelphia: The Blakiston Company and predecessors, 1921 to 1948).
4. R. Pratt, R. and H. W. Youngken, Jr. *Pharmacognosy* (Philadelphia: J.B. Lippincott Company, 1951), 644 pp.; N. M. Ferguson *A Textbook of Pharmacognosy* (The Macmillan Company, New York, 1956), 374 pp.; E. P. Claus, *Gathercoal and Wirth Pharmacognosy* (Philadelphia: Lea & Febiger, 1956), 731 pp.; E. Ramstad, *Modern Pharmacognosy* (New York: McGraw-Hill Book Company 1959) 480 pp.
5. See table of contents pages for *Journal of Natural Products (Lloydia)*, 1980 to current date. Papers dealing with isolation and structure determination of new, naturally occurring compounds dominate during this period.
6. Dietary Supplement Health and Education Act of 1994, 103d Congress, 2d Session, Senate Report 103-410, 49 pp.
7. Anon.: Washington Wire: DSHEA Summary, *Herb Research News* Spring, 4-5 (1995).
8. V. E. Tyler, "Herbal remedies," *J. Pharm. Technol.* 11(1995): 214-220.
9. V. E. Tyler, "The overselling of herbs," in *The Health Robbers: A Close Look at Quackery in America*, S. Barrett and W. T. Jarvis, eds.(Buffalo, NY: Prometheus Books, 1993), pp. 213-24.
10. R. E. Schultes, "The heritage of folk medicine," in *Medicines From the Earth*, W. A. R. Thomson, ed.(New York: McGraw-Hill Book Company, 1978), pp. 137-38.
11. M. Blumenthal and P. King, "Ma Huang: Ancient herb, modern medicine, regulatory dilemma," *HerbalGram* No. 34(1995): 22-26, 43, 56-57.
12. E. N. Brandt, Jr., and L. A. Larsen, "Minutes of the Special Working Group on Food Products Containing Ephedra Alkaloids of the FDA Food Advisory Committee," Washington, D.C., October 11-12, 1995, 8 pp. (unpublished).
13. A. K. Jain, R. Vargas, S. Gotzkowsky, and F. G, McMahon, "Can garlic reduce levels of serum lipids? A controlled study," *Am.J. Med.* 94(1993): 632-35, and S. Phelps and W. S.

Harris, "Garlic supplementation and lipoprotein oxidation susceptibility, *Lipids* 28(1993): 475-77.

14. D. W. Gordon, G. Rosenthal, J. Hart, R. Sirota, and A. L. Baker, "Chaparral ingestion: The broadening spectrum of liver injury caused by herbal medications, *J. Am. Med. Assoc.* 273(1995): 489-90.

15. This assertion may be verified by perusal of an excellent series of articles on drug development that appeared in *Pharmaceutical News* in 1994 and 1995. The key articles are: B. B. Molloy, D. T. Wong, and R. W. Fuller, "The discovery of fluoxetine," *Pharm. News* 1, no. 2 (1994): 6-10; C. R. Ganellin, "Case histories of drug design," *Pharm. News* 1, no. 4(1994): 21-25 ; D. Cavalla, "Case histories of drug design," *Pharm. News* 2, no. 3(1995): 31-33 ; H. Schwartz, "The discovery of fluconazole," *Pharm. News* 2, no. 4(1995): 9-12 .

16. V. E. Tyler, "Herbs and health care in the twenty-first century," *Proceedings of Herbs '95,* Tenth Annual National Conference of the International Herb Association (Chicago, 1995), pp. 1-8.

17. V. E. Tyler, *Herbs of choice: The therapeutic use of phytomedicinals,* (Binghamton, NY: Pharmaceutical Products Press,1994), 209 pp.

18. V. E. Tyler, "Plant drugs, healing herbs, and phytomedicinals," *HerbalGram* No. 33 (1995): 36-37, 44-46.

19. J. M. Riddle, and J. W. Estes, "Oral Contraceptives in Ancient and Medieval Times," *Am. Scientist* 80 (1992): 226-33 .

Pharmacology:
Current and Future Trends

by George A. Condouris

P HARMACOLOGY is a biomedical science that deals with the <u>effects</u> of chemicals on the body and the <u>mechanisms</u> by which they produce these effects. Pharmacology is now on the verge of an explosive discovery of new types of drug and novel mechanisms of action. This explosion is an outcome of the remarkable advances made over the last two decades by pharmacology, molecular biology, molecular genetics, and other biomedical disciplines. The discoveries have produced a sharper view of the normal and pathological functions of the body, which provides pharmacology with a vast number of new tissue and cellular sites where new drugs can act to control cellular functions. The task confronting pharmacology is formidable, since many of the newly discovered sites for potential pharmacological intervention are buried deep in the cell architecture where they are protected by successive layers of biological barriers. Drugs modeled after the products formed when genes are activated in the cell nucleus, for example, are mainly macromolecules such as proteins. The massive size of these gene products, or their synthetic counterparts, pose new problems relating to pharmacokinetic factors that affect the movement of drugs from the site of administration to their intended receptor targets.

A major goal of pharmacologic research in the near future is to provide drugs with greatly enhanced pharmacologic specificity and maximum safety. The vision of Paul Ehrlich's early twentieth century "magic bullet," with which each disease will have a specific and unique remedy, seems to be closer to reality.

Pharmacological research is dominated by interest in drugs for therapeutic use, although pharmacologists also have significant interest in studying the toxicology of substances derived from environmental or manufacturing processes. In the early history of pharmacology (the middle of the nineteenth century), drugs were derived primarily from natural sources, i.e., from plants and animals. Eventually, this road to drug development advanced to the use of semi-synthetic modifications of natural products, and ultimately to completely synthetic drugs. The therapeutic drugs currently in use are actually derived from all three sources. It is interesting to note that the design of certain entirely new kinds of drugs are again rapidly focusing on natural animal substances.

Receptors in Pharmacology

Pharmacology is on the threshold of uncovering totally new drug entities. This exciting situation comes about because of the extraordinary advances made by the fields of biotechnology, molecular genetics, pharmaceutical sciences, and other biomedical disciplines, which have provided many new biochemical and physiological sites for pharmacological intervention. In 1995 there were 234 biotechnology drugs in clinical trials, up 64% from 1993.[1] A key element in the exploitation of these new discoveries is the concept of *drug receptors*.

Nearly 100 years ago Paul Ehrlich, an imaginative and persistent physician and scientist, postulated that in order for a drug to exert its action, it must first combine with a specific chemical constituent on the tissues. He called this constituent a *receptor*, and even scratched out a diagram of this concept (**Fig. 1**).[2] This event ushered in the *receptor doctrine*, which has

George A. Condouris, Ph.D., is Adjunct Professor of Pharmacology and Toxicology, and Chairman Emeritus at the New Jersey Medical School, UMDNJ, in Newark, New Jersey. He received a M.S. in Pharmacology from Yale University Medical School, Ph.D. in Pharmacology from Cornell University College of Medicine, and was a Visiting Investigator in Neurophysiology from 1955 to 1957 at Rockefeller University. Dr. Condouris's research interests include neuropharmacology, cardiovascular pharmacology, mechanisms for pain relief, and local and general anesthetics.

Dr. Condouris is a member of the American Society for Pharmacology and Experimental Therapeutics, and a charter member of the International Association for the Study of Pain. His current national professional activities include serving on the Pharmacology-Morphology Advisory Committee of the Pharmaceutical Research and Manufacturers of America Foundation, Inc. (1981-present); Member and Chairman of the Scientific Review Panel for the Foreign Faculty Fellowship Program in the Basic Medical Sciences, sponsored by the Educational Commission for Foreign Medical Graduates (1982-present); Secretary for the Association for Medical School Pharmacology (1993-present); and an active member of the American Society for Regional Anesthesia. He has been active on committees developing educational programs in medical school pharmacology, and has served on several scientific review panels, including NIH panels.

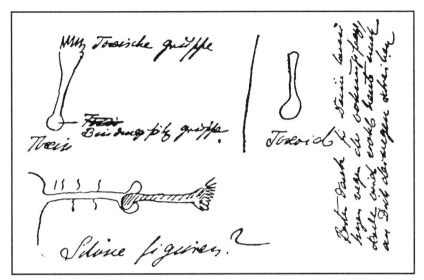

Fig. 1. The first sketch by Ehrlich of his concept of the interaction between a drug or antibody with a cell receptor, in a letter to Carl Weigert, 1898. (From Bruno Heymann, "Zur Geschichte der Seitenkettentheorie Paul Ehrlichs," Klinische Wochenschrift *7 (1928): 1307.)*

guided the development of pharmacology ever since. During the past twenty years, receptor science in the United States and abroad has developed at an extraordinary rate, fueled largely by the generous financial support of biomedical research by the Federal government following World War II. Drug-receptor interactions have been characterized with greater definition and the actual isolation of many cellular receptors has been accomplished. Up to about the late 1960s a drug receptor was correctly conceived as a functional entity described as "a pattern of physico-chemical forces on cell membranes that is complementary to a pattern of forces on the drug molecule." But the actual physical and chemical composition of drug receptors remained essentially unknown.

Today's highly sophisticated technology for receptor isolation has succeeded in the isolation and cloning of a wide array of receptors for just about every class of current drugs. In fact, success has been so great that we no longer speak of a solitary receptor for a given drug, but use such phrases as "receptor superfamily" and "receptor subtypes". For example, the receptor for the neurotransmitter dopamine as well as for certain psychotropic drugs interacting at the same cellular sites, is now a family of receptors containing five subtypes. Other receptor families have as many as seven or eight subtypes, and the lists keep growing.

CASCADE OF MEDIATORS IN ASTHMA

ALLERGEN
↓
RECEPTOR ON MAST CELL MEMBRANE
↓
HISTAMINE
↓
H-1 RECEPTOR ON BRONCHIOLAR SMOOTH MUSCLE
↓
CONTRACTION OF SMOOTH MUSCLE
↓
CONSTRICTION OF BRONCHIOLES
↓
WHEEZING, ETC.

Fig. 2. A classical, but outmoded view of the mechanisms involved in the development of an asthmatic attack.

Drug receptors are large protein molecules with sugars and other chemical moieties attached. Many are embedded within cell membranes, and some, such as the ionic channel receptors can even span the membrane, bringing the cell interior in contact with the extracellular environment. The biotechnology of cloning either a whole receptor, or a biologically active small sequence, has even allowed the recent isolation of so-called "orphan receptors" or receptors having similar, but not identical, molecular composition (homology) with a natural receptor. The orphan receptor interacts poorly with certain known drugs that interact with the natural receptor (like morphine for the opiate receptor), but has no known endogenous ligand, and may have effects that differ somewhat from the expected one. An example of an orphan receptor is an opiate receptor subtype, ORL_1 [opioid receptor-like], which recently has been isolated and cloned. Paradoxically, it appears to involve an hyperalgesic action instead of a pain-relieving (analgesic) effect. A peptide known as nociceptin or orphanin FQ has also recently been discovered, which may be an endogenous ligand for this receptor. When injected into laboratory animals, it causes an increase in pain response (pro-nociception) instead of an analgesic effect.[3] The role of this new receptor-ligand system on the body economy remains to be explored.

Drug receptors, thus, are the key to initiating a particular pharmacological action. The development of new, more specific and less toxic drugs is within reach as a consequence of the plethora of drug receptors uncovered by biotechnology.

CASCADE OF MEDIATORS IN ASTHMA

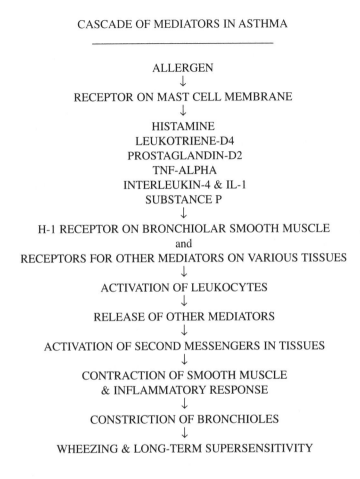

ALLERGEN
↓
RECEPTOR ON MAST CELL MEMBRANE
↓
HISTAMINE
LEUKOTRIENE-D4
PROSTAGLANDIN-D2
TNF-ALPHA
INTERLEUKIN-4 & IL-1
SUBSTANCE P
↓
H-1 RECEPTOR ON BRONCHIOLAR SMOOTH MUSCLE
and
RECEPTORS FOR OTHER MEDIATORS ON VARIOUS TISSUES
↓
ACTIVATION OF LEUKOCYTES
↓
RELEASE OF OTHER MEDIATORS
↓
ACTIVATION OF SECOND MESSENGERS IN TISSUES
↓
CONTRACTION OF SMOOTH MUSCLE
& INFLAMMATORY RESPONSE
↓
CONSTRICTION OF BRONCHIOLES
↓
WHEEZING & LONG-TERM SUPERSENSITIVITY

Fig. 3. A contemporary view of the pathophysiology of an asthmatic attack. The initial event invokes the sequential activation of a series of cytokines and second messengers that ultimately results in the symptoms and pathology of asthma.

Second Messengers and Receptors

The drug-receptor interaction, however, is only the first step leading to a pharmacological response. The interaction may actually generate a whole cascade of sequential intermediate steps before the drug-receptor interaction is translated into a cellular response. What is vital to the appreciation of impending explosion in new drug development is the fact that each step in the cascade also involves biologic entities, which themselves have receptors with unique specificities. The number of target sites for drug intervention is growing in an exponential fashion.

The pharmacotherapeutic management of asthma illustrates the involvement of multiple receptor-mediated steps. A classic, but simplistic view of the mechanism of asthma (**Fig. 2**) proposes that an allergen like pollen interacts with receptors on the cell membrane of mast cells found in lung tissue. The mast cells release the unbound and active form of histamine into the extracellular space where it interacts with the H1 subtype of the histamine receptor resident on the smooth muscle of the bronchioles, thereby causing a contraction of the muscles with consequent constriction of the bronchiole, and emergence of the wheezing symptoms of acute asthma. Treatment consists of using several different drugs: histamine antagonists (antihistaminics), which block histamine at the H1 receptor; a beta adrenergic receptor agonist such as albuterol to relax the muscle; or theophylline to blunt the strength of muscle contraction. The contemporary view of asthma is considerably more complex (**Fig. 3**). The allergen not only releases histamine, but also a number of other endogenous chemicals. Some of theses chemicals, called cytokines, interact with membrane receptors on certain white blood cells to cause them move into the area invaded by the pollen or other offending agent (chemotaxis). These leukocytes, in turn, release additional chemicals, which interact with their own unique receptors to cause further tissue damage and to invoke the inflammatory response. The initial allergen-mast cell interaction has now been amplified into many receptor-mediated interactions. The continual activation of this complex system may, over time, convert acute asthma into a chronic state. The number of sites for pharmacological intervention has now been greatly increased.

Once cell membrane-bound receptors are activated, a new set of intracellular chemicals with their own complement of receptors carry the message to the final biologic response. As of the moment, there are approximately two dozen steps in the cascade of "second messengers."

Drugs have been developed at the experimental stage that block at just about each of the receptor sites for the cytokines and the second messengers. Some are in clinical trial. For example, an Interleukin-1 receptor antagonist (Antril®; anakinra) to be used in asthma is in Phase I/II clinical trials.

Chiral Drugs or Right-Hand Left-Hand

Louis Pasteur, in 1848, with laborious and persistent effort examined pure crystals of racemic acid (tartaric acid) from grapes and discovered that the crystals existed in left- and right-handed forms. That is, they were mirror images of each other. In solution, the two forms imparted certain physical differences. This discovery opened the important field of stereochemistry and has profound importance to biology in general, and to pharmacology specifically. Many drugs also have left and right handed forms, and often only one form possesses the pharmacological effect. The term chiral (from the Greek word for "hand") is associated with drugs or chemicals having "handedness." In the manufacturing process chiral drugs usually exist as both forms in approximately 50-50 ratios. Since drug receptors almost always have a predilection for one form of "handed" drugs (antipode or enantiomorph), an aggressive line of research today involves the preparation of only the geometric form carrying the desired action. The bonuses derived from this manipulation are the enhancement of drug specificity and the elimination of undesirable effects. For example, in the pain-relieving drug propoxyphene (Darvon®), only the right-handed form has the analgesic action. But the left-handed form, while lacking significant analgesic action, does have cough-suppressing action. The latter's trade name is Novrad®, or Darvon® spelled backwards. Chiral technology for the selective synthesis of one or the other form of drugs is presently in a highly advanced state and is expected to generate significantly better drugs.

Gene Therapy

Molecular genetics has provided the means for entirely new concepts in drug design. As hinted above, we can go back to natural substances as models for new drugs. Genes and the products of genes offer virtually unlimited models for developing new drugs.

With the mention of "gene therapy," the first notion that comes to mind is the idea that genes can be introduced into a person's genetic code to either replace a vital missing gene, or to replace a defective gene with a competent copy. This technology is currently widely used in laboratory research using "transfected" cells or "transgenic" animals. Human investigations have also been started. There were seventeen drugs involving gene therapy in clinical trials in 1995.[4] Considerable publicity has been given to gene therapy for cystic fibrosis, a condition in which there is a defect in the gene controlling the biosynthesis of the receptor that modulates the movement of chloride ions across membranes in the respiratory tract and other organs. The cloned receptor, Cystic Fibrosis Transmembrane Conductance Regulator (CFTR), has been tried in early clinical studies with some success.[5]

There is, however, another aspect of gene therapy that is more readily amenable to pharmacological intervention. This has to do with the subject of gene control or gene regulation.

Briefly, the rationale is as follows (**Figs. 4 & 5**). Genes must be activated or "turned on" in order to "express" their genetic capacity. Gene activators generally are proteins. Some genes are already "turned off" by "repres-

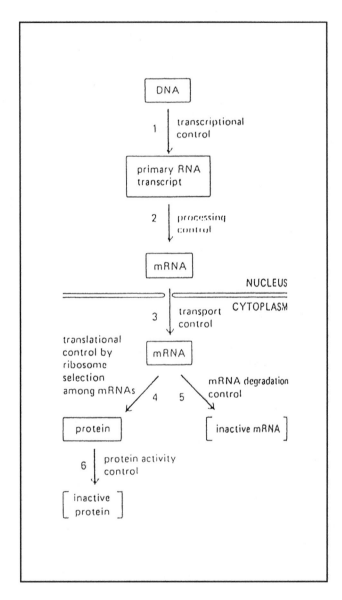

Fig. 4. Major steps in the mechanisms for gene expression showing sites for potential pharmacological intervention. (From Alberts, et al., "Control of gene expression," in Molecular Biology of the Cell, *3rd ed. (NY: Garland, 1994), 403.)*

PHARMACOLOGY AND GENE THERAPY

- BLOCK OF GENE ACTIVATION, OR REPRESSION

- BLOCK OR DISRUPT FORMATION OF GENE MESSAGE

- BLOCK MESSENGER TRANSPORT OUT OF NUCLEUS

- BLOCK DELIVERY OF THE GENE MESSAGE (ANTISENSE)

- BLOCK THE GENE PRODUCT (PROTEIN ANTAGONISTS)

Fig.5. Potential actions of drugs in modifying the mechanism of gene expression and products of gene expression.

sor" chemicals and must be de-repressed to be activated. An activated gene then expresses its function, which generally is to manufacture proteins. It accomplishes this by transcribing a coded message to messenger ribonucleic acid (mRNA). All this is carried out within the cell nucleus. The mRNA must then be actively transported out of the nucleus into the cytoplasm where machinery exist for making proteins. In the cytoplasm, the messenger delivers

ANTISENSE DRUGS IN CLINICAL TRIAL-1995

TRIAL PHASE	DRUG NAME	INTENDED USE	MANUFACTURER
Phase I	Isis 2302	Inflammatory diseases	Isis Pharm.
Phase I	LR-3001	Leukemia	Lynx Therap.
Phase II	Afovirsen	Genital warts	Isis Pharm.
Phase II	GEM 91	HIV & AIDS	Hybridon
Phase III	ISIS 2022	Cytomegalovirus	Isis Pharm.

Fig. 6. Five antisense drugs were in clinical trials in 1995.

the message to make a specific protein which is then transported out of the cell to its target tissue, or which may even act within the same cell to start another cycle of gene activation. Every step in this process involves highly selective receptors that are vulnerable to pharmacological attack. An example of this is offered by the use of antisense drugs.

Molecular biology technology has the ability to strip down the molecular structure of gene regulatory proteins into the smallest possible amino acid sequence. Once the truncated sequence is known, small nucleotides can be made that have a nucleotide sequence that is complementary to the essential sequence in mRNA or its precursors. These small nucleotides are called antisense oligonucleotides. They can combine with the complementary structure in the mRNA or precursor RNA transcripts to block the execution of the genetic message for making new proteins in the cytoplasm. Five antisense drugs were in clinical trials in 1995 (**Fig. 6**). The first antisense drug injected into humans was given to treat genital warts (Afovirsen). It had shown favorable properties against the causative virus in preclinical laboratory studies, and progressed to clinical studies up to Phase II. However, in December 1995, its manufacturer voluntarily withdrew the drug from further clinical investigation because patients would not accept the discomfort of the three injections per week that were required to attain clinical effectiveness.[6] A second antisense drug, also developed by the same company, is in the advanced stage of clinical testing (Phase III). The drug was developed to block the replication of Human Cytomegalovirus (HCMV), which causes devastating infections in immunocompromised patients where the mortality rate from pneumonia is up to forty percent. Moreover, about one percent of live births in the United States have congenital infections with this virus. Five to ten percent of these have severe neurological problems.[7]

A major problem confronting the pharmacological utilization of this technique is the difficulty of delivering the macromolecular antisense drugs and synthetic gene regulators to their targets deep in the cell interior. What pharmacologists have known for years is now being encountered by biotechnologists, namely, that macromolecules are notoriously difficult to deliver to their targets. However, significant progress is being made in the development of new drug delivery systems. (An informative article on the subject of gene therapy appeared recently in *Scientific American*.[8])

Drug Delivery Systems

A fundamental goal of pharmacological research is to improve the delivery of drugs to their target sites. Even contemporary drugs with their small molecular sizes can experience difficulties in reaching their sites of action. As an example, only ten percent of an oral dose of L-Dopa gets to the brain where it exerts its antiparkinson effects. The body has layers upon layers of biological barriers that impede the movement of drugs. Fortunately, a large amount of information exists for overcoming these barriers with chemical manipulations of the drug molecules. For example, drugs can be made less ionic or charged, which makes it easier to get through biologic membranes. Or, as in the case of L-Dopa mentioned above, its rapid metabolism by enzymes outside the brain can be prevented by the concomitant administration of an inhibitor of the enzyme (carbidopa). This expediency leads to a smaller dose requirement for L-Dopa, which reduces its adverse effects.

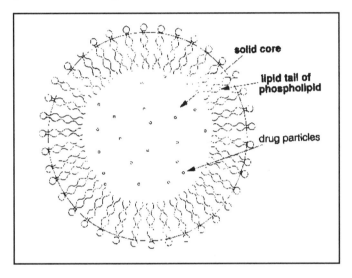

Fig. 7. An example of a liposome prepared to deliver a local anesthetic (bupivacaine) for extended action. This "liposphere" is microscopic in size, about 15 micra. (From Condouris and Green, "Local anesthetic action of bupivacaine-impregnated lipospheres," The Pharmacologist, *June 1993 (abstract).)*

With therapy using gene products, which are protein molecules hundreds of times larger than conventional drugs, the problems of drug delivery become formidable. But pharmacology and the pharmaceutical sciences have undertaken solutions to these problems. The question is how to get these massive molecules from the blood, for example, to the cytoplasm of cells, or deeper, into the nucleus.

One intriguing success story relates to an antisense oligonucleotide designed to inhibit the growth of human (KB) cultured cells by blocking the receptor for an essential growth factor, Epidermal Growth Factor (EGF). The

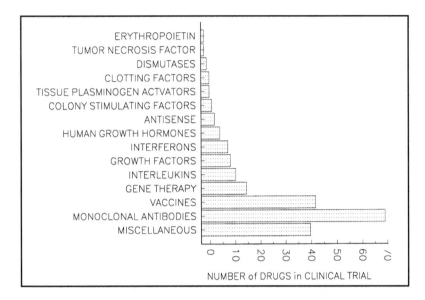

ERYTHROPOIETIN
TUMOR NECROSIS FACTOR
DISMUTASES
CLOTTING FACTORS
TISSUE PLASMINOGEN ACTVATORS
COLONY STIMULATING FACTORS
ANTISENSE
HUMAN GROWTH HORMONES
INTERFERONS
GROWTH FACTORS
INTERLEUKINS
GENE THERAPY
VACCINES
MONOCLONAL ANTIBODIES
MISCELLANEOUS

NUMBER of DRUGS in CLINICAL TRIAL

Fig. 8. Biotechnology medicines in development in 1995. (Adapted from Biotechnology Medicines in Development. 1995 Survey.*)*

antisense molecule, unfortunately, failed to penetrate the cell membrane. But the cells were tricked into gobbling up (endocytosis) the antisense drug that had been embedded within a liposphere whose outer coat was covered with the vitamin folic acid. (A diagram of one type of liposphere is shown in **Figure 7.**) Folic acid itself is actively pumped into the cell via a receptor-mediated process. The folic acid coat fools the cells into pumping the antisense-ladened liposheres through the cell membrane. Once at its site of action, the oligonucleotide was released, blocked the EGF receptor (EGRF), and successfully inhibited cell growth.[8]

Conclusion

The issues described in this overview represent only the tip of the iceberg. Important and far-reaching discoveries occur daily. The future of new therapeutics is bright. **Figure 8** shows the numbers of drugs derived from molecular genetics and molecular biology that were in clinical trials in 1995.[10]

There is a caveat that needs to be raised in the face of this enthusiasm. Many of the discoveries are made utilizing stripped down biological systems such as cells in culture. The story can change when these findings are examined in the whole subject, which possesses so many processes that resist external forces. The liver, kidney, and scores of enzymes are ready to counteract the changes. There are adverse effects that cannot be discerned from in vitro studies. This is where the crucial pharmacologic studies come in. The numbers of scientist being trained in traditional pharmacology is diminishing in favor of training in the more fundable areas of molecular biology and molecular genetics. This has the potential of causing a lag in the future development of these new and sophisticated drugs. The problem has been recognized and attempts at rectifying the situation have been started.

References

1. *Biotechnology Medicines in Development:. 1995 Survey* (Presented by the Pharmaceutical Research and Manufacturers of America, Washington, DC).
2. For a rewarding insight into Ehrlich's thought processes, see P. Ehrlich, "Address delivered at the dedication of the Georg-Speyer-Haus"(1906), in *Readings in Pharmacology* , ed. L. Shuster (Boston: Little, Brown and Co., 1962), pp. 233-43.
3. J. C. Meunier, C. Mollereau, L. Toll, C. Suaudeau, C. Moisand, P. Alvinerie, J. L. Butour, J. C. Guillemot, P. Ferrara, B. Monsarrat, H. Mazargull, G. Vassart, M. Parmentier, and J. Costentin, "Isolation and structure of the endogenous agonist of opioid-like ORL_1 receptor," *Nature* 377(1995): 532-35. R. K. Reinscheid, H. P.Nothacker, A. Bourson, A. Ardarti, R. A. Henningsen, J. R. Bunzow, D. K. Grandy, H. Langen, F. J. Monsma, Jr., and O. Civelli, "A neuropeptide that activates an opioid-like G protein-coupled receptor," *Science* 270(1995): 792-794.
4. *Biotechnology Medicines in Development* (n. 1).
5. J. Zabner, B. W. Ramsey, D. P. Meeker, M. L. Aitken, R. P. Balfour, R. L. Gibson, J. Launspach, R. A. Moscicki, S. M. Richards, T. A. Stanaert, J. Williams-Warren, S. C. Wadsworth, A. E. Smith, and M. J. Welsh, "Repeat administration of an adenovirus vector encoding Cystic Fibrosis Transmembrane Regulator to the nasal epithelium of patients with cystic fibrosis," *J. Clin. Invest.* 97, no. 6 (1996): 1504-11.
6. L. M. Fisher, "Isis drops human trials of a genetic drug," *New York Times*, December 29, 1995.
7. R. F. Azad, V. B. Driver, K. Tanaka, R. M. Crooke, and K. P. Anderson, "Antiviral activity of a phosphorothionate oligonucleotide complementary to RNA of the human cytomegalovirus major immediate-early region" *Antimicrobial Agents & Chemotherapy* 37, no. 9 (1993) : 1945-54.
8. "Special Report: Making gene therapy work," *Scientific American* 276, no. 6 (1997): 95-120.
9. S. Wang, R. J. Lee,G. Cauchon, D. G. Gorenstein, and P. S. Low, "Delivery of antisense oligodeoxyribonucleotides against the human epidermal growth factor receptor into cultured KB cells with liposomes conjugated to folate via polyethylene glycol" *Proc. Natl. Acad. Sci. USA* 92(1995): 3318-22.
10. *Biotechnology Medicines in Development* (n. 1)

Current and Future Trends in Medicinal Chemistry

by John A. Montgomery

T HE use of drugs for the treatment of human illnesses has roots in antiquity, when herbs and herbal concoctions were used therapeutically. For centuries, accidental discoveries and empirical observations provided the remedies used, and although the first correlation between structure and biological activity was announced in 1869 by Alexander Crum Brown and Thomas Fraser, it was almost ten years later that the concept of drug receptors was formulated by James Langley. Paul Ehrlich greatly clarified Langley's ideas. He coined the name "receptor" and defined it as a chemical group, normally active in a cell's metabolism, which, on combining with a drug, triggers the observed response. Emil Fischer developed the "lock and key" concept of enzyme specificity and A. R. Cushney proposed that the shape of a drug molecule can be crucial to its activity and that a part of the molecule must fit a structure complementary to it. Gradually, other ideas important to drug discovery began to emerge, such as the demonstration by A. J. Clark that the action of drugs on receptors quantitatively followed the Law of Mass Action, and findings by Edgar Stedman in 1929 that some receptors are actually enzymes, which eventually led to Donald Woods' concept of antimetabolites in 1940. Despite these slow (but very important) advances in our understanding of drug action, most drugs in use today were discovered more or less empirically. That is to say, lead compounds were found by screening a large number of synthetic chemicals or natural products for a desirable effect in some test system that might, or might not, be a good model for the human illness under study. This screening is inherently repetitious and time-consuming. Once an active (lead) compound has been identified, it is usually possible to improve on its activity or to reduce side effects by systematic molecular modifications.

The process of developing drugs by structural modification of a lead compound requires only that the structure of the compound be known. It is not necessary to know the structure of the target or even what the target is. As with screening, however, the process is primarily one of trial and error even though the probability of success is much greater than a purely random process and a number of approaches streamlining the process in many different ways have been developed.

Most illnesses affecting humans have been identified by their clinical manifestations, but modern biologic approaches, mostly based on molecular biology, have made it possible to study these illnesses at the molecular level and to identify the processes responsible for the clinical observations. Test systems can then be developed based on the underlying cause(s). This giant step forward resulted in the development of a number of drugs—such as captopril by Miguel Ondetti and David Cushman, and cimetidine by Robin Ganellin and Sir James Black—that have come to market in the last fifteen to twenty years. However, molecular modification was still done essentially blind, even though educated guesses—based, for example, on the mechanism of an enzymatic reaction—have been helpful.

Metabolism and Drug Design

A somewhat different approach led to the design of fludarabine phosphate, a new antileukemic agent. Fluorine is an interesting atom to introduce into a biologically active molecule since it is about the same size as the hydrogen it replaces but, being one of the most electronegative atoms, it can make a large change in the chemical properties of a molecule. For this reason,

John A. Montgomery retired as Senior Vice President of Southern Research Institute in February of 1990 and is now a Distinguished Scientist of the Kettering-Meyer Laboratory where for the past forty years, he has carried out research on drug discovery and development. He and his associates are responsible for the development of two new classes of anticancer agents—the nitrosoureas and the imidaxoletriazines. Two other anticancer agents, fludarabine and cladribine, were recently approved by the FDA for the treatment of human leukemia, while two others, clomesone and mitopterin, are in Phase II trials. He is also Executive Vice President and Director of Research of BioCryst Pharmaceuticals, Inc., a company devoted to structure-based drug design; a Senior Scientist in the Comprehensive Cancer Center, and Associate Director of the Center for AIDS Research, both at the University of Alabama at Birmingham. Dr. Montgomery has received numerous awards including the Herty Medal, the Southern Chemist Award, the T.O. Soine Award, the Cain Award, the Alfred Burger Award, the Madison Marshall Award, and the Smissman Bristol-Myers Squibb Award. He received a Distinguished Alumnus Award from the University of North Carolina and served eight years as a member of The President's Cancer Panel of the National Cancer Institute.

it was inserted into adenosine, an important nucleoside that is a component of nucleic acids. The resulting 2-fluoroadenosine was extremely toxic and a useful biologic probe. However, it was designed as an anticancer agent and yet it killed normal body cells and cancer cells equally well. Adenosine is normally rapidly converted to inosine in the body by an enzyme called adenosine deaminase. Cytarabine, a useful drug for the treatment of human leukemias, contained a different sugar from adenosine suggesting the synthesis of 2-fluoro-9-b-D-arabinofuranosyladenine (fludarabine). The corresponding adenine nucleoside, the antiviral agent vidarabine, is rapidly deaminated by adenosine deaminase and showed very little anticancer activity in experimental animal systems, unless it is protected from adenosine deaminase. Fludarabine, as predicted, was resistant to adenosine deaminase and cured animals with experimental leukemias. It is now widely used in the treatment of adult leukemias in humans. It was converted to the phosphate, a prodrug form, to increase its water solubility for human use. Relatives of fludarabine, such as cladribine, recently approved for the treatment of hairy cell leukemia, and CFDA, are also showing promise.

Structure-Based Drug Design

Little definitive information has been available on the three-dimensional structure of the receptor targets (which may be the active sites of enzymes). Two techniques have only recently provided this much-needed and long-sought-after information: X-ray crystallographic analysis and newer nuclear magnetic resonance (NMR) techniques. Both approaches have their limitation. Although molecular biology has for the most part provided pure proteins that are not readily available by isolation in sufficient quantities for crystallization, it is still not possible to crystallize all proteins. Membrane-bound receptors are a particular problem. NMR, on the other hand, does not provide the same precise information and has only been applied to relatively small proteins or polypeptides, but it does not require crystals and measurements in solution are possible. The use of NMR in conjunction with X-ray crystallography is a promising approach.

In any event, it is now possible to design potential drugs based on the three-dimensional structure of a receptor. A recent example is the development of potent inhibitors of purine nucleoside phosphorylase (PNP), an enzyme that catalyzes the cleavage of purine nucleosides to the purine base and a sugar phosphate. Interest in PNP arises from its critical role in purine nucleoside metabolism, which affects T, but not B, cell function. Children lacking PNP activity exhibit severe T cell immunodeficiency. Proliferating T cells have been implicated in the origin and development of various autoimmune diseases including rheumatoid arthritis, systemic lupus erthematosus, psoriasis, and type I diabetes. PNP inhibitors, which should shut down T cell proliferation, might be effective in the treatment of these diseases. Other uses for such a drug might be the treatment of T-cell leukemia and lymphomas, and the prevention of organ transplant rejection.

The three-dimensional structure of PNP, isolated from human blood, was determined by X-ray crystallographic analysis. The active site, where the enzyme catalyzes the reversible phosphorolysis of certain nucleosides was characterized from the binding of substrate analogues (enzyme inhibitors).

The iterative drug design scheme involved both conventional enzyme inhibition data and X-ray crystallographic analysis for evaluation of new inhibitors. A combination of these data with molecular modeling laid the foundation for the design of the next round of target molecules. Proposed structures were screened by modeling the enzyme-inhibitor complex using interactive computer graphics and AMBER-based molecular energetics. Monte Carlo/energy minimization techniques were used to sample space available to potential inhibitors docked in the active site. The results of these analyses led to proposed modification of existing compounds and to the identification of new target structures.

Crystallographic analyses and inhibition data led to the selection of 9-

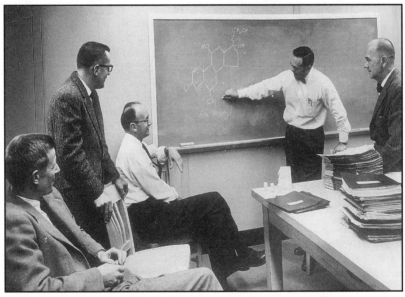

Structural modifications of chemical entities often yield new drugs. Here the members of the Upjohn Co. research team who developed a new corticosteriod, methylprednisolone, discuss its molecular configuration (c. 1960). (Courtesy Drug Topics Collection, American Institute of the History of Pharmacy.)

deazaguanine derivatives as candidate PNP inhibitors. The first 9-deazaguanine derivatives prepared were clearly more potent than the most potent known inhibitor. Further work led to the identification of several families of potent membrane-permeable inhibitors of PNP. From these compounds, 9-(3-pyridylmethyl)-9-deazaguanine (BCX-34, peldesine) was chosen for development. This drug is orally bioavailable, a potent inhibitor of human T cell proliferation, an effective PNP inhibitor in animals, and of low toxicity. Phase I/II clinical studies with peldesine have shown that a dermal formulation of the drug is safe and efficacious in the treatment of cutaneous T-cell lymphoma.

The design of potent PNP inhibitors by means of X-ray crystallographic analysis is one of several examples of the utility of this approach to the design of enzyme inhibitors. The success of early clinical trials indicates that it is also a useful approach to the discovery of new drugs. Other examples of the use of X-ray crystallography are the design of inhibitors of influenza neuraminidase, of HIV protease for the treatment of AIDS, inhibitors of thymidylate synthetase for cancer, and inhibitors of carbonic anhydrase for glaucoma. It is not unreasonable to suggest that serendipity, which has played a major role in drug discovery in the past, may be relegated to a minor role in the future.

Nuclear magnetic resonance (NMR) is the only other experimental technique that can provide structural details of proteins at atomic resolution. High quality crystals, which can be difficult to obtain, are not required and solution measurements can have some advantages. On the other hand, there are limitations on the size of the proteins that can be studied and the data obtained with NMR is not as precise as that which is possible with X-ray crystallography. The two approaches can provide complementary information.

A good example of the use of NMR is the study of the binding of cyclosporin, a clinically-used immunosuppressant, to one of its receptors, cyclophilin A. Using uniformly-labeled ^{13}C-cyclosporin A bound to cyclophilin, its conformation in the bound state was found to be very different from the conformation of the uncomplexed drug determined by X-ray crystallography and NMR. The NMR studies also revealed the portions of cyclosporin that interact with cyclophilin. The data are consistent with the structure-activity relationships that indicate the important cyclosporin residues for binding and immunosuppressant activity. Future developments are expected to improve the speed and accuracy in the determination of three-dimensional structures by NMR.

Combinatorial Chemistry

The search for new drugs or lead structures from natural sources— plants, marine organisms, and so forth—has been going on for many years, but the idea of the synthetic organic chemist purposefully creating a mixture of many organic molecules to identify a lead is a new one. It stems from the expense and time required to synthesize new compounds that are pure and well-characterized for screening against some biologic target, with the knowledge that the vast majority of these compounds will turn out to be worthless. In contrast, one can generate literally millions of compounds rapidly and very cheaply, but this approach requires a rapid and cheap screening technique, preferably automated, and depending on the approach, a way to identify and characterize a "hit"—a biologically-potent compound in these synthetic mixtures. The first libraries constructed were peptide and oligonucleotide libraries, which are relatively simple to design and prepare, even though most drugs on the market are small molecules. This is a rapidly-moving field in which new methods are being developed almost daily to prepare all kinds of small molecule libraries, to assure chemical diversity, to identify the library contents, and to speed up the whole process. It is as yet too early to critically evaluate the impact combinatorial chemistry will make on drug discovery, but clinical candidates are already forthcoming and enthusiasm is high.

Computational Chemistry

The use of computational chemistry in drug design had its beginning in the concept of quantitative structure-activity relationships (QSAR), which began with an equation published in 1868 relating physiological activity and chemical structure (Crum Brown and Fraser). Today, it embraces not only all the various approaches to improved equations relating biologic activity to structure (the ultimate goal of which is the accurate prediction of the tightness of binding of a drug to its receptor), but all the approaches to defining receptor active sites when they have not been determined by X-ray or NMR analysis, to fitting molecules into receptor sites, to designing molecules to fit receptor sites (whether or not the structures of the sites are known), to the development of programs to search databases, and to convert two-dimensional databases to the more useful three-dimensional databases; and, of course, all the computer-modeling programs. All these approaches are leading to the rational design of new drugs replacing systematic modification of a lead structure with the resulting reduction in time for, and cost of, producing a new drug. The importance of being first to the marketplace with a novel drug cannot be over-emphasized (from a drug company's point of view).

New Types of Drugs

Changes in the approaches to the development of new drugs described above have resulted in new types of molecules being developed as drugs.

However, these new types of drugs are also a result of the continual search for greater selectivity of drug action. The following new types of molecules have appeared in the last few years and at least one of them has been approved for use in humans.

Peptidomimetics

The great therapeutic potential of proteolytic enzyme inhibition, as demonstrated by captopril and related compounds, remains largely unfulfilled, primarily because peptidal inhibitors are hampered by their generally poor pharmacological properties such as low oral bioavailability, metabolic instability, and unfavorable pharmacokinetics. Many modifications of the normal peptide amide bond structure have been investigated leading to a new class of potential drugs called peptidomimetics. Two such inhibitors of HIV protease have recently received FDA approval for the treatment of AIDS in humans, although neither compound has ideal small molecule drug properties and both are expensive to manufacture. No doubt, improvements will result from continuing work on these and other protease inhibitors.

Oligonucleotides

At its most elementary level, rational drug design is a search for specificity, and specificity is the appeal of oligonucleotides, despite the difficulties they present. Simply put, oligonucleotides containing 11-15 units should be able to selectively bind to a single RNA species in a cell, preventing the synthesis of a single disease-related protein rather than inhibiting its action. The difficulties in the development of oligonucleotides as drugs are similar to those of peptides and peptidomimetics, although perhaps more severe. The myriad of potential applications of an effective drug with such specificity are too numerous to recount here, but the application to the many forms of cancer and to viral diseases, including AIDS, is particularly noteworthy.

Biological Response Modifiers

Even though a number of the new approaches to cancer treatment do not involve drugs in the usual sense of the word, some mention of these approaches should be made. Most of them are based in immunology. Examples are monoclonal antibodies, chimeric monoclonals, monoclonals attached to radioactive nuclides or toxins, interferons interleukins, interleukins used with tumor infiltrating lymphocytes (TIL) and with genetically-engineered TIL cells. All of this work seems to be pointing ultimately to the development of therapeutic vaccines.

Prodrugs for Gene Therapy

Gene therapy encompasses an extremely wide range of techniques and applications. It includes any technique to introduce DNA into cells for a therapeutic purpose. This discussion is confined to the gene therapy approaches to cancer treatment, which is an attempt to obtain greater selectivity—and therefore, less toxicity—than can be obtained with the currently-used anticancer drugs. Genes that sensitize cells to drugs that are normally non-toxic represent a new approach to selectivity. They are chosen to create artificial differences in sensitivity between normal and malignant cells. Most genes currently under investigation mediate sensitivity by encoding a viral or bacterial enzyme that metabolizes inactive forms of a drug ("prodrug") into a toxic antimetabolite capable of killing cells by inhibiting nucleic acid synthesis. Many techniques are under investigation for the introduction of these genes into neoplastic cells exclusively, a key to this approach.

One of the first genes studied was the herpes simplex thymidine kinase gene, followed by treatment with the antiherpes drug, ganciclovir. Ideally, ganciclovir is then converted to its toxic form only in cancer cells containing the herpes gene. This treatment has been demonstrated to work in rodent test systems and clinical trials are planned. Other examples of this technique are the use of bacterial cytosine deaminase followed by treatment with 5-fluorocytosine, an unctuous compound that is converted to the anticancer drug, 5-fluorouracil only in the target cells, and the bacterial gene for purine nucleoside phosphorylase that cleaves non-toxic purine nucleosides to their toxic purine bases in cells transfected with the enzyme.

Summary

Discoveries in recent years have changed the practice of medicinal chemistry dramatically. This is best illustrated by what may be the most active areas of drug discovery research in the world today: The search for effective inhibitors of HIV protease, an enzyme essential to replication of the AIDS virus. Most of the recently-developed techniques discussed in this review have been applied to this problem by a number of research groups. First, molecular biology was used to sequence the entire HIV genome and to express and characterize most of the viral proteins, eventually leading to the identification of the protease as a drug target. This work made it possible to produce enough enzyme for crystallization, which was necessary to determine the three-dimensional structure of the enzyme active site and the structure of complexes of over 200 inhibitors bound in the active site. All the powers of computational chemistry have been brought to bear, including searches of 3-D databases for lead compounds (high through-put screens have also been employed in the search for leads). Molecular modeling has been used extensively. This work exemplifies better than any other the modern approach to medicinal chemistry, and has led to the discovery of clinically-active agents, two of which have already been approved for human use by the FDA, in a relatively short time frame.

Small molecules will continue to play a very important role among drugs of the future. Structural biology based on information provided by X-ray crystallographic and NMR analyses, and aided by site-directed mutagenesis, is becoming the bedrock of the discovery of this type of drug. Molecular biology, essential to the small-molecule approach, will also continue to add macromolecules to the list of new therapeutics. One thing is clear: The development of new drugs is today, as never before, a team effort to be shared equally by medicinal chemists and biologists, molecular and otherwise. The "genius in the attic" is a thing of the past.

Suggested Readings

1. Burger's *Medicinal Chemistry and Drug Discovery*, fifth ed., vol. 1: Principles and Practice, Manfred E. Wolf, ed. (John Wiley and Sons, Inc., New York, NY).
2. Recent volumes of *Annual Reports in Medicinal Chemistry*, James A. Bristol, ed. (New York: Academic Press, Inc.).
3. Goodman and Gilman's *The Pharmacological Basis of Therapeutics*, ninth ed., J. G. Hardman, L. E. Limbird, P. B. Molinoff, R. W. Ruddon, and A. G. Gilman, eds. (New York: McGraw-Hill).

Recent Trends and the Future of Pharmaceutics

by George Zografi

T HE history of drug therapy in the nineteenth and twentieth centuries is most often thought of in the context of major drug discoveries, such as those of the alkaloids, antimicrobials, insulin, antipsychotics, and immunosuppressants. Indeed, central to the improvement of health care through drug therapy in the future will be the need to continue to uncover new chemical entities in a wide range of therapeutic areas such as infectious disease, cardiovascular disease, mental disorders, and cancer. A simplistic perception of the drug product development process might suggest that once a potentially useful drug is uncovered, it can merely be dissolved in water or mixed with inert ingredients into a "pill" and be administered to the patient. A recently observed example where such is often not the case is in the use of DNA recombinant technology to produce therapeutically active proteins. Dissolving proteins in a buffer and injecting them intravenously into patients would seem to be a simple process. However, very many proteins in aqueous solution denature and lose their potency during the period of manufacture, storage, and use without changing chemically. What steps are needed to overcome such problems? Who is trained to do this? In a broader perspective, because of such issues the process of drug product development, after drug discovery, and the approval of such products for distribution to the public for clinical use, generally involve a series of steps that can take years to complete. These include: biological safety assessment; development of chemical analytical procedures; characterization of physical properties of various materials; formulation into dosage forms, and optimization of large-scale manufacturing procedures. Central to the process of drug product development today also is the need to develop standards of chemical purity, biological safety, and therapeutic efficacy within a reasonable time period and in a cost-effective manner.

195

With this general picture in mind, we can define the discipline of pharmaceutics as that branch of the pharmaceutical sciences that is concerned with the development of dosage forms or drug delivery systems that insure proper therapeutic effects in a cost-effective manner. To reach such goals requires attention to at least four major issues: 1) reproducible manufacture at minimal cost; 2) the retention of physical and chemical stability of dosage form components during the entire period of manufacture and storage; 3) the provision of reproducible therapeutic performance through appropriate attention to temporal and spatial release of the drug (biopharmaceutics), as well as a proper understanding of the absorption and disposition of the drug after release (bioavailability and pharmacokinetics); and 4) assurance of proper patient acceptance, compliance, and convenience in the administration of the drug.

To accomplish such objectives today three components must be integrated into a pharmaceutical product: the active ingredients, the inactive ingredients (known as excipients) and the packaging. Excipients, although not therapeutically active themselves, play an important role in all of the factors listed above. They are included to facilitate the manufacturing process; to maintain chemical and physical stability including antimicrobial preservation; to optimize drug release and therapeutic efficacy; and to proved aesthetic qualities and patient convenience. Often, however, the use of excipients for one function can present other problems. Let us consider, for example, the excipient magnesium stearate, used as a lubricant in tablet formulation because of its fat-like qualities and poor adhesion properties. In relatively small amounts, it tends to cover the powders and granules that will be used to form tablets by compaction under high pressures. By coating the powders and the steel punches and dies used in tableting, magnesium stearate reduces adhesion to the punches and dies and prevents "sticking" of the tablet so that it remains intact upon completion of the compaction process. However, the presence of this somewhat fat-like material that prevents adhesion also can impart to the system a tendency to prevent aqueous fluids from penetrating the tablet after administration, in essence, acting like a waterproofing agent, resulting in reduced disintegration time and reduced release rate of the drug. In the case of a chemically unstable drug like aspirin, the presence of magnesium stearate also has been shown to promote chemical degradation. Hence, the choice of excipients becomes a problem of balancing desired functionality with un-

George Zografi is Professor of Pharmaceutics at the University of Wisconsin-Madison. Since receiving his B.S. in pharmacy from Columbia University in 1956 and Ph.D. in pharmaceutics from the University of Michigan in 1960, he has been a member of the faculties of Columbia, Michigan, and Wisconsin. In 1975-1980 he served as dean of the University of Wisconsin-Madison, School of Pharmacy.

desired incompatibilities.

Packaging, too, presents interesting challenges to the drug product development process. Typically, a package is merely used to contain the product so as to make handling of the drug convenient, while also protecting it against adverse environmental conditions, such as relative humidity, oxygen, or light. In other cases, packaging is designed to deliver the drug accurately and conveniently, as in the case of ocular drug delivery (eye drops), intravenous injection (syringes), or pulmonary delivery (oral metered dose inhalers). In such cases, the package is an integral part of the entire drug delivery system with a significant effect on therapeutic efficacy. In many cases, however, packaging materials, such as glass, polymers, or rubber can interact with drugs to render the product ineffective or even toxic. Consequently, we can conclude that the field of pharmaceutics exists to ensure that rational drug product development occurs from the moment the drug itself is prepared to the point at which it is administered to the patient. It requires individuals, therefore, strong in the physical and chemical sciences but also aware of the complexities associated with drug absorption and disposition *in vivo*.

Recent Trends in Pharmaceutics

Any assessment of the research and technological issues currently being addressed in the area of pharmaceutics can be divided into two major components: the need for continued improvement of conventional or traditional dosage forms, and the need to develop new concepts in drug delivery and drug delivery systems. Conventional dosage forms typically have been designed to provide immediate release of a dose of drug for either systemic or local effect. Conventional dosage forms include: oral solids, such as capsules and tablets; oral liquids, such as syrups and elixirs; sterile solutions or suspensions, such as with injectables or ophthalmic preparations; and topical products administered to the skin, nose, lung, rectum, or vagina. The major challenge with such dosage forms is to be able to manufacture them reproducibly with optimal stability and therapeutic effect. This is particularly important today as the pharmaceutical industry faces greater pressures to reduce the overall time for drug product development and approval, while still insuring high quality. For this purpose, those working in the pharmaceutics area continue to be very concerned with technological issues such as new chemical and physical forms of drugs, new excipients, more sophisticated packaging, and more economical methods of manufacturing and quality control.

For the past twenty-five years, it has become increasingly recognized that superior control of how drugs are delivered to the patient can greatly improve drug therapy through better patient compliance and a reduction in biological side effect. In this time there has been an enormous effort made in the pharmaceutics field to develop new concepts in drug delivery, going beyond the conventional dosage forms discussed above. Although there have been some notable successes, expectations have often exceeded final results. Such concepts of controlled drug delivery can be divided into three groups with increasingly greater complexity. In the first and simplest approach, dosage forms are designed along conventional lines, but with materials that allow for a slow release of one dose of the drug over a period of hours to years. This can be in the form of tablets or capsules that release the drug in the gastrointestinal tract over a period of twelve to twenty-four hours, intramuscular injections, or transdermal patches that can provide drug release over days and weeks, and polymeric implants that can provide release over a period of years, as in the case of the Norplant contraceptive. Such products are now on the market and continue to be developed with increasing control built in.

In the second approach to drug delivery, the dosage form is designed to be administered by injection and to be directed to specific organs and cells, e.g., heart, brain, or kidney. We may think of this as "spatial" drug delivery to very specific locations, just as one might expect from the proverbial "magic bullet." Here scientists attempt to define the properties of diseased tissues or cells that might be specifically attractive to the drug delivery system. For example, one can develop an antibody for a particular cancer cell line and attach this antibody to the surface of the drug delivery system or directly to the drug. Besides finding such antigen-antibody combinations, the greatest challenge currently facing scientists in pharmaceutics is the ability to attach the antibody and to maintain its stability during processing. Such "site-specific" targeting of drugs would appear to be of particular importance in the future treatment of cancer, AIDS, and in the growing area of gene therapy wherein genetic material is delivered into the nucleus of specific cells for the purpose of treating various genetic diseases.

In the third approach to controlled drug delivery, we can design a delivery system that is temporally controlled so as to deliver drug only when needed. Thus for example, when pain, infection, or inflammation are most severe, a given amount of drug release would occur as a response to the intensity of the disease. The triggering mechanism might be tied to a change in pH or to the local concentration of certain molecules associated with the disease, i.e., enzymes associated with inflammation. In the case of diabetes, a sensor placed in the body might be able to respond to elevated glucose levels and trigger the release of insulin from a reservoir. Indeed, such devices are now in well advanced stages of development.

Summary

The field of pharmaceutics has and will continue to play and important role in the drug development process. During the past forty years, remarkable improvement in the design of cost-effective, stable, and therapeutically active drug delivery systems have come about by the linking of basic sciences and technology through academic and industrial research. By continuing to work towards the development of more sophisticated spatial and temporal drug delivery systems described above, pharmaceutics is well-positioned to make major contributions to significant health care needs in areas such as cancer, AIDS, gene therapy, etc. Because of the importance of drug delivery and the significant problems to be overcome, pharmaceutics will have to continue to attract scientists that are creative and energetic, along with the necessary investment of financial support. Traditionally, the large pharmaceutical companies have devoted extensive resources to new research and development in pharmaceutics through the establishment of programs within the company and support of academic research. In recent years, however, there is clearly a trend toward a reduced direct involvement of these companies in such research and toward an increasing number of smaller companies devoted entirely to various aspects of drug delivery. Such changes appear related to the increasing global competition among larger companies and a greater attention to shortening the drug development process with reduced costs. Thus, it would appear to me that the major advances in drug delivery in the future through basic research and development will come from more highly specialized laboratories, and even academia, leaving the larger global companies as the sources of new drug entities for these systems, as well as the vehicle for large-scale manufacturing, marketing, and product distribution. In the beginning of the next century, I anticipate that it will be possible to enhance the systemic absorption of large molecules, such as proteins and DNA. We also will have made greater progress toward more sophisticated and cost-effective spatial and temporal drug delivery systems. Meanwhile, in the short term, the bulk of pharmaceutical scientists working in pharmaceutics will continue to develop conventional dosage forms of high quality, decreased cost, and optimal therapeutic effects by improving processing methods as well as through the use of new and more effective excipients and packaging making up the total dosage form.

Clinical Trials: New Developments and Old Problems

by Mark Parascandola

T HE story of the clinical trial as we know it typically begins with British medical statistician Sir Austin Bradford Hill (1897-1991). In 1946 Hill designed a "rigorously planned investigation with concurrent controls" for the United Kingdom Medical Research Council to evaluate streptomycin as a treatment for pulmonary tuberculosis. The trial, results of which were published in 1948 in the *British Medical Journal*,[1] has been recognized as the first randomized double-blind controlled clinical trial and acted as a model for subsequent trial design. Hill's *Principles of Medical Statistics*,[2] first appearing as a series of articles in *The Lancet* in early 1937, had previously discussed the potential value of and theory behind such an experimental design. Having statisticians work alongside physicians in carrying out experiments was still a new and not fully accepted practice at the time, but it has since become routine.

The randomized controlled clinical trial has become the "gold standard" for testing new medicines for safety and efficacy. The development of standards for experimental design was given impetus from the vast growth of the pharmaceutical industry and the introduction of new classes of medicines in this century. Drug related disasters provided further pressure for formal regulation. The Kefauver-Harris Amendments of 1962, in response to the Thalidomide disaster, required more extensive information from drug manufacturers about precautions and side effects, as well as requiring proof of efficacy. Evidence from "adequate and well-controlled clinical investigations" is now required by the Food and Drug Administration for new drug approval.[3] The establishment of the discipline of clinical pharmacology also played an important role in the development and promotion of clinical trial methodology, and Harry Gold, "the father of clinical pharmacology," was a powerful early advocate of carefully controlled blinded trials in the United States.[4]

However, the identifying features of the modern clinical trial have not gone unchallenged or remained unaltered. While the basic structure appearing in the streptomycin trial remains, both in scientific theory and in regulatory practice, new developments have helped it to evolve. I will address some challenges raised against central elements of the modern clinical trial. While I conclude that these arguments ultimately fail, they prompt clarification of the goals and limitations of the clinical trial. Much of the recent history of clinical experimentation initially appears to indicate a progressive dismantling of Hill's model trial, but I will argue that the central elements present in that trial continue to guide theory and practice. I will discuss in turn control, randomization, and blinding, and will conclude with a more general discussion of the empirical status of the clinical trial.

Control

A controlled trial is one in which the experimental medicine is compared against another treatment or the absence of treatment. Such comparative experimentation is not a recent development. In 1747 aboard the H.M.S. *Salisbury* British navy surgeon James Lind divided sailors suffering from scurvy into several groups; those given fruits were cured within days, while those given other traditional medicines showed no improvement. In contemporary controlled trials patients are typically divided into two groups, one is given the experimental medicine and the other either a standard treatment, a placebo (a supposedly inactive treatment, such as a sugar tablet), or no treatment at all. The former is referred to as the experimental group and the latter as the control group.

The reason for comparing treatments is that investigators want to know more than just whether the patients get better; they want to know whether they get better *because* of the experimental drug. A cause is something that makes a difference; hence, one can make inferences about causes from observing differences in outcomes. If it is the drug that *causes* patients to re-

Mark Parascandola holds an M.Phil. in History and Philosophy of Science, and a Ph.D. in Philosophy from Cambridge University, UK. He is currently the DeWitt Stetten, Jr., Memorial Fellow in the History of Twentieth-Century Biomedical Research and Technology at the National Institutes of Health, and has worked as a Research Associate with the *Medicines: The Inside Story* project. His research interests are focused on the philosophy and methodology of biomedical research.

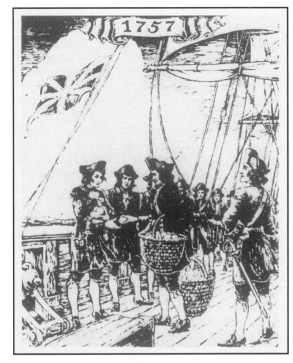

British navy surgeon James Lind hands out oranges to sailors aboard the H. M. S. Salisbury. In an early comparative trial, Lind divided sailors suffering from scurvy into several groups and gave each group a different treatment.

cover from the disease, then it is likely that there will be more patients in the group that received the experimental drug who recover.

However, there may be other differences between the two groups that account for the differences in recovery rates. Suppose the control group has an unusually large percentage of regular smokers and that the experimental group has none. Suppose also that smoking aggravates the condition being investigated; it might be the case that those in the control group fail to recover because of their smoking, and not because they are lacking the experimental drug. Smokers must be distributed equally so that such relevant factors are balanced between the groups. Researchers ultimately want two groups identical in all relevant respects, excepting the difference in treatment being studied.[5]

Use of controls is considered to be an essential element in modern trial design, but this use has not been free of controversy. Some researchers have argued that while efforts should be made wherever possible to achieve adequate controls in medical experiments, in some situations this may be unacceptable for ethical reasons. The World Medical Association Declaration of Helsinki, first adopted in 1964 and based on the earlier Nuremberg Code, sets out basic standards for ethical conduct in experiments using human subjects. The Declaration states that "[c]oncern for the interests of the subject must always prevail over the interest of science and society."[6] However valuable the results of a particular experiment might be for human health, the argument goes, individuals should not be used as mere means to that end. Hence, in medical studies is it is unethical to withhold treatment from those who need it or to knowingly give an inferior treatment.

The use of placebo controls in particular has generated substantial debate. It is unethical to leave some patients without treatment for the purposes of experimental design when a known effective treatment exists.[7] However, in cases of scientific uncertainty, which are many, ethical decisions are not so easy. Those appealing to the Declaration have noted that its wording leaves little room for interpretation.[8] However, others have responded that this very lack of flexibility is reason for rejecting the Declaration, developed in the wake of Nazi atrocities, as a set of necessary requirements for ethical clinical experiments.[9]

Sometimes information that the experimental treatment is more effective or safer becomes clear during the course of a trial, and a data monitoring committee may (using so-called "stopping rules") halt the trial so that both groups can receive the better treatment. A trial may also be halted if harmful side effects are discovered.[10] This move away from rigid experimental design is a recent development, largely in response to pressure for cures for rapid life-threatening diseases such as AIDS. A trial of AZT for AIDS, started in February of 1986, was prematurely terminated in September of that year when substantial improvements were seen in the experimental group, allowing all trial participants to receive the drug. At the time the drug was available only to trial participants in the experimental group, and no other effective therapy existed. The following year AIDS activist groups, such as Act Up, increased pressure for greater access to therapies still in the early testing stages. The result has been more inclusive trial designs and an increase in "compassionate use," allowing patients with serious debilitating conditions greater access to experimental therapies.[11]

Randomization

A randomized trial is one where patients are randomly allocated to either an experimental or control therapy. This differs, say, from distributing patients based on their occupation or placing all female patients in the control group. Those non-randomized methods of allocation can lead to clumping of patients with certain characteristics into one of the two groups, possibly distorting results. The aim of randomization is to reduce bias in allocation so that groups are balanced with regard to relevant factors. While some basic factors, such as age or sex, may be easily monitored for control, there are innumerable potentially relevant differences between patients that go unacknowledged in experimental practice. Because of the complexity of biological organisms it is not possible to formally control for every potentially relevant variable. By giving each individual an equal chance of being assigned to a particular group, randomization helps to equally distribute relevant factors between the groups. However, for the technique to be effective, the groups must be large enough that the chance of unbalanced distribution is very low; it is often stated that a trial must have at least 200 participants for randomization to be effective.[12]

British statistician Sir Ronald Aylmer Fisher (1890-1960) is generally credited with being the first to advocate the use of randomization in experiments. Fisher applied randomization to agricultural experiments at the Rothamsted Experimental Station in England from 1923, and, more influentially, advocated the practice in his *The Design of Experiments*, first published in 1935.[13] Bradford Hill also discussed randomization in his 1937 book. But randomization was not so readily accepted by the majority of experimenters and statisticians,[14] and it was somewhat later before the practice was introduced into experimental design in clinical medicine. In 1948 British medical statistician Major Greenwood (1880-1949) wrote that Fisher's ideas were "applicable far beyond the bounds of soil research."[15] In that same year the report of Hill's streptomycin trial was published, the first to allocate patients to experimental and control groups using random sampling numbers.[16] The report stated that "[d]etermination of whether a patient would be treated by streptomycin and bed-rest (S case) or by bed-rest alone (C case) was made by reference to a statistical series based on random sampling numbers drawn up for each sex at each center by Professor Bradford Hill."[17]

Arguments provided by early advocates of randomization were far more optimistic than what most investigators currently believe. Fisher wrote that "the simple precaution of randomisation will suffice to guarantee the validity of the test of significance, by which the result of the experiment is to be judged."[18] Fisher claimed randomization would *guarantee* the statistical inference through ensuring comparable groups. This, however, is unrealistic, as there are types of differences that randomization cannot control for, such as differences correlated with treatment. Suppose some contingent part of the handling process the experimental medication has gone through affects how it works inside the patient—for instance, maybe it was stored near a source of radioactivity. Here the effect is correlated with the treatment, even though it is not caused by the substance under study. Conclusions drawn about the substance itself will be misleading, as they will not apply to samples of the same medication that went through a different handling process. There may be countless other such differences correlated with a particular treatment, though many will not make plausible confounders; for example, suppose that there are different physicians for the two groups, and the color of the attending physician's eyes is relevant to the effects of the medicine. Such factors, of course, can be safely ignored as irrelevant in most cases, but in doing so trial organizers must use judgment based on current medical knowledge, rather than relying on theoretical guarantees.

In the 1970s, Bayesian statisticians began to question the use of randomization in clinical research, arguing that it is not essential for a well-designed trial and that it can sometimes even be harmful.[19] Most Bayesians believe that probabilities are always merely measures of subjective degrees of belief, and that in making inferences based on statistical data from a trial investigators must also take into account their prior personal and theoretical beliefs.[20] Bayesians remain in the minority, and randomization has become standard. As Ian Hacking has noted, "the broad mass of routine empirical experimenters take randomized design for granted and suppose that their employers would fire them if they did not."[21] However, some groups have linked their methodological arguments to ethical and policy issues, and have thereby gained increasing visibility.

Bayesian statisticians have noted that individual judgment must be used to determine which factors must be randomized and which can be safely ignored, exposing, in Colin Howson and Peter Urbach's words, "yet another essentially personal element in what purports to be a purely objective account of scientific inference."[22] Such judgment precludes the need for actual randomization, because once a factor has been recognized as relevant to the outcome it can be controlled for. Since Fisher, the most important selling point of randomized experimental design has been the objective measure of effectiveness it supposedly provides, a radical improvement over earlier reliance on the subjective judgments of individual physicians. The Bayesian arguments appear to throw this vision into doubt, but I will maintain that their rationale for rejecting randomization ultimately fails.

Randomization is not, it is clear, the universal guarantee of inference that Fisher claimed it was, but it is, most researchers maintain, necessary for achieving the most reliable experimental design. David Byar and colleagues, writing in 1976, responded to early criticism of randomization. "Although randomization does not ensure that the treatment groups are 'comparable' for all factors that may affect prognosis, the validity of significance levels based on randomization does not require this unachievable assumption."[23] Randomization significantly increases the *probability* of having balanced groups by controlling for innumerable potential confounders. Current advocates of randomization defend it not as a guarantee of inference, but as insurance in the long run against substantial accidental bias.[24] Moreover, admitting a role for judgment based on prior theoretical beliefs does not invalidate the benefits of the clinical trial, as I will argue in the concluding section.

The most persuasive arguments against randomization are ethical and policy-oriented rather than methodological; these arguments show that randomization is sometimes undesirable in practice. A physician has a special responsibility to the particular patient, and this responsibility precedes any interest in knowledge gained from research. However informative an experiment might be, it ought not be performed at the expense of human individuals. Hence, the "uncertainty principle;" a physician will only recommend a patient for participation in a randomized trial if she is uncertain about which treatment would be better for the patient's health, or if the relative value of a treatment is in dispute.[25] But if she is convinced that either the experimental or control treatment is significantly better for that patient, it is unethical to recommend randomized assignment. Because of this and similar concerns, requiring randomization across the board without room for exceptions is problematic.

Randomization remains desirable, both ethically and methodologically, in many situations. For many experimental therapies it is not clear what the better treatment is for some individual. With new diseases for which there is no effective cure, such as AIDS, there is frequently significant scientific uncertainty. And bad experimental design may also be unethical, as there is no reason to perform an experiment at all if it will not provide reliable information. An advocate of extensive use of randomization might also cite the Declaration of Helsinki in their defense in response to ethical criticism, as it requires that "[b]iomedical research involving human subjects must conform to generally accepted scientific principles."

However, it is important to recognize that a study is not wholly invalidated if not randomized; randomization is necessary to achieve the most reliable design possible, but it is not necessary for a more modest level of reliability. Since 1988 regulatory authorities have taken a more flexible view of trial design, especially in dealing with promising treatments for life-threatening diseases. Patients are also allowed more choices and a greater level of participation in their treatment, with the result that randomization is not always strictly required.[26]

Blinding

In a blinded trial participants do not know which group, experimental or control, any particular patient has been assigned to. This information is only revealed during the trial if a patient develops harmful symptoms. In Hill's streptomycin trial researchers diagnosed patients without knowing which group they were in; "[t]he films have been viewed by two radiologists and a clinician, each reading the films independently and not knowing if the films were of [control] or [experimental] cases."[27] Experimental and control medicines may be made to look identical, distinguished only by a coded number revealed after the trial is over, so that neither the patient nor the researcher can discover which is being given in any particular case. In clarifying its requirement for "adequate and well-controlled clinical investigations" in 1970 the FDA specified the need "[t]o perform studies blind whenever feasible, as a means of avoiding patient and physician response bias and selection bias."[28]

Blinding is employed to prevent forms of bias that cannot be eliminated through randomization or explicit controls. Suppose a clinician favors the experimental therapy; she may unknowingly record observations or make judgments in a way that supports that therapy. Such effects may be very subtle and may go unnoticed even by a conscientious trial participant. Patients may also report their symptoms to favor a specific therapy, and they may actually "feel" better if they are aware that they are receiving the therapy they favor. Blinding is the only means for reducing these forms of bias. However, as with other forms of bias protection, blinding is never foolproof in practice. Participants may break the code or find other ways to distinguish between the different therapies. For this reason the success of blinding procedures may be checked during the trial. For example, patients may be asked which treatment they *believe* they are receiving; if the distribution of answers given differs greatly between the two groups then it is likely that the blinding procedure has failed.

There are three levels of blinding: single-blind, double-blind, and triple-blind. In a single-blind study patients are not informed which group they are in, but researchers are. In a double-blind study neither patients nor researchers know which patients are in which group, assisting in more accurate reporting of results by researchers who may be unknowingly biased. In a triple-blind study statisticians analyzing initial results also do not know which group is the experimental and which the control; the trial is unblinded only in the final stages of analysis. Triple-blinding helps prevent possible bias of epidemiologists and statisticians from distorting the conclusions.

The success of blinded trials is one element of clinical trial design that has been called into question within debates over the strength of evidence for the efficacy of homeopathic remedies. Homeopaths work with micro-doses of substances that have been through many stages of dilution; sometimes the end product is so diluted that investigators can be certain that not a single molecule of the active ingredient is left in the solution. A century ago homeopaths argued that conventional testing methods were not applicable to their therapies, but recently advocates of alternative medicines have increasingly pushed for the use of double-blind placebo controlled studies to validate their treatments. Since 1980 reports of several such trials, which previously would have appeared only in homeopathic publications, have appeared in mainstream medical journals, mainly British.[29] These studies, and their places of publication, have generated significant debate. Conclusions from these trials remain weak at best, but the debates surrounding them are revealing of attitudes towards contemporary clinical trial design.

Those who rejected the conclusions of studies favoring homeopathic treatments blamed bias in statistical analysis for these "unbelievable" results. One commentator, in a 1993 letter to *The Lancet* commenting on a review study by a Dutch group, asked "I wonder how often we are presented with only the lowest of several possible p values in medical research articles? Probably this happens most of the time, when the choice favors the innovation."[30] The implication here is that double blinding is not sufficient, especially in testing such controversial claims. Hence, statistical analysis should, as far as possible, be carried out blinded, though this also is no guarantee.

In 1994 David Reilly and colleagues in Glasgow published the results of a study designed to test the reproducibility of earlier results, which they claimed provided support for the effectiveness of a homeopathic therapy for asthma. They offered a dilemma; either we are forced to accept that there is reproducible evidence in favor of homeopathic therapies or "we must ask if the technique of randomised controlled clinical trials is fundamentally flawed, and capable of producing evidence for effects that do not exist . . . To question the tool which has built most of today's pharmacological practice is no less perplexing than asking whether homeopathic treatments are active."[31] They suggested, rhetorically, that the clinician's expectation of outcome might be transmitted by "subtle effects that circumvent even double blinding." In this case the statistical analysis was not challenged, so that any bias present must act in spite of double blinding. Blinding, of course, is not foolproof in practice, and there are, as discussed above, sources of bias that cannot be controlled for. Yet, this admission is no reason for abandoning the clinical trial as an effective, indeed the most effective, means of evaluating medical therapies. I will take up Reilly and colleagues' challenge as a way into discussing some broader epistemic concerns about clinical trials in the final section.

Theory and Experiment

Reilly and colleagues offer the option of accepting the capacity of the clinical trial to produce false positives, results favoring a hypothesis that is false. Yet we have *already* admitted this much. In practice randomization does not guarantee that the experimental and control groups are balanced in all relevant ways, and blinding is not foolproof. There are no guarantees in the empirical sciences, particularly in the biomedical sciences where the complexity of organisms and their environment provides countless potential confounding variables and other sources of bias.

The interpretation of experimental data throughout the empirical sciences requires the use of judgment based on theory and previous experience. In this much the Bayesians are right. For example, informal guidelines for causal inference in epidemiology recommend that conclusions be "biologically reasonable;"[32] even if a correlation is observed between, for example, patient recovery and attending physician's eye color, the inference to a direct causal relationship would be highly implausible. However, the Bayesians also cannot provide any guarantee of balanced treatment groups, relying solely on personal judgment based on limited knowledge to say which factors can be ignored and which must be controlled for. Moreover, they offer no viable alternative to randomization for avoiding hidden confounders. Bayesians urge us to make use of our prior theoretical beliefs because of our weak epistemic situation, but if our position is such then we ought to make use of *all* the tools we have, including randomization.

The worries raised by the Bayesians are merely the old "induction problem." The problem is that regardless of how many experiments are run, there is always some possibility that an important part of the story is missing, that not all relevant variables have been controlled for. Unique features of the experimental apparatus or local factors in the laboratory or clinic may be responsible for the observed phenomena, as numerous studies in the history and philosophy of science have shown in recent years.[33] However, these are worries for all of the biological sciences, and indeed for all of empirical science, and to use such skeptical claims against the randomized clinical trial in particular is unjustifiable.

Philosopher of science Karl Popper's anti-inductivist program has had an unhealthy influence on methodological thinking in the life sciences, and some investigators have explicitly argued against randomized clinical trials through worries about inductive inference. Debate in Germany in the 1980s over ethical and legal implications of controlled trials provides one such example; one team asserted that "[s]cientific conclusions that go beyond the trial groups are in fact inductive, and as such scientifically untenable, as is generally agreed—at least in Germany—on the basis of Popper's theory of knowledge. In particular, it is not possible to use induction or statistical inference to conclude from the findings of a trial as to which is the best possible treatment for a particular new patient."[34] Yet, clearly, every time a physician prescribes a medicine for a child she uses induction, inferring from past observations of safety and efficacy that the medicine will be safe and effective for this particular child. Giving up induction would leave us not only without scientific research, but without health care either.

So what sorts of judgments are investigators warranted in making based on data from clinical trials? Is it fair to require understanding of a mechanism of action before making a causal inference? Reilly and colleagues stated that "asking 'how?' before asking 'if?' is a bad basis for good science when dealing empirically with things that may as yet evade explanation."[35] The mechanism by which smoking causes cancer is still poorly understood, but it is a paradigm instance of a good causal inference. Yet an editorial in *Nature,* replying to "those of supernatural inclinations" who would accept the claims of homeopathy, maintained that "[t]he principle of restraint which applies is simply that, when an unexpected observation requires that a substantial part of our intellectual heritage should be thrown away, it is prudent to ask more carefully than usual whether the observation may be incorrect."[36]

What is needed is a balance between theory and evidence. It is right that evidential standards should differ relative to their context. We accept the tobacco and cancer link not only because there is such a vast quantity of clinical evidence, but also because it is consistent with current biological theory. The evidence for homeopathic therapies, however, remains weak and is strongly in conflict with fundamental theory. But to cling too tightly to theory is not good science either. The value of the tools of conventional modern science, such as the clinical trial, is that they are not inherently tied to any *particular* theory.[37] It is this potential for radical revision that distinguishes conventional science from the rigid, dogmatic approach of homeopathy and other "alternative" systems. This flexibility is what continues to make the clinical trial a valuable tool.

While the essential structure of the randomized clinical trial remains, in recent years, a more flexible approach has been taken towards trial design itself, especially in the regulatory context. There are limits, both ethical and methodological, to strict trial design, but these limits are not practical liabilities. The move to more flexible experimental design is not a move away from the randomized double-blind clinical trial, but simply part of its evolution as a tool for medical research. It remains the best tool we have for evaluating new medicines, and its fundamental structure will remain a model for good experimental design into the future.

Notes and References

1. "Streptomycin treatment of pulmonary tuberculosis: A medical research council investigation," *British Medical Journal*, October 30, 1948, pp. 769-782. See also Hill's personal account in his "Memories of the British streptomycin trial in tuberculosis: The first randomized clinical trial," *Controlled Clinical Trials*, 11(1990):77-79.
2. *Principles of Medical Statistics* (London: The Lancet Ltd., 1937).
3. The May 8, 1970 Federal Register Statement (21 CFR 314.111) provides several criteria for determining whether this requirement has been met. See also *General Considerations for the Clinical Evaluation of Drugs* (Washington, DC.: Food and Drug Administration, 1977).
4. Duncan E. Hutcheon, "Harry Gold, M.D., F.C.P., 1889-1972," *The Journal of Clinical Pharmacology* 12(1972):303-305; Walter F. Riker, Jr., "Harry Gold: December 25, 1899 - April 21, 1972," *The Pharmacologist* 14(1972):104-105; Harry Gold, "Clinical pharmacology— Historical note," *The Journal of Clinical Pharmacology*, 7(1967):309-311. For a comprehensive historical account of the introduction of clinical trials in the United States, see Harry M. Marks, *The Progress of Experiment: Science and Therapeutic Reform in the United States, 1900-1990* (New York: Cambridge University Press, 1997).

5. Abraham M. Lilienfeld, "*Ceteris Paribus*: The evolution of the clinical trial," *Bulletin of the History of Medicine*, 56(1982): 1-18. For example, see A. B. Hill, "The clinical trial" *The New England Journal of Medicine*, 247(1952):113-119; R. Peto, *et al.*, "Design and analysis of randomized clinical trials requiring prolonged observation of each patient: I. Introduction and design" *Brit. J. Cancer*, 34(1976): 585-612; David A. Lilienfeld and Paul D. Stolley, *Foundations of Epidemiology*, 3rd. ed. (New York: Oxford University Press, 1994), p. 156.

6. As amended by the 29th World Medical Assembly, Tokyo, Japan, 1975.

7. James H. Jones' historical study of the forty-year experiment that deliberately left 400 African American men with syphilis untreated provides a disturbing example of unethical experimental practice; see James H. Jones, *Bad Blood: The Tuskegee Syphilis Experiment* (New York: The Free Press, 1981). For a discussion of earlier ethical controversies over the use of humans in research see Susan E. Lederer, *Subjected to Science: Human Experimentation in America before the Second World War* (Baltimore: The Johns Hopkins University Press, 1995).

8. For example, see Kenneth Rothman quoted in Gary Taubes, "Use of placebo controls in clinical trials disputed," *Science*, 1995, 267:25-26, and Kenneth J. Rothman and Karin B. Michels, "The Continuing unethical use of placebo controls," *The New England Journal of Medicine*, 331(1994):394-398.

9. See Taubes, "Use of placebo controls" (n. 3), and Louis Lasagna, "The Helsinki Declaration: Timeless Guide or irrelevant anachronism?" *Journal of Clinical Psychopharmacology*, 15(1995):96-98.

10. Stuart J. Pocock, "When to stop a clinical trial," *British Medical Journal*, 305(1992):235-240.

11. For more details of the story of the FDA and AIDS drugs see James Harvey Young, "AIDS and the FDA" in Caroline Hannaway, Victoria A. Harden, and John Parascandola, *AIDS and the Public Debate* (Amsterdam: IOS Press, 1995), and James J. Eigo, "Expedited drug approval procedures: Perspectives from an AIDS activist," in *Food, Drug, and Cosmetic Law Journal*, 45(1990):384.

12. For example, Sheila M. Gore, "Assessing clinical trials—Why randomise?" *British Medical Journal* 282(1981):1958-1960.

13. *The Design of Experiments* (Edinburgh/London: Oliver & Boyd, 1935). See also Ian Hacking's "Telepathy: Origins of randomization in experimental design," *Isis* 79(1988):427-451, which traces some curious earlier uses of randomization as a tool for experimentation under theoretical uncertainty.

14. See Joan Fisher Box, *R. A. Fisher: The Life of a Scientist* (New York: Wiley, 1978), and on the development of Fisher's ideas see her "R. A. Fisher and the design of experiments, 1922-1926," *The American Statistician*, 1980 34(1980):1-7.

15. Major Greenwood, "The statistician and medical research," *British Medical Journal*, Sept. 4, 1948, 467-468.

16. However, it was not without precursors. See H. Corwin Hinshaw and William H. Feldman, "Evaluation of chemotherapeutic agents in clinical trials: A suggested procedure," *Amer. Rev. Tuberculosis* 50(1944):202-13. They advocated use of chance and described their own experiments where patients were assigned to either an experimental or control group by flipping a coin.

17. "Streptomycin treatment of pulmonary tuberculosis" (n. 1), p. 770.

18. R. A. Fisher, *The Design of Experiments* , p. 21. Note that Hinshaw and Feldman, "Evaluation of chemotherapeutic agents,"(n. 16), p. 205, to their credit, did not justify chance-based selection as a guarantee of significance tests, but urged its use "so that all accessory factors

which bear on the prognosis should be balanced as accurately as is possible in the two groups."

19. David A. Harville, "Experimental randomization: Who needs it?" *The American Statistician* 29(1975): 27-31; Milton C. Weinstein, "Allocation of subjects in medical experiments," *the New England Journal of Medicine* 291(1974): 1278-1285; Peter Urbach, "Randomization and the design of experiments," *Philosophy of Science* 52(1985): 256-273. However, some Bayesians have argued in favor of randomization; for example, see D. B. Rubin, "Bayesian inference for causal effects: The role of randomization," *Annals of Statistics*, 6(1978):34-58.

20. F. P. Ramsey, "Truth and probability," *The Foundations of Mathematics and Other Logical Essays* (London: Routledge and Kegan Paul, 1931); L. J. Savage, *The Foundations of Statistical Inference* (New York: Wiley, 1962).

21. Ian Hacking, "Telepathy" (n. 13).

22. Colin Howson and Peter Urbach, *Scientific Reasoning: The Bayesian Approach*, 2nd. ed. (Chicago: Open Court, 1993), p. 270.

23. David P. Byar, *et al.*, "Randomized clinical trials: Perspectives on some recent ideas," *The New England Journal of Medicine*, 295(1976):74-80, p. 76.

24. Byar, "Randomized Clinical Trials"(n. 23); Gore, "Assessing Clinical Trials"(n. 12); Kenneth F. Schaffner, "Clinical trials and causation: Bayesian perspectives," *Statistics in Medicine* 12(1993):1477-1494.

25. David P. Byar, *et al.*, "Design considerations for AIDS trials," *The New England Journal of Medicine* 323(1990): 1343-1348.

26. Thomas C. Merigan, "You *can* teach an old dog new tricks: How AIDS trials are pioneering new strategies," *The New England Journal of Medicine* 323(1990):1341-1342; Institute of Medical Ethics Working Party on the Ethical Implications of AIDS, "AIDS, ethics, and clinical trials," *British Medical Journal* 305(1992):699-701.

27. "Streptomycin Treatment of Pulmonary Tuberculosis"(n. 1), p. 770.

28. As stated in the FDA's *General Considerations for the Clinical Evaluation of Drugs*. (n. 3).

29. R. G. Gibson, *et al.*, "Homeopathic therapy in rheumatoid arthritis: Evaluation by double-blind clinical therapeutic trial," *British Journal of Clinical Pharmacology* 9(1980): 453-459; David Taylor Reilly, *et al.*, "Is homeopathy a placebo response?: Controlled trial of homeopathic potency, with pollen in hayfever as model," *The Lancet* , October 18, 1986, 881-886; E. Davenas, *et al.,* "Human basophil degranulation triggered by very dilute antiserum against IgE," *Nature* 333(1988):816-818; Peter Fisher, *et al.*, "Effect of homeopathic treatment on fibrositis(primary fibromyalgia)," *British Medical Journal* 299(1989):365-366; Michel Labreque, *et al.*, "Homeopathic treatment of plantar warts," *Canadian Medical Association Journal*, 1992, *146*:1749-1753; David Reilly, *et al.*, "Is evidence for homeopathy reproducible?" *The Lancet* 344(1994):1601-1606. A controversial meta-study using 107 previously reported experiments from various sources was carried out by Jos Kleijnen, *et al.*, "Clinical trials of homeopathy," *British Medical Journal* 302(1992):316-323.

30. Peter C. Gøtzsche, "Trials of homeopathy" (letter) *The Lancet* 341(1993):1533, commenting on Jos Kleijnen, *et al.*, "Clinical trials of homeopathy" (n. 29).

31. Reilly, *et al.* "Is evidence for homeopathy reproducible?" (n. 29), pp. 1605-1606.

32. Sir Austin Bradford Hill, "The Environment and disease: Association or causation?" *Proceedings of the Royal Society of Medicine* 58(1965):295-300; Alfred S. Evans, "Causation and disease: The Henle-Koch postulates revisited," *Yale Journal of Biology and Medicine* 49(1976):175-195; David E. Lilienfeld and Paul D. Stolley (rev.), *Foundations of Epidemiology* 3rd. ed. (New York: Oxford University Press, 1994), pp. 265-66.

33. On the epistemology of experiments see, for example, Harry Collins, *Changing Order: Rep-*

lication and Induction in Scientific Practice (Chicago: University of Chicago Press, 1992) and Ian Hacking, *Representing and Intervening: Introductory Topics in the Philosophy of Natural Science* (Cambridge: Cambridge University Press, 1983).

34. R. Burkhardt and G. Kienle, "Basic problems in controlled trials" *Journal of Medical Ethics*, 9(1983):80-84, p. 81.
35. Reilly, *et al.* "Is evidence for homeopathy reproducible?" (n. 29), p. 1606.
36. Editorial, "When to believe the unbelievable," *Nature* 333(1988): 787.
37. It is helpful to recall here Hacking's "Telepathy" (n. 13), which discusses the use of randomization in psychic research.

Section 4.

From Medicines to Market and Patient

MEDICINES are a complicated commodity. After the application of the most advanced science and technology, drugs need to go through developmental stages where they are transformed into products manufactured, distributed, and consumed.

During the last twenty years perhaps no area of commerce has changed as much as the health care sector. As a physical commodity, medicines have attracted a great deal of attention from insurance companies and governmental officials looking to cut costs. Louis Lasagna argues that the high profits of pharmaceutical firms is reasonable when balanced against the tremendous risks involved. In his view, we need to protect this vital industry.

In the area of medicines, the United States Food and Drug Administration has worked long and hard to protect the public. A major boon to this effort came in 1962 with the passage of the Kefauver-Harris amendments that mandated that medicines be not only safe, but effective. The fight for effective medicines goes back long before 1962. John Swann describes the broad effort among various agencies and organizations to ensure the quality of medicines sold and consumed. Along the way he relates some interesting tales about how opinions can change about the usefulness of medicines.

No matter how effective drugs are, they must be marketed. Mickey Smith uses the four "P's" of marketing—product, price, place, and promotion—as a discussion outline for this topic. He concludes that "good marketing makes good medicine." With the great changes in communications technology taking place now and probably in the future, marketing of medicines will look much different in the next century.

In the end, a medicine works as well as the physician-pharmacist-patient relationship allows. If communication is stifled between any two members of this triad, the therapy may fail. Paul Ranelli analyzes these interactions using the current model of pharmaceutical care. His prescription for success is more involvement among all players in this relationship.

It is most fitting, after looking at the microcosm of the physician-pharmacist-patient interaction, to conclude the symposium and this volume with a broad overview of medicine use. As the former head of the Centers for Disease Control and one involved in several international efforts to reduce or eradicate disease, William Foege brings both a practical and a philosophical voice to the topic.

Recent Trends in Drug Development

by Louis Lasagna

This past century—especially the last six decades—has witnessed a veritable pharmacotherapeutic revolution. Antibiotics have made it possible to cure previously untreatable infections. Psychiatric illnesses ranging from anxiety states and mania to schizophrenia and psychotic melancholia have yielded to new therapies. Elevated blood pressure can be brought to normal by drugs. Hormonal therapy has dramatically altered the physician's ability to deal with such deficiencies of glandular function as myxedema, diabetes mellitus, and Addison's disease. Immunosuppressants have made organ transplants a realistic option. Acute leukemia in children, once a sentence of death, can be cured. New treatments for arthritis, peptic ulcer, parkinsonism, pernicious anemia, and Hodgkin's disease have dramatically altered the course of those diseases. Vaccines have eliminated smallpox from the planet and essentially wiped out poliomyelitis in North America. We have a multiplicity of approaches to preventing unwanted pregnancies.

Therapeutic and preventive progress in the twentieth century has, therefore, been dramatic. But equally impressive are the problems remaining unsolved. AIDS, our newest plague, is as yet incurable. Cancers not removable by surgery or radiotherapy are only amenable to chemotherapy in a minority of cases. The dementias are barely treatable. A number of degenerative neurologic and muscular diseases resist attempts at amelioration. And even when treatments *are* available, they are imperfect, since not all patients respond satisfactorily; serious adverse events are not rare, and troublesome side effects are all too common. Patients and physicians, therefore, have reason both to be grateful for the fruits of the research and development efforts of the past and frustrated by the many unmet needs of the present.

A major role in bringing new drugs to market has been that played by

217

the international pharmaceutical industry. The industry has not done it without help, to be sure, because federally supported research, in countries all over the globe, has often provided building blocks upon which a therapeutic edifice could be built. Intramural and extramural NIH funds, thus, have in a very real sense represented an indirect subsidy to this industry.

More recently, the nascent biotechnology industry has enlarged the playing field, by raising venture capital to support the search for new products (originally proteins, more recently other categories such as peptides, nucleotides, cells, and even low molecular weight synthetics) mostly unlike the small molecule new chemical entities (NCEs) that have been the traditional products of the older, more traditional pharmaceutical industry. There are now 1300 such small biotechnology firms in the United States, but most have no stream of income generated by marketed diagnostic or therapeutic products of their own, and only about 220 are involved in human clinical trials.

In this century, the international pharmaceutical industry has been, for the most part, very profitable. This profitability needs to be assessed and quantified in a special way, however, because the considerable amount of money plowed back yearly into research and development (R & D) does not usually result directly in sales income in the calendar year in which the investment was made. Rather, there is a lag of considerable duration between

Louis Lasagna was appointed Dean of the Sackler School of Graduate Biomedical Sciences at Tufts University in July of 1984. Prior to that, he was Chairman of the Department of Pharmacology and Toxicology from 1970-1980 and Professor of Pharmacology and Toxicology and of Medicine at the University of Rochester School of Medicine and Dentistry until his move to Tufts University in 1984. Before moving to Rochester, he spent sixteen years at the Johns Hopkins University School of Medicine where he started the first academic group devoted solely to clinical pharmacology. Dr. Lasagna received his M.D. from Columbia University in 1947.

Dr. Lasagna has worked and written extensively in the areas of clinical trial methodology, analgesics, hypnotics, medical ethics, and the placebo effect. He serves on a number of editorial boards and has been a consultant to several of the National Institutes of Health as well as the Food and Drug Administration. He was a member of the Commission on the Federal Drug Approval Process which examined the drug development and approval process and reported its findings to Congress in April 1982. Dr. Lasagna served on the General Accounting Office's Health Advisory Committee, Human Research Division, and was Chairman of the National Committee to Review Current Procedures for Approval of New Drugs for Cancer and AIDS, which operated under the aegis of the President's Cancer Panel. In 1990, Dr. Lasagna was appointed to Secretary Sullivan's "Blue Ribbon Panel," which was commissioned to examine the Food and Drug Administration. In 1995, Dr. Lasagna served with three former FDA Commissioners on the so-called "Rogers Group" to prepare an agenda for legislative reform of the drug regulatory process.

investment and return, making the drug industry akin to the natural gas and petroleum industry, where the "dry holes" far outnumber "the gushers," and return on investment is delayed for an unpredictable period of time. Estimates of how much it takes to bring a new chemical entity to market require not only the tracking of both successful candidates and failures, but the "cost of money" as well, since in addition to out-of-pocket expenses one has to add in the money that *could* have been earned by "safe" investments yielding an eight to ten percent return. The average cost of bringing an NCE to market is variably estimated at present to be a third of a billion dollars or more.

While profitable by and large up until now, however, the drug industry of the twenty-first century faces a number of threats that have surfaced in the last decade. One such threat is generic substitution, i.e., the prescribing and dispensing of less expensive equivalent versions of patented drugs sold by non-innovative manufacturers who are able to compete with the innovator product because patent exclusivity has expired. Money diverted from innovators by this means represents funds that are not available to search for new drugs.

A second threat is therapeutic substitution, wherein a hospital or HMO formulary committee (for example) threatens to substitute a similar but not identical drug (often a less expensive generic) for a patent-protected drug unless the latter's manufacturer provides the hospital or HMO with a considerably discounted product. This represents an effective way to get around pricing that would otherwise be determined by patent exclusivity.

A third threat is the increasing cost and complexity of drug development. It now usually takes ten to fifteen years from drug discovery to drug marketing, and there has been a gradual increase in the data submitted to achieve new drug approval by the FDA: more trials per new drug application (NDA), more patients per trial, and more procedures per patient. How much of this is justifiable and indeed necessary and how much is waste, a response to unreasonable demands, or a reflection of incompetence and inefficiency, is not at all clear.

A fourth threat is the pressure all over the world for holding down the cost of health care. In all developed countries, the population is "graying," with increased health care needs, but governments everywhere are demanding that health care costs be "capped" at some arbitrary percentage of gross national product. While some of this concern can be mitigated by cutting out indefensible expenses (such as unneeded drugs or lab tests or procedures or surgery), science will continue to come up with new ways to spend health care dollars. Some innovations may achieve net savings by diminishing other health care expenses, but most probably will not.

A fifth (and related) threat is the market's demand for "outcomes research," i.e., persuasive pharmacoeconomic data that justify using a new pharmaceutical in preference to older marketed products. Everyone would

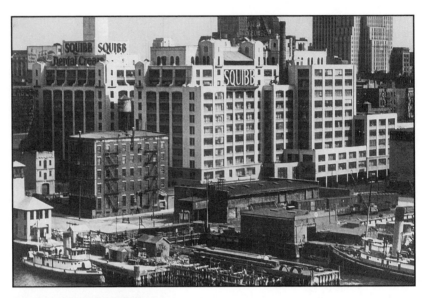

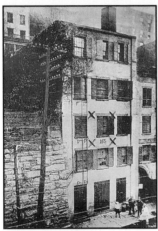

The changes in size of the manufacturing laboratories of E. R. Squibb and Sons, in Brooklyn, New York, between 1858 (shown to the left) and 1958 (above) mirror the expansion of the American drug industry during this same period. (Courtesy Drug Topics Collection, American Institute of the History of Pharmacy.)

prefer "breakthrough" drugs to "me-too" drugs, but the search for successful unique approaches is almost by definition more difficult, longer, and more expensive than for a drug only slightly different from what is already available. But third party payers increasingly demand comparative data to justify use of a new drug and reimbursement for it. Is the drug at launch persuasively better, or safer, or more convenient or cheaper?

A sixth threat (although some could argue that it is not) is the frequency of mergers of drug houses. Some have predicted that eventually the world may only have ten international giants sharing most of the global market. The rationale for such mergers involves the addition of complementary product lines and the cutting of costs by eliminating unnecessary jobs. One such merger was followed by a twenty-five percent down-sizing of the work force globally, and a combined R & D budget that was no larger than the budget of the larger company alone before the merger. Are such moves really cost-effective? Will they increase the flow of products in the development pipeline?

And is such merger or acquisition activity the only way out for most biotechnology firms, i.e., to be acquired by either a traditional pharmaceutical company or by one of the few successful biotechnology firms before the absorbed firm runs out of venture capital (since many are "betting the company" on one approach)? Are there any possible remedial responses to these threats? Let me propose a few for consideration:

- We need to cut the time and expense for bringing new drugs to market by increasing the dialogue between the regulators and the regulated, with collegial interaction from the beginning to the end of the process, and with an effective appeals mechanism to resolve disputes, so that the ultimate NDA becomes essentially self-reviewing because all the right questions have been asked and answered.

- Our society must realize that the public health requires a healthy drug industry—one that is profitable enough to justify shareholders' investment in an increasingly expensive and risky business.

- We need to focus on the treatment of individuals rather than what Nietzche would have called "the herd." To get a drug on the market requires evidence of efficacy in a *group* of treated subjects when compared to a control group of some kind, but the pioneer clinical trial expert A. Bradford Hill wrote thirty years ago (and it is still true today) that such controlled trials do not tell physicians what they want to know, which is how best to treat Mr. Jones or Mrs. Smith without engaging in trial-and-error prescribing. Such an improvement in our predictive ability would not only benefit patients and physicians, but could conceivably help drug companies by identifying subpopulations uniquely well treated by Drug X or Drug Z, the drug thus deserving to be used and remuneration for the drug to be unquestioned.

- We need to get cooperation between the best scientific brains, wherever they may be—industry, academe, or government—in the search for new remedies or vaccines, because the tough disease nuts left to be cracked are not likely to yield without such cooperation. An excellent example was the cooperation between all three sectors in the development of AZT (zidovudine) for AIDS; we need more such efforts. Gene therapy is exciting in its potential, and it will be difficult at best to implement, even with the best brains at work, but unlikely to succeed without them. (Luck is also needed; serendipity has often been the way to a new remedy, but as Pasteur pointed out, chance favors only the prepared mind.)

- In trying to save health care dollars, we must not be penny wise and pound foolish. For example, cutting back on drug expenditures has resulted at times in net increases in expenditures by increasing hospitalization days. Health care needs to be thought of in its totality, not in bits and pieces of the puzzle.

- Finally, how much of our GNP should we spend on health? I do not see any reason to fix on any one arbitrary percentage. Our national dollars pay for all sorts of things: health care, defense, highways, education, construction, and so forth. Shouldn't our citizenry be making the decision as to how much should go where? I suspect that most citizens would agree to an increase in health care expenditures to avoid rationing even if it required a concomitant decrease in other spending areas. And if so, why not? Gaucher's disease now can be treated with enzyme replacement therapy at a cost of $100,000 to $400,000 per year per patient. To my knowledge, third party payers are reimbursing for this, but what if this disease were not a rare one, but afflicted millions? Would we decide it was unaffordable?

And what about the increasingly prevalent Alzheimer's dementia, which Elie Wiesel has compared to a book whose pages fall out, one by one, leaving at the end nothing but dusty covers? This cruel disease—cruel to families as well as the victims—cries out for cure, or prevention, or at least a halting of the degenerative process. If we do come up with really effective therapy that is very expensive, will we pay for it? If we succeed in finding a gene therapy for cystic fibrosis but it costs a million dollars per patient, will it be deemed "too costly"? I have no glib answers to these questions, but suggest that they deserve debate.

Sure Cure: Public Policy on Drug Efficacy Before 1962

by John P. Swann

T HE movement to reform the Food and Drug Administration and the laws that agency is charged to uphold includes an element that most of us associate with the Kefauver-Harris drug amendments of 1962, an element that many consider to be a cornerstone of drug regulation in this country—drug effectiveness. For example, Congressman Joe Barton of Texas, chairman of the House Subcommittee on Oversight and Investigations of the Committee on Energy and Commerce, which controls two-thirds of the federal budget, including FDA's, recently had this to say about drug efficacy:

> As an engineer, I think you can come up with a standard definition or repeal the efficacy requirement altogether and let the market determine efficacy and let the FDA continue to regulate safety, because health care professionals are not going to prescribe or use things that don't work. Certainly, a qualified, competent, ethical doctor or health care professional is not. So you can make the argument from a market or philosophical perspective that you don't need [FDA] to even determine efficacy—just make sure that it doesn't hurt people.[1]

This would seem to be an especially ripe time to present some historical perspective on drug efficacy, because a long line of laws, agencies, institutions, and individuals throughout the twentieth century and before have sought to elevate therapeutics, to ensure that Rep. Barton's market serves the best interest of the patient. In the first part of this essay I will characterize efforts, private and public, to promote and regulate drug efficacy: from the early work of the Committee on Scope of the *United States Pharmacopoeia* and the U. S. Post Office Department, to the efforts of the Hygienic Laboratory of the U. S. Public Health Service and the deliberations of the Council of

223

Pharmacy and Chemistry of the American Medical Association, to the laws themselves that mandated drug efficacy, both explicitly and by inference.

The second part will address the FDA's emerging link of drug safety with drug efficacy, culminating in two case studies in the 1950s and early 1960s that were defining episodes in this history. The first concerned the new drug application for Hepasyn, a cancer treatment sponsored by the San Francisco College of Mortuary Science, and the second dealt with the withdrawn approval of a new drug application for the antimicrobial agent, Altafur. *How* one would determine efficacy is an important issue that has been debated for decades. However, in light of current considerations of even *whether* there should be a mandate for efficacy, a more focused investigation into the construction of specific efficacy standards is better left to another historical inquiry.

As early as 1813, the Vaccine Act authorized a federal agen to ensure that "genuine matter" be supplied for citizens receiving smallpox vaccinations. It is unclear how successfully this law was enforced. Later, the Import Drugs Act of 1848 required that medicines imported in the United States be examined for their "fitness for medical purposes," and if they failed to meet the potency identified in the United States Pharmacopoeia or several other drug compendia named in the law, they would not be allowed into the country. The law worked well in the beginning, but analytical capabilities could not keep pace with adulteration suterfuge. Also, some inspection post assignments were made increasingly on the basis of political patronage. Thus, the venerable Edward R. Squibb observed that the law was a virtual dead letter by 1860.[2]

A Reference Standard for Effective Drugs, I: USP

The *United States Pharmacopoeia* (USP) was one of the earliest venues in this country where, at least to some degree, effective drugs were distinguished from others. Though in truth, throughout much of the history of the

John P. Swann received his Bachelor's degree in Chemistry and History from the University of Kansas, and his Ph.D. in the History of Science and Pharmacy from the University of Wisconsin. Thereafter he was named a post-doctoral fellowship at the Smithsonian Institution, and later became a senior research assistant at the University of Texas Medical Branch. His publications have focused on the history of drugs, biomedical research, the pharmaceutical industry, and regulatory history. In 1989 he received the Edward Kremers Award from the American Institute of the History of Pharmacy for his book, *Academic Scientists and the Pharmaceutical Industry: Cooperative Research in Twentieth-Century America.* Since 1989 he has been an Historian at the U.S. Food and Drug Administration.

USP, one could say with some accuracy that if a drug were in the USP, it was not necessarily effective, and if it were not in the USP, it was not necessarily ineffective. According to the first USP (1820), the function of a pharmacopoeia was "to select from among substances which possess medicinal power, those, the utility of which is most fully established and best understood; and to form from them preparations and compositions, in which their powers may be exerted to the greatest advantage."[3] Nevertheless, the first USP included both a primary list of materia medica, "articles of decided reputation or general use," and a secondary list of medicines, "the claims of which are of a more uncertain kind."[4] The former included belladonna, camphor, opium, and cinchona, as well as olive oil, musk, and cinnamon. The secondary list included carrot, black snake root, and wild lettuce.[5] This binary approach continued until USP VI of 1882, which combined both into a single section of preparations.[6]

The Committee of Revision for USP VII (1893) made it known that the USP did not wish to be a standard of reference for the therapeutic value of any drug listed or unlisted. Rather, it existed "to fix the identity, and the standard of quality, purity and strength of medicinal substances commonly prescribed by physicians."[7] Indeed, despite the nascence of pharmacology and other basic pharmaceutical sciences by this time, inert and therapeutically worthless drugs persisted in the *Pharmacopoeia*.[8]

In 1901, Committee of Revision chairman Charles Rice established the Subcommittee of Scope, which he charged with surveying professional opinion to inform the selection process. But through the first half of the century the subcommittee served as a lightning rod for the ongoing differences between pharmacists and physicians—both of whom were represented on the revision committee—over the appropriate scope of the USP. Basically, physicians wanted the *Pharmacopoeia* to be a tool for therapeutic decision-making, whereas pharmacists wanted it to be a tool for drug-making.[9] Consequently, the former scheme would be more exclusive, but the latter approach would provide guidance for the wider variety of products one would likely need to dispense.

Rice assured his committee that the *National Formulary* would happily accept therapeutically wayward drugs cast off from the USP,[10] yet the Committee of Revision often overrode recommendations from the physician-dominated scope subcommittee. This frustrated one member of the latter to blast the revision committee for equating efficacy with popularity. Ironically, exclusivity mandated by long-standing rules of the *Pharmacopoeia* kept many therapeutically valuable drugs out of the USP because they were proprietary products, such as aspirin and adrenalin.[11]

By the early 1930s the Committee of Revision's criteria for admission to the USP remained the following: drugs of therapeutic value, products not privately controlled, and frequently prescribed drugs. However, USP XII of

1942 no longer considered the patent or trademark status of a drug for admission, and in 1950, during the deliberations for USP XV, the scope subcommittee based its admissions policy primarily on efficacy, and only incidentally on frequency of use. In 1965, following the federal mandate that approved drugs be safe and effective, the USP Board of Trustees—partly out of a concern that FDA might usurp the *Pharmacopoeia's* standard-setting function—advocated that the USP admit all FDA-approved single-entity products. The revision committee, however, chose to retain its selection function.[12]

Attack on Quackery Masquerading as Efficacy, I: The Post Office

Before the Bureau of Chemistry began cracking down on manufacturers making false claims of efficacy for their products, and before the Hygienic Laboratory became concerned with efficacy of biological products that it regulated, the Post Office Department, operating under the postal fraud law of 1872, cracked down on those using the mails to defraud the public, including manufacturers of ineffective remedies. The 1872 law, broadened in 1895, permitted the Postmaster General to issue a "fraud order" if a party used the mails to obtain money through false or fraudulent pretenses. The fraud order

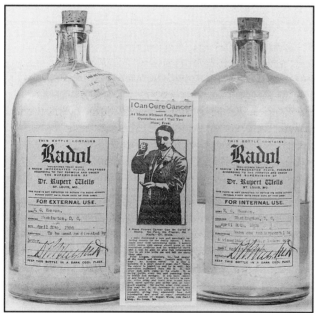

Trying to tap into the fascination with radioactivity, Radol claimed to cure cancer with a radium-impregnated fluid, a hoax that Samuel Adams exposed in Collier's in 1906. The Post Office Department secured a fraud order against the manufacturer.

enabled all mails sent to the offending party to be intercepted, stamped "Fraudulent," and returned to the sender.[13]

The law was passed mostly with security fraud in mind, but beginning about the turn of the century the Post Office began to interdict worthless nostrums that claimed to cure tuberculosis, restore lost manhood, straighten kinky hair, and so on. For assistance in analyzing some of these questionable products, the Post Office turned to the Public Health Service[14] and, particularly, to the Bureau of Chemistry of the U. S. Department of Agriculture, which at that time employed most of the chemists in the federal government.[15]

One postal action had a significant impact on future cases. Around 1900 postmaster J. M. McAnnulty of Nevada, Missouri, initiated a fraud order against the American School of Magnetic Healing, which advertised through the mails that, for a fee, it could heal any illness telepathically. The company appealed the Post Office fraud order, eventually to the Supreme Court, which found in favor of the American School. Justice Peckham ruled that, since the usefulness of medical treatments is usually just a matter of opinion and not an absolute truth, the efficacy of any particular treatment is not for the Postmaster General to decide. Peckham qualified his ruling, though, in saying that efficacy could be a material fact, demonstrated scientifically, in cases where medicine has progressed beyond an empirical stage. (It had not, according to this interpretation, in the case of the effect of the mind on disease.) Also, if an efficacy claim simply were completely unrestricted, promising a cure in every case, fraud could be established.[16]

The door was left slightly ajar, so, as James Harvey Young has shown, "choosing its cases with care, the Post Office Department developed an excellent statistical record of success."[17] Action, typically with the Bureau of Chemistry's analytical assistance, was taken against the dregs of nostrumiana, those egregious cases in which vendors guaranteed cures for blindness, cancer, epilepsy, and other diseases. In 1908 the bureau analyzed fifteen alleged cancer cures for postal fraud violations. One such cure, Radol, supposedly was made radioactive by exposure to radium. In fact, the fluorescence of the product had nothing to do with radium. The promoter suffered not only a fraud order from the Post Office Department, but liability under the Food and Drugs act as well—which cost him $100.[18]

In fact, there were cases in which the Post Office could step in where other agencies were powerless or otherwise hamstrung to deal with false therapeutic claims. Such was the fate of Tuberclecide, a worthless treatment for tuberculosis. In 1916 the Bureau of Chemistry lost a decision against this nostrum; the discoverer claimed ignorance of *how* his treatment cured tuberculosis—only that it did. The judge was not convinced that fraudulence had taken place (this not atypical reasoning is explained later on). However, twelve years later a federal circuit court upheld a postal fraud order against

Tuberclecide in the light of greater scientific knowledge.[19] Similarly, the bureau failed in a number of cases against cures for drug habits that contained the very ingredient responsible for the addiction, while the Post Office successfully secured fraud orders against these operations. Such was the case with Habitina, a drug cure that contained both morphine and heroin.[20] The postal fraud law, therefore, offered another means of differentiating effective from ineffective drugs—albeit applicable only to some highly blatant examples.

The Hygienic Laboratory and the Efficacy of Biologics

Regulations for the 1902 Biologics Act did not at first mandate efficacy. Rather, products sampled in the open market had to be "potent"; manufacturing methods had to be in place that would not impair the potency; and labeling had to include an expiration date.[21] Otherwise, the Hygienic Laboratory would withhold the license required of the firm to distribute such an agent. The Division of Pharmacology of the Hygienic Laboratory (the precursor of the National Institutes of Health) devised or adapted standards to determine the potency of biologics.[22] Efficacy was not an explicit requirement until 1934, but that did not prevent some firms early on from using licensure as a guarantee of therapeutic performance in their advertisements, which was perfectly legal.[23]

To be sure, the Hygienic Laboratory considered efficacy when licensing manufacturers for specific biologics long before 1934. This was a move long championed by the American Medical Association, which in 1915 supported an amendment to the 1902 law that would prevent the interstate commerce of worthless biologics, with the burden of proof placed on the manufacturer.[24] In 1923 John Reichel, director of laboratories at H. K. Mulford, a leading firm, testified to Congress that companies had understood "for years" that no matter how clean your operation, a license would be withheld if there were "lack of proof that [the biologic] has any real merit."[25]

According to George McCoy, Hygienic Laboratory Director from 1915 to 1937, "it was the intention of Congress to restrict the use of preparations coming under [the 1902] law to such as had therapeutic or prophylactic activity."[26] For example, the laboratory rejected a license application for an alleged typhus vaccine after pharmacologists could not establish any effect of the vaccine on experimental typhus. Several cases in which licenses were sought for tuberculosis treatments that had no therapeutic value prompted denials from the laboratory. Yet, in the case of license requests for treatments of colds and the flu, where the laboratory was unable to develop experimental therapeutic models to ascertain efficacy,[27] the laboratory typically granted the license, reasoning that, even though the product probably was not effective, it was also probably harmless.[28] Similar reasoning drove FDA's policy on safe yet ineffective drugs prior to the 1962 amendments (discussed later).

Muckraking journalism, one of the key forces behind the 1906 Food and Drugs Act, once again helped expose the dregs of a medical industry. Norman Hapgood, former editor of *Collier's* when that magazine was publishing attacks on the patent medicine menace in the early twentieth century, continued the assault on bogus medicines as editor of *Hearst's International*. In the early 1920s Paul DeKruif published a series in Hapgood's journal on questionable claims by some biologics manufacturers.[29] Soon Congress attempted to bring some legislative relief by amending the Biologics Control Act to include control of biologics advertising. During the acrimonious hearings on this bill between February and May 1924, proponents invoked a mantra that Secretary of Health, Education, and Welfare Abraham Ribicoff would echo nearly forty years later during the Kefauver hearings: that hogs, sheep, and cattle were protected against worthless biologics, but humans were not. In 1913 the Bureau of Animal Industry of the U. S. Department of Agriculture issued regulations for livestock requiring that a biologics license be withheld if the product were "advertised so as to mislead or deceive the purchaser or... misleading in any particular." However, the 1902 law and the Hygienic Laboratory's regulations afforded no such protection for humans.[30]

The many opponents of the bill countered that the regulation of biologics advertising would retard scientific investigations; that the proposed bill would keep important drugs like Salvarsan, typhoid vaccine, and diphtheria antitoxin off the market during testing to establish their efficacy; that existing legislation—the mail fraud laws, the 1902 act, and the 1906 act with its Sherley amendment—sufficed for advertising control; that regulation of a product that was principally advertised directly to physicians was an interference in the practice of medicine (an argument that anticipated by decades some of the rhetoric in the control of off-label drug use); and that such an effort would put far too much power in the hands of a small group of government officials.[31] McCoy was concerned, not with the attempt to corral advertising abuses, but rather with the way Congress proposed going about it; under the bill, the Hygienic Laboratory would have to monitor advertising and issue statements of disapproval to accompany any ad for a biologic that claimed prophylactic or therapeutic value without the laboratory's approval. McCoy, sensitive to the need to control worthless treatments, proposed a different amendment whereby the Hygienic Laboratory (through the Secretary of the Treasury, who oversaw the 1902 act) could deny or suspend a license if that were in the "public interest."[32]

McCoy's modification eventually was discarded, the final permutation of the bill simply prohibiting the advertising of any biological agent "under any false or misleading representation as to its nature, origin, composition, physiologic reaction, or therapeutic effect."[33] Industry representatives in the hearing promised to support the bill if the medical profession appeared to want it. However, when the *Journal of the American Medical Association* offered its "enthusiastic and wholehearted support" for the amendment, opponents offered scores of letters and editorials from clinics, associations, and individual practitioners denouncing the *Journal* and the bill.[34] The Hygienic Laboratory's support by this time had waned, too, with the prospect of the additional responsibility without any promise of a concomitant increase in staffing or budget.[35]

In the end, the attempt to amend the Biologics Act failed. However, in 1934 the Hygienic Laboratory—by then known as the National Institute of Health—formalized its long-standing policy on ineffective vaccines, serums, and other biological products by promulgating a regulation that "licenses for new products shall not be granted without satisfactory evidence of therapeutic or prophylactic efficiency."[36] At last humans and livestock were on a more equal footing.

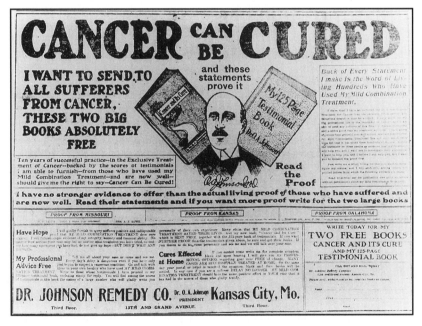

The case involving Dr. Johnson's cancer cure redefined the sense of "false therapeutic claims" following the Supreme Court's interpretation of an element in the 1906 Food and Drugs Act.

Attack on Quackery Masquerading as Efficacy, II: The Bureau of Chemistry

Regulation of efficacy was considerably more restricted under the next federal law addressing therapeutic agents, the Food and Drugs Act of 1906. The closest the law itself came to the issue was under the description of misbranding, defined as any statement on the label regarding the product or its ingredients that was "false or misleading in any particular."[37] The Bureau of Chemistry interpreted this to apply to false therapeutic claims. Thereafter, some manufacturers tempered their claims voluntarily, and others abided by the bureau's interpretation of misbranding only after judicial intervention, resulting in the removal of many labeled claims—if not advertised ones or the patent remedy itself. Nearly one hundred such cases were successfully prosecuted by 1911.[38]

However, the case involving Dr. Johnson's Mild Combination Treatment for Cancer was resolved quite differently. In 1911 the U. S. Supreme Court rendered a decision against the government in its case against this treatment that claimed to cure cancer. Oliver Wendell Holmes and the majority of the court ruled against the connection between false labeling and a manufacturer's curative claims, believing the law addressed the statement of identity of the product rather than "inflated or false commendation of wares." Moreover, on the issue of leaving the bureau to decide a question of therapeutic effect, the court believed the bureau was a likely source to determine composition, "but hardly so as to medical effects." Apparently Justice Holmes and his five colleagues believed jurists were more capable on the latter count! Finally, Holmes invoked the McAnnulty decision to buttress his argument that therapeutics is an area of widely diverging opinions.[39] Charles Evans Hughes and two other justices dissented.

President Taft responded that the Johnson decision rendered moot over 150 pending cases "involving some of the rankest frauds by which the American people were ever deceived," and he encouraged Congress to apply legislative relief.[40] The court had made it clear that any attempt to control mere expressions of opinion would fail again, so Congress passed a bill, introduced by Kentucky Congressman Swagar Sherley, that was couched as severely as members believed possible.[41] It prohibited any statement "regarding the curative or therapeutic effect of such article or any of the ingredients or substances contained therein, which is false and fraudulent."[42]

But the "joker" in the amendment was "fraudulent," which necessitated proof that the manufacturer intended to defraud the consumer. Unscrupulous firms that chose to fight, the Bureau of Chemistry later discovered, often escaped by professing belief that their products were effective. In 1922 a retired court reporter who sold a liniment made of turpentine, ammonia, formaldehyde, oils of mustard and wintergreen, and raw eggs took the bureau to court.

The agency had seized his product for mislabeling because he claimed it would cure tuberculosis. However, the jury was persuaded that the reporter believed in the efficacy of his treatment, and found in his favor.[43]

This was also the case with "Lee's Save the Baby," which the agency seized in 1929 for misbranding. Expert medical testimony during the trial concurred with the agency's conclusion that nothing in this product could competently treat colds, cough, croup, bronchitis, laryngitis, tonsillitis, pneumonia, and so on, which the labeling claimed. However, the judge in this case ruled in favor of the personal testimony and testimonial letters offered on behalf of this product.[44]

Similarly, a former shirt salesman promoted Banbar, an extract of the horsetail weed, as an effective treatment for diabetes. For $12 a pint patients could take Banbar orally rather than the injections required of insulin, which Banting and his colleagues at the University of Toronto recently had introduced in 1923. The principal government witness during the court proceedings, Elliott P. Joslin, was *the* internationally recognized authority on diabetes. On the basis of the 12,000 diabetic patients he saw every year, Joslin testified that insulin—combined with diet and exercise—was the only effective treatment for this disease. The defense offered hundreds of testimonial letters on behalf of Banbar. The jury found in favor of the defense, despite the fact that the government presented death certificates—attributed to diabetes—for individuals who had submitted these testimonials.[45] During the deliberations to write a new law to replace the 1906 act, FDA chief Walter Campbell made it clear to Congress that "what we are seeking to do here is put the courts on notice... that it is the purpose of Congress to have consideration given therapeutic claims."[46] Indeed, the 1938 Food, Drug, and Cosmetic Act left no doubt that false claims of efficacy constituted misbranding.

A Reference Standard for Effective Drugs, II: The AMA

The American Medical Association was one of the interests that Harvey Wiley had helped to amalgamate to pass the 1906 act. From the turn of the century on, the AMA was probably the leading private group that tried to effect policies that would foster the availability and prescribing of efficacious drugs, in many ways. As early as 1849, two years after its founding, the association adopted a resolution to found a board to analyze and publicize nostrums; unfortunately, the matter of funding got in the way of this enterprise.[47]

In 1908 the association's journal reported the poor state of affairs in prescribing practice among the profession, perhaps a reflection of the minimal education many physicians received in materia medica. The association editorialized for more rational therapeutics through no less an authority than Torald Sollmann, the eminent pharmacologist at Western Reserve University Medical School. The AMA established continuing education courses on drug use and action through local medical societies; by 1909, two hundred societies were offering the course. The AMA published commentaries on effective therapeutics. *Epitome of the United States Pharmacopeia and National Formulary*, which ran from 1907 to 1955, addressed products of therapeutic value in these compendial standards and pointed out listed drugs of dubious merit. Similarly, *Useful Drugs* (1913 to 1952) compiled core products from the above and other compendia with which the medical student and practitioner needed to be familiar.

Arthur Cramp's publications for the AMA's Propaganda Department were much more basic, and certainly aimed at a wider audience—much like the work of Samuel Hopkins Adams and other muckraking journalists that preceded his own. Cramp publicly excoriated the worthlessness and danger of patent medicines (many if not most still quite legal) in *Nostrums and Quackery*, the first edition of which appeared in 1911. The AMA also helped organize pharmacological and clinical investigations of the efficacy of drugs, the former through the Committee on Therapeutic Research, established in 1912, the latter through the Therapeutic Trials Committee, which began in 1945 and continued after 1950 as the Committee on Research. Thus, the AMA early on tried to promote informed prescribing of therapeutically useful drugs in many different ways.[48]

Perhaps the most significant AMA effort to promote drug efficacy, though, was through its Council on Pharmacy and Chemistry. This originated as a joint AMA and American Pharmaceutical Association concern with ridding the landscape of the nostrum evil by forming a federal bureau to certify pharmaceuticals, funded by what we would now call user fees. This idea faltered within the AMA, but in 1905 the organization's Board of Trustees unilaterally established the council, recommending the publication of a book of council-approved pharmaceuticals not in the USP.[49] Its fifteen members— pharmacologists, chemists, pharmacists, and a bacteriologist and pharmacognosist—represented academe, the AMA, the Hygienic Laboratory, and the Bureau of Chemistry. From the outset the Bureau cooperated with the council; for example, the Drug Division performed analyses until the council received a laboratory of its own, and there was ongoing Bureau representation on the council.[50]

No pharmaceutical would be admitted to *New and Nonofficial Remedies*, the council's official compendium of accepted drugs, that had "unwarranted, exaggerated or misleading statements as to therapeutic value." But no matter what the claim, useless drugs were unacceptable. Also, companies had to play entirely by council rules. A product could be denied acceptance if a firm derived substantial earnings from other products not in compliance with those directions.[51] The council, which depended heavily on the advice of outside expert consultants,[52] evaluated the evidence a manufacturer submitted to support the efficacy and any claims made for a drug. Inclusion in *NNR* entitled the manufacturer to label the product with the "accepted" seal of the council and have advertising access to AMA, state medical, and other journals. Conversely, rejected drugs were denied access to these journals, and the council published a notice of the denial in the AMA journal. Of course, this was a private venture, and there was no legal obligation for manufacturers to secure council acceptance of their products.[53]

In 1955 the council did away with the acceptance program, a move that Harry Dowling attributed to a combination of apathy and depleted cash reserves.[54] Thereafter the council used *New and Nonofficial Remedies* to publish its evaluations of pharmaceuticals simply for the record, a reference to the actual therapeutic value of a drug; the proscriptive function of the council ceased. Strangely enough, the *Journal of the American Medical Association* might carry an advertisement with a claim directly contradicted by *NNR*.[55] The council continued to rely on the reviews of industry-submitted data by consulting experts. But with the club of the old program removed, council reviewers typically had to extend their search for relevant data beyond whatever evidence a firm might submit.[56] The AMA council's drug evaluation program continued after 1962, in large part because *New and Nonofficial Drugs* (the new name for *NNR* after 1958) and its successor, *New Drugs*, were a resource on the relative efficacy of one drug compared to another, something FDA did not consider under the efficacy provisions of the new law.[57]

Before leaving the AMA's impact on the efficacy issue, it is worth considering where the association stood on the role of the practitioner in estimating a drug's usefulness. In 1944 the Council on Pharmacy and Chemistry stated that the average physician certainly was trained to observe clinical responses. However, they questioned if this person possessed the detailed knowledge of pharmacology and other background sciences to determine "which patients might have recovered without drug intervention, which preparations are unnecessarily complex, which contain agents that are incompatible, which may have lost part of their effectiveness because of partial absorption into the container or by oxidation, and the host of other factors that must be considered."[58] A year later the secretary of the council advised FDA that it was "in the interest of the medical profession to have provided an amendment [to the 1938 act] whereby the members of the profession will be assured of continually potent and effective penicillin or derivatives thereof."[59]

In 1954 the AMA Board of Trustees said "the average physician has neither the time nor the facilities to experiment with new drugs in order to determine their proper indications for use," a reservation that Louis Goodman, the esteemed co-author of *The Pharmacological Basis of Therapeutics*, echoed and elaborated on some time later.[60] However, eight years later the association testified during the Kefauver hearings that "a drug's efficacy varies from patient to patient... hence any judgment concerning this factor can only be made by the individual physician who is using the drug to treat an indi-

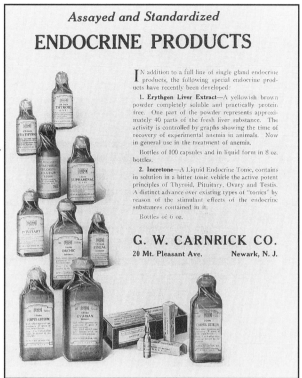

Assayed and Standardized

ENDOCRINE PRODUCTS

IN addition to a full line of single gland endocrine products, the following special endocrine products have recently been developed:

1. Erythgen Liver Extract—A yellowish brown powder completely soluble and practically protein free. One part of the powder represents approximately 40 parts of the fresh liver substance. The activity is controlled by graphs showing the time of recovery of experimental anemia in animals. Now in general use in the treatment of anemia.

Bottles of 100 capsules and in liquid form in 8 oz. bottles.

2. Incretone—A Liquid Endocrine Tonic, contains in solution in a bitter tonic vehicle the active potent principles of Thyroid, Pituitary, Ovary and Testis. A distinct advance over existing types of "tonics" by reason of the stimulant effects of the endocrine substances contained in it.

Bottles of 6 oz.

G. W. CARNRICK CO.

20 Mt. Pleasant Ave.   Newark, N. J.

FDA took a dimmer and dimmer view of the value of orally administered hormones, such as the pituitary, orchic, pineal, and other preparations pictured here (from American Druggist Year Book and Price List, *1929).*

vidual patient."[61] Despite their long collaboration on many issues of drug regulation, dating back to the association's support of the 1906 act, it seemed federally mandated drug efficacy went too far for the AMA by the early 1960s.

"Efficacy" in the Statutes before Kefauver-Harris

Efficacy per se did not appear in federal law for the first time in 1962. A number of earlier statutes explicitly required effectiveness for several specific drugs, and one law came close to including this as a requirement for all drugs. In addition, as early as 1939 the FDA began to raise regulatory concerns with certain types of drugs that lacked efficacy yet allegedly contained therapeutically active ingredients.

In December of that year FDA advised the industry that some oral preparations of ovary extracts lacked any ingredients that would have estrogenic or progestational activity. In such cases the article would be deemed adulterated and misbranded. However, one year later the agency backed off a bit; if some physicians wanted to employ inert products such as oral ovarian extracts, the 1938 act would not stand in their way. However, the law required material facts on the label, and in this case the agency considered the lack of therapeutic effect, based on scientific evidence, material. Thus, one year later FDA advised manufacturers that oral or otherwise inert ovary, suprarenal, pituitary, prostate, pineal, and mammary extracts should be labeled with the statement that such an article "does not contain any known therapeutically useful constituent of the glands mentioned."[62]

FDA did not invoke the connection between lack of efficacy and safety in the case of the glandular extract regulations, but this link was very much behind the insulin, penicillin, and later antibiotic amendments of the 1940s and 1950s. The Insulin Amendment of 1941, passed one day before the expiration of the University of Toronto's patent on insulin—and thus regulation over production standards—charged FDA to certify each batch of insulin produced as to its strength, quality, and purity "to adequately insure safety and efficacy of use."[63] Floor discussion of the amendment in the House reflected the need for an effective preparation of standardized potency in light of insulin's narrow margin of safety.[64]

The insulin law served as the basis for the Penicillin Amendment of 1945 and the similar antibiotic laws that followed; the wording of the efficacy requirement was lifted directly from the 1941 law.[65] In September 1943 the War Production Board had organized a plan for FDA to certify military supplies of penicillin for efficacy and purity.[66] The Administrator of the Federal Security Agency apprised Speaker of the House Sam Rayburn of the importance of having a certified, effective preparation: "Penicillin is administered in cases of extreme illness. Sometimes the physician must wait as long as 12 hours before its effects become manifest in the patient. If the product administered is lacking in the expected potency, the patient may pass beyond human aid before the fault of the drug is recognized by the physician."[67] Like the insulin law, the penicillin legislation and the antibiotic certification laws that followed passed Congress without incident. The same could not be said, though, of the short-lived attempt to include efficacy in the Durham-Humphrey Amendment of 1951.

Early versions of the 1951 law that defined prescription and nonprescription drugs originally included the provision that drugs ineffective for use without the supervision of a physician or dentists would have to be dispensed under a prescription. Later versions indicated that the Federal Security Administrator, based on the generally-held opinions among scientific experts, would determine which drugs would be unsafe and ineffective for use without the supervision of a physician or dentist.[68] However, pointed floor debate in the House, objection by affected interests such as industry, and a less than enthusiastic endorsement by FSA Administrator Oscar Ewing—not necessarily in that order—felled the efficacy provision.[69]

During the debate over Durham-Humphrey, one member who supported the efficacy provision said that even though the law probably would exclude it, Congress would have to define the meaning of drug safety.[70] However, FDA had already begun defining it in some cases as a function of drug efficacy. For example, the agency relied heavily on efficacy data when serious diseases such as pneumonia were involved, as in the review of new drug applications for sulfapyridine from October 1938 to March 1939.[71] But the defining case, the case the agency eventually intended to be a precedent-setting case in the link between efficacy and safety, began to unfold about the same time Congress was debating the efficacy provision of Durham-Humphrey.

Hepasyn and the Search for Efficacy

Arginase, a liver enzyme that helps hydrolyze the amino acid arginine, was discovered by Albrecht Kossell and Henry D. Dakin in 1904.[72] By the early 1930s various workers noticed that cancerous tissue bore an unusually high concentration of arginine, and that arginine appeared to accelerate cell division in tumor tissue. Despite difficulties in replicating these observations, interest in the therapeutic application of this discovery grew.[73] Researchers achieved little success when administering the natural lysing agent of arginine, arginase, to control tumor growth, though there was a notable exception.

Ved Vrat, a former graduate student at Stanford who became chief assistant at the Electronic Medical Foundation's[74] American Institute of Radiation (AIR) in suburban San Francisco around 1950, reported the following year that arginase effected complete control of tumor growth in mice with concomitant histological changes.[75] By that time the Permanente Medical Foundation had taken over the institute, and in the latter half of 1951 the foundation tested Vrat's arginase on ten terminal cancer patients. The clinician in charge of the trials concluded it did not benefit his patients in any way, and he strongly suspected that Vrat's results were questionable—a conclusion echoed by Vrat's superior at Permanente.[76] The Permanente Foundation thus ceased its clinical trials with arginase, but by this time scores of patients already had received the enzyme in a nearby but completely independent venue.

Vrat's laboratory chief at the radiation institute and fellow arginase researcher, dentist Wesley G. Irons, had been investigating arginase long before his short-lived and explosive venture with Vrat.[77] He first became interested in cancer after his father died of the disease in 1939, and he began work on arginase when he was on the faculty at the University of California at San Francisco Schools of Pharmacy and Dentistry as an anatomist, from 1943 to 1949; he received research support from the university for one year, and in the mid-1940s he published some initial results of his success with arginase in mice.[78]

After the university refused to renew his contract, Irons moved to the institute to continue the arginase work. But before Permanente absorbed AIR, Irons agreed to an offer from an individual he had met during his days of securing cadavers for anatomy instruction—Leo Hosford, president of the San Francisco College of Mortuary Science. Hosford told Irons he could continue his work at the college, which had an unused laboratory and a $25,000 research fund. In exchange, any practical result from the research would become the property of the college.[79]

Hosford again used his undertaking connections to arrange for clinical trials of Hepasyn, the trade name the San Francisco college selected for arginase. The Chief of Staff of Hollywood Presbyterian Hospital, E. Forrest Boyd (known as "Frosty" Boyd since his days on the Stanford University football team),[80] had a patient who served as attorney to and an officer for the Forest Lawn Cemetery in Pasadena. The attorney knew Hosford from mortuary conventions, and he alerted Boyd to the San Francisco college's interest in testing Hepasyn. Favorably impressed with Hosford and the Hepasyn operation, and having secured permission and general investigational guidelines from the research committee of Hollywood Presbyterian Hospital, Boyd began testing Irons-manufactured Hepasyn in November 1950.[81]

Within a year Boyd had treated about 100 patients with Hepasyn.[82] By the Summer of 1951, when Vrat's articles on experimental therapeutics with arginase appeared and reports of Boyd's success with Hepasyn were coming out of Los Angeles, the Cancer Commission of the California Medical Association began to investigate. The Permanente Foundation issued a public letter in October responding to rumors of a cancer cure by indicating that "no encouraging response" had been derived from arginase.[83]

About the same time, the Cancer Commission alerted the National Research Council's Committee on Cancer Diagnosis and Therapy—the organization to which Irons and Vrat had sought support during their collaboration—to the situation in California. On October 22d the NRC committee requested Boyd to submit to them any animal or clinical data he might have. At the same time, the committee requested FDA to provide any information the agency might have about arginase in the treatment of cancer.[84] This was not the first time the agency had heard of arginase, but it did prompt FDA to inspect the manufacturing facilities of the San Francisco College of Mortuary Science.[85] However, since Hepasyn had not moved in interstate commerce, the inspectors could do little but note some manufacturing problems that, in years to come, would continue to plague Hepasyn production.

March and April of 1952 was a tumultuous time for the Hepasyn collaborators, and yet the mortuary school was still over a year away from filing a new drug application. Irons and Boyd published promising results of Irons' animal work in *Arizona Medicine*; eventually Boyd reported similar findings with his clinical cases. The authors claimed that Hepasyn significantly attenuated tumor growth, caused the encapsulation of tumors to afford neat surgical separation from healthy tissues, disorganized tumor activity at the cellular level, and deposited calcium in the tumor material.[86] In the popular press, Irons claimed the preliminary clinical results were hopeful enough to continue the trial.[87]

The research committee of Hollywood Presbyterian Hospital was less impressed; they suspended Boyd's clinical investigations pending the outcome of independent tests to confirm the animal studies. The Sloan-Kettering Memorial Institute for Cancer Research concluded that Hepasyn did not retard tumor growth and that tumors in treated and untreated animals were virtually indistinguishable.[88] Moreover, a damaging series of articles by science writer Milton Silverman appeared in the *San Francisco Chronicle* in late April that catalogued the negative reaction to this work by many in the clinical and biomedical communities.[89] Thus, by this time state medical officials lambasted the results, recognized experts in argisine biochemistry could not duplicate either Irons or Vrat's results, the clinical trials at the hospital where the lead investigator was chief of staff were suspended by his colleagues, and the whole disagreeable affair had been paraded in the media. So naturally the

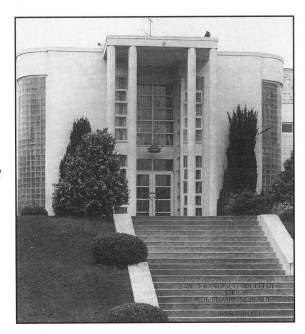

The San Francisco College of Mortuary Science (est. 1930), which Leo Hosford headed as the founding director, produced Wesley Irons' liver extract under the brand name Hepasyn and served as E. Forrest Boyd's clinic where ambulatory cancer patients received this drug (San Francisco History Center, San Francisco Public Library).

San Francisco College of Mortuary Science proceeded to submit a new drug application for Hepasyn!

Even though the school sent the NDA to their Washington attorney on 25 June 1953, the application was not actually filed by the attorney for over five months.[90] Another FDA inspection of the Hepasyn manufacturing facility at the San Francisco college revealed ongoing production concerns, such as the fact that sterility testing was done organoleptically on this parenteral drug. Also, with Hollywood Presbyterian Hospital no longer allowing clinical trials of Hepasyn, the college of mortuary science instituted their own clinic in April 1953, with Boyd traveling to San Francisco once a week to administer the drug to ambulatory patients.[91]

Boyd claimed that he treated 175 patients with Hepasyn, yet he submitted results for only ten "typical" patients in the NDA, covering a variety of cancers: brain, lung, bone, breast, and so on.[92] The patients, according to the NDA, did not experience any harm or complications from the therapy. Quite to the contrary, tumor masses were densely encapsulated, most of the patients reduced their pain medication, they all developed a sense of euphoria, most gained weight, and the patients experienced no metastases from the cancer after beginning treatment. It was, as he said, "convincing evidence that something unusual has transpired in these patients." Even the three patients who died had shown improvement.[93] The NDA avoided using the word "cure," yet the results clearly claimed that Hepasyn "benefited" patients in several specific ways. This distinction would be important to the FDA's defense of its actions on Hepasyn three years later.

The FDA, perhaps not surprisingly, regarded the application as incomplete and therefore officially not filed with the agency. For example, pertinent publications and reports were not part of the NDA, reports that perhaps not coincidentally reflected negatively on the value of Hepasyn in animal studies. Moreover, the agency informed the San Francisco college that "10 case histories can hardly be regarded as full reports of investigations made, when 175 case histories are said to be available." Labeling for physicians was lacking, as well as quality control procedures to be used in the manufacturing. Finally, the college had failed to indicate how the activity and potency of Hepasyn would be specified. This last issue was especially important, as the FDA reviewing pharmacologist indicated to his superior: "It seems to me that without some measure of activity of the product, it is impossible to establish an *effective* dose and therefore impossible to establish a *safe* dose."[94] Commissioner George Larrick made it clear to the college that it was indeed in their best interest to complete the NDA, because based on the information thus far available, the therapeutic value of their drug seemed dubious. Hepasyn, albeit safe, had to be of some benefit as well if sold for cancer, and the agency was prepared to let the federal courts settle the issue if necessary.[95]

Meanwhile, the mortuary college was trying to recover from the recent departure of Irons, who said he left principally because of Hosford, a man he characterized as avaricious and unethical, singularly responsible for rushing the NDA for Hepasyn. In fact, Irons appears to have left before the NDA was actually filed.[96] He did not give up on arginase, though. In February 1954 he moved his production to another San Francisco area location and began manufacturing arginase for clinical tests at the Arenac Osteopathic Clinic of the Marilyn Memorial Osteopathic Hospital in Au Gres, Michigan. The three osteopaths at the Arenac Clinic, using homeopathic concentrations of arginase,[97] treated about seventy patients within six months with what they described as most efficacious results, pending follow-up. But they endeavored to halt the investigations if their initial promising results began to sour.[98]

Why the group abandoned arginase is not clear, though Irons' contract with Hosford gave the San Francisco college exclusive commercial rights to Irons' work.[99] For whatever reason, their work shifted abruptly, because in May 1955 Arenac Laboratories of San Leandro (the first of three names Irons gave his manufacturing operation during the history of this new drug application) filed a new drug application for Acutalyn, a liver extract for the treatment of arthritis.[100] This extract, according to the sponsors, worked on arthritis through a mechanism analogous to that claimed for arginase's action against cancer. Irons and his colleagues believed the base, guanidine, was closely involved in the etiology of arthritis, and that Acutalyn reduced guanidine *in vitro* to urea.[101] Physicochemically, arginase and Acutalyn were very similar—so much that Irons submitted his animal work with arginase to establish that "no adverse effects have *ever* [emphasis in original] been noted" with Acutalyn. The latter, the NDA stated, was the active component of the compound he had been investigating since 1940 as arginase;[102] a rather casual dismissal of Irons' 15 years of allegedly promising results with argisine in cancer.

The agency had an incredulous reaction to the claim of complete freedom from adverse reactions with this parenterally administered product, particularly because there was no documentation to support it. The evidence for clinical safety and efficacy was questionable as well, since the sponsors submitted data in the form of summaries and averages; individual case histories, they said, were available on request. The above, coupled with other data lacking in the application such as manufacturing controls, not surprisingly led the new drug branch to regard the NDA as incomplete.[103] Irons and the osteopaths responded instead with testimonials; in fact, in September 1955 one of the osteopaths admitted that in the case of outpatients—who made up many of the test subjects—there were no records of their treatment. Only a month earlier he had assured the FDA that they had records of over 200 cases of different types of arthritis "successfully controlled" with Acutalyn.[104]

By the Spring of 1956, having grown tired of waiting for the FDA to move on the NDA, Irons and his attorney drew up a point-by-point rebuttal to the agency's insistence that the NDA was incomplete, in need of additional data. For example, responding to the agency's desire to see stability data on Acutalyn, Irons and his attorney said the new drug branch did not understand organic chemistry because they should know that Acutalyn could easily have an expiration date of 150 years; they used a six-month expiration instead "just as a protection to user and recipient."[105] The new drug branch reminded Irons that he still failed to supply the additional data to complete the application. However, FDA allowed Irons to file the application over the branch's protest anyway, under recent regulations the agency had proposed for cases in which the agency and NDA sponsor differed over the completeness of an application. On 3 October Irons withdrew the Acutalyn NDA rather than proceed to a hearing on the application's merit.[106] When he persisted in distributing Acutalyn through normal commercial channels under the guise of investigational status, FDA took Irons to court for marketing an unapproved drug, to which Irons pleaded no contest and was fined $600. Irons' liver extract had a third life, as Heparamine, also an arthritis treatment. Though the FDA took no action in this case, the California State Department of Public Health arrested Irons in 1960 for violating state drug laws. He passed away seven years later.[107]

Returning to Irons' former partners in the Hepasyn saga, the manufacturing problems with the drug worsened when the mortuary college expanded the variety of dosage forms: supposedly enteric-coated tablets, suppositories, and an ointment, all intended for self-medication use at home after the eight-week course of Hepasyn injections. Inelegant and untested for potency or dissolution or anything, widening the range of dosage forms perhaps was not the most appropriate direction for the company to take. The stability of the injectable product was still unknown, and the sterility testing was grossly inadequate as far as the agency was concerned.[108] The organization of clinical work changed by August 1954, presumably prompted by Boyd needing to cut back his trips to San Francisco. The Hepasyn clinic was moved from the mortuary college to another San Francisco location, on Ellis Street, where two physicians carried out the work under Boyd's directions.[109]

As glaring as the manufacturing problems were, the agency focused on the clinical evidence because this was the key to establishing the link between efficacy and safety. The mortuary college appeared ready to oblige the agency, a fact that perturbed the secretary of the college who believed his colleagues were "laying too much stress upon efficacy when it is safety that is involved under the New Drug section of the law."[110] Barring more convincing clinical studies, the FDA believed arginase ineffective in the treatment of cancer.

However, as long as the mortuary college operation remained local in scope and did not promote Hepasyn to attract patients from outside California, then FDA was willing to bypass regulatory action. These circumstances were in direct contrast with the agency's experience with the infamous Hoxsey cancer cure.[111] Still, stringing the "incomplete NDA" along in search of more clinical evidence and manufacturing data did not sit well with the pharmacologist who reviewed the original NDA submission: "I believe we are contributing to the delinquency of a cancer quack (pseudo-scientific variety) by considering this New Drug Application. As long as we continue to negotiate with this outfit about an NDA they continue under the guise of a scientific investigation in the treatment of cancer patients."[112]

Boyd submitted additional case evidence, reiterating the earlier claims for improvement afforded by Hepasyn. But FDA still regarded the NDA incomplete because it lacked full reports of investigations to demonstrate Hepasyn's safety; for example, the application lacked pathological evidence to document the product's therapeutic value.[113] But by October 1955, nearly two years after the original data were filed, the agency believed the mortuary college had submitted sufficient information to complete the NDA, and informed the college that its review would require the full six-month period allowable by law.[114] In effect, the FDA launched an investigation into the safety-efficacy issue:

> We have given considerable thought to the proper handling of this application and have decided in conjunction with [General Counsel William] Goodrich that since this preparation is ineffective in the treatment of malignant disease its use is not safe in such situations. In other words, while section 505 does not refer to efficacy we are going to try and take the position that efficacy is so intimately bound up in the use of this material that the lack of efficacy will make it unsafe for use.[115]

During the remainder of the year the agency began to marshall evidence on the assumption that the San Francisco College of Mortuary Science, if their NDA were denied at least in part on the basis that it was ineffective against cancer, would appeal the decision in a formal hearing. Indeed, some agency officials close to the case believed Hepasyn—the pyrogenicity problem connected to its manufacture aside—was relatively non-toxic.[116]

The key, of course, was its use in a life-threatening condition for which other therapies offered bona fide relief. Thus, field personnel began tracking down Boyd's patient records at Hollywood Presbyterian Hospital and at the Hepasyn clinics in San Francisco. Possible expert witnesses were approached, those familiar with both the animal studies and the clinical performance of Hepasyn. The handful of other physicians besides Boyd who were involved in the clinical work were interviewed. Other individuals familiar with the studies at Hollywood Presbyterian became potential sources, such as representatives from Cutter Laboratories, which had considered investing in the Hepasyn work early on but quickly backed out. The agency even looked

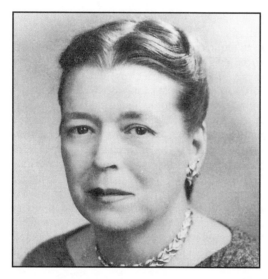

FDA medical officer Barbara Moulton organized the agency's case against Hepasyn in anticipation of a hearing with the San Francisco College of Mortuary Science (courtesy of Sally Brewster Moulton).

into the Permanente Foundation's experience with argisine.[117]

In late December 1955 Commissioner Larrick advised the college that the agency planned to deny the NDA on the grounds that 1) "Safety has not been proven because of lack of proof of efficacy in diseases that are invariably fatal unless treated with adequate efficacious means," 2) "The manufacturing and control procedures are inadequate," and 3) "There is evidence of untrue statements and misleading omissions of material facts." Unless the NDA were withdrawn, a notice of hearing would be issued next month.[118] The college, still unprepared to go to a hearing, chose to withdraw the NDA instead, with the intention of resubmitting it when they felt their evidence was adequate to stand up in a hearing.[119]

In the following months the college attempted to resubmit the Hepasyn NDA twice, and despite the agency's claim that it was incomplete, the college insisted that the NDA be considered as "filed;" their own preparations for the anticipated hearing apparently were ready. Thus, the countdown to a formal hearing began on 9 January 1957.[120] With the hearing only a few months away, Albert Holland, medical director at FDA, recognized that Hepasyn "may well be a precedent-establishing case no matter which way the courts decide it," that this would be "one of the most significant contests that has faced the Administration."[121]

The agency's strategy would be ill-served, according to Barbara Moulton, the principal medical investigator for the case, if they relied on proof that Hepasyn did not cure cancer; the mortuary college never said it would. Rather, it was necessary to establish that each one of the therapeutic claims for Hepasyn was unproven: that it produced marked pain relief, prolonged useful life, produced visibly smaller tumors, yielded x-ray and biochemical evidence of healing, and effected encapsulation of tumors for facile surgical removal. Each of these claims had to be destroyed because the agency had already approved other cancer treatments, much more toxic than Hepasyn, that afforded limited relief, such as hormones, antimetabolites, and radioisotopes.[122]

District offices in California continued with the earlier efforts to secure details of Boyd's patients; an inspector copied over 11,000 pages of records at Hollywood Presbyterian Hospital.[123] Work continued on a witness list, with various members of the physician staff at Hollywood Presbyterian added. Other district offices in home states of Hepasyn patients tracked the outcome of therapy, which Boyd had not included in the NDA. A final inspection of the Hepasyn production facility would check if control procedures had improved.[124] On April 8th FDA issued a notice that a hearing would be held in one month because of the agency's decision to prevent the NDA for Hepasyn from becoming effective.[125]

One week later Boyd resigned from the Hepasyn project, in part because of mounting pressure from the California Medical Association and other physicians, and in part because of his personal belief that physicians and court cases did not make for good publicity.[126] A week after that the agency and the mortuary college met in a pre-hearing conference and the college was presented with some of the clinical evidence FDA had discovered. There were scores of inconsistencies and omissions between the NDA and the actual clinical case record; the pre-Hepasyn status of many patients was misstated; and the pathological evidence did not support any therapeutic claim for Hepasyn.[127] Three days later the San Francisco college withdrew its NDA rather than go through with the hearing, which prompted Commissioner Larrick to inform the college that their data were "thoroughly discredited" and would not support any future new drug application.[128] The story, however, was not quite concluded.

Nothing in the Food, Drug, and Cosmetic Act made unlawful the submission of false statements in a new drug application, but the United States Code subjected anyone who "knowingly and willingly" falsified or concealed material facts in any matter within the jurisdiction of any agency to a fine of up $10,000 and imprisonment of up to five years. Of the three principals, Moulton believed Irons was the least culpable since he departed shortly before the NDA was first filed. Hosford, over whose signature the NDA was submitted, was legally responsible, though Moulton believed he could easily plead that he was an innocent victim of others' fraud, too ignorant of medical matters.[129] Moulton placed the greatest blame on Boyd, based on the clinical records she reviewed and the fact that he was a good surgeon yet knew he was "associating with individuals who were qualified neither in research, medical training, or moral standing."[130] Eventually the agency decided it would be impossible to prove that any of the principals "knowingly or willingly" falsified the NDA;[131] shades, perhaps, of the Sherley amendment.

Efficacy on Trial: Altafur

The Hepasyn case never went to a hearing, but two years after those proceedings were supposed to begin, Eaton Laboratories, a division of the Norwich Pharmacal Company, submitted a new drug application that FDA eventually opposed largely on the basis of lack of efficacy. And that case *did* proceed to a hearing. Following the 1936 report by pharmacologist Chauncey Leake of the University of California at San Francisco that furan derivatives appeared to have bactericidal properties, researchers at Eaton began to develop the nitrofurans as a broad-spectrum class of antibacterial agents in the mid-1940s.[132] Altafur (furaltadone) was a product of Eaton's nitrofuran program, and the firm submitted a new drug application for Altafur tablets to

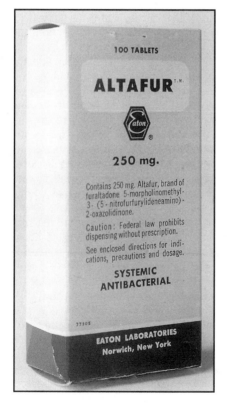

Altafur (furaltadone), a systemic antibacterial agent introduced by the Eaton Laboratories division of Norwich Pharmacal Company in 1959, led to the safety-efficacy hearing that never materialized in the Hepasyn case.

Once Altafur's efficacy came into question, particularly vis-à-vis the rising adverse reactions associated with this drug, FDA objected to Eaton Laboratories' promotion of Altafur as a drug of first choice.

*ALTAFUR effected 78% favorable results (129 cures, 57 improvements) among 240 patients previously treated unsuccessfully with other antibacterial agents.

Christenson, P. J., and Tracy, C. H.: Current Therapeutic Research 2 :22, 1960.

Altafur®

brand of furaltadone

tablets of 250 mg. (adult) and 50 mg. (pediatric), bottles of 20 and 100

Note: Each dose should be taken with food or milk. Alcohol should not be ingested in any form during ALTAFUR therapy and for one week thereafter.

a therapy of first choice in

- **bacterial pneumonias** ■ **bronchiolitis**
- **bronchitis** ■ **tonsillitis** ■ **otitis media**
- **soft tissue infections** ■ **cellulitis and abscess** ■ **surgical wound infections**
- **infected lacerations**

■ perorally effective against the majority of common pathogenic bacteria, including the antibiotic-resistant staphylococci ■ decisive bactericidal action ■ development of significant bacterial resistance has not been encountered ■ side effects minimal or avoidable ■ does not destroy normal intestinal flora or encourage monilial overgrowth (little or no fecal excretion)

THE NITROFURANS — a *unique* class of antimicrobials

EATON LABORATORIES, NORWICH, NEW YORK

FDA on 1 May 1959. The agency requested some additional chemical data on the product, but the application was made effective on 9 September.[133]

By late October Eaton received thirty reports of reversible circulatory and neurological side effects associated with the consumption of alcohol in patients using Altafur. The firm alerted practitioners to these reactions with a "Dear Doctor" letter that included word of the "very impressive" therapeutic results achieved so far with Altafur.[134] By late May 1960 practitioners reported several cases of double vision with Altafur—without any alcohol involvement.[135] Soon news of adverse reactions increased; more visual disturbances and serious circulatory disorders.

In July the agency met with Eaton to discuss Altafur's toxicity, particularly with respect to what FDA believed were "meager and unconvincing data" for the drug's efficacy.[136] FDA's concern with the latter stemmed from a recommendation by a National Research Council committee, headed by Phillip Miller of the University of Chicago. HEW Secretary Arthur Flemming commissioned this group to review the policies, procedures, and decisions of FDA's Division of Antibiotics and the New Drug Division of the Antibiotic Branch in the wake of the Henry Welch affair. The committee evaluated over two dozen NDAs that FDA had preselected as important or controversial; Altafur was among this group of applications, and committee member Wesley Spink of the University of Minnesota inspected that NDA around the time FDA notified Eaton about the agency's efficacy concerns. According to Commissioner Larrick, the Miller committee recommended FDA to reconsider Altafur. In its report of 27 September 1960 to Secretary Flemming, the first of eleven recommendations made by this committee was that FDA should be given statutory authority for drug efficacy as well as safety, because the latter could depend on the former.[137]

Eaton believed FDA was treating Altafur unfairly compared to chloramphenicol, the effective broad-spectrum antibiotic that had been known since the early 1950s to cause fatal blood dyscrasias in some patients. However, FDA's focus on evidence for the therapeutic value of Altafur suggested the difference between the two cases. Specifically, the agency's concern with the nitrofuran addressed 1) the many serious infections Eaton claimed Altafur could treat, such as endocarditis and osteomyelitis; 2) the fact that Eaton promoted Altafur as a drug of first choice in a range of infections that included bacterial pneumonias, surgical wound infections, and bronchitis; 3) the claim that Altafur worked against antibiotic-resistant staph infections, though the *in vitro* studies upon which this claim was based required a minimum inhibitory concentration of Altafur well above the plasma level attainable even with triple the recommended dosage; and 4) the paucity of reports on Altafur from clinical researchers experienced with antibiotic therapy and infectious diseases.[138]

FDA threatened to suspend the new drug application, but agreed to continue it on a conditionally effective basis for three months. Eaton agreed to cease promoting Altafur and revised the labeled indications drastically: for use only in those infections untreatable with other drugs. During the interim period FDA would reconsider the extant data on Altafur, examine any additional information Eaton might submit, and secure the opinions of experts in the treatment of infectious diseases.[139]

The company submitted additional case studies to FDA, as well as interpretations of all the clinical cases in the NDA by four investigators. All suggested that Altafur appeared to occupy a therapeutic niche, though three urged more study. FDA concluded its study somewhat differently: the marketing of Altafur should be discontinued at once, and if the firm wanted to review clinical data with the agency further, it would best be done in the venue of a hearing to decide the suspension of the Altafur NDA.[140] This was based partly on the neurological, hematological, gastrointestinal, and dermatological reactions with Altafur, but the thrust of the agency's objections stemmed from their interpretation that Altafur simply wasn't efficacious to justify its toxicity. Again, here was the link between safety and efficacy.[141]

The hearing, conducted by examiner Edward E. Turkel of the Social Security Administration, began on 23 January 1961 and lasted several weeks. It took Turkel several months after that to sort out the considerable testimony by each side and their witnesses. Those testifying for Eaton included a physician who first reported the deleterious effects of Altafur on vision. FDA's witnesses included one of the four physicians whom Eaton had used to interpret their final submission of clinical evidence. Eaton, represented principally by the celebrated food and drug law specialist Vincent Kleinfeld, argued strenuously that efficacy was irrelevant in the consideration of the Altafur NDA and immaterial as far as the hearing was concerned; the law required safety only. But Turkel allowed the efficacy testimony, which ran hundreds of pages in the hearing transcript.

In the end, it was the efficacy issue that decided the hearing in FDA's favor. Turkel was persuaded particularly by the testimony of Maxwell Finland of Harvard and George Jackson of Illinois, which strongly disputed any therapeutic value of Altafur; Finland had been a member of the Miller committee of the National Academy of Sciences.[142] Turkel contrasted this with the methodologically flawed clinical results of Eaton's witnesses, which included the simultaneous use of Altafur with antibiotic drugs and with other therapies without employing clinical controls, and failure to identify causative organisms. The weight he assigned to the different results derived largely from the examiner's distinction between clinical research and medical and even medical specialty practice: "Procedures followed in clinical research with drugs are different than the procedures followed in the ordinary practice of medicine. In evaluating the toxicity and efficacy of a new drug a whole variety of in vitro and in vivo work is done in clinical research which is not done in the private practice of medicine."[143] Here, Turkel's explanation simply echoed what the American Medical Association had argued.

Turkel reasoned that, to whatever extent Altafur might be of some value in lesser infections, its toxicity did not justify its use, especially given that other, less toxic antibacterial drugs were available. Therefore, based on his findings that efficacy was a relevant issue to this case, that the evidence indicated Altafur was ineffective, and that the treatment of serious conditions could not be delayed, Turkel concluded that Altafur was not safe for the conditions indicated in the labeling and ordered the NDA suspended.[144] It was analogous to the argument for penicillin certification in 1941.

Eaton appealed the issue, but the agency upheld the examiner's decision and suspended the NDA for Altafur on 16 August 1962, less than two months before Congress passed the 1962 drug amendments. The firm did not press its case in court.[145] Ironically, six days after the final ruling on Altafur, FDA approved a new drug application from Eaton Laboratories for furaltadone. However, this was under the trade name Valsyn Gel, a treatment for staphylococcal mastitis in cows.[146]

It is little wonder that former Commissioner of Food and Drugs Arthur Hayes, Jr., said the 1962 amendments did not invent drug efficacy evaluations; they merely codified them.[147] By the time Senator Kefauver began the hearings that ultimately ended with a new drug law that embraced efficacy, the latter was already an established component of public health in America. We can see this witnessed in many institutions: in the early nineteenth century it was an important part of the founding principles of what would be our official drug compendium, federal agencies enforced it since the administration of Teddy Roosevelt, it was the basis of voluntary certification by a professional society for half of this century, Congress wrote it explicitly into federal drug law by the early 1940s, and it served as a key criterion in the evaluation of new drug applications for selected products years before the Kefauver-Harris amendments. When we begin to think about rolling back efficacy standards, history might help us remember why we had them in the first place.

Notes and References

Acknowledgment: I am indebted to Frances Kelsey for her comments and suggestions.

1. "Abolishing GMPs and Other Plans for FDA," *Dickinson's FDA Review* 3, no. 2 (February 1996): 23.
2. Vaccine Act of 1813, 2 *U. S. Stat.* 806: Peter Barton Hutt, "The Transformation of United States Food and Drug Law," *Journal of the Association of Food and Drug Officials* 60, no. 3 (1996): 18; Import Drug Act of 1848, 9 *U. S. Stat.* 237 (26 June 1848) (quotation); and James Harvey Young, *Pure Food: Securing the Federal Food and Drugs Act of 1906* (Princeton: Princeton University Press, 1989), 3-17. I thank Peter Barton Hutt for bringing the efficacy elements of these two laws to my attention.
3. *Pharmacopoeia of the United States of America* (Boston: Charles Ewer, 1820), 17.
4. USP (1820), 21, quoted in Glenn Sonnedecker, rev., *Kremers and Urdang's History of Pharmacy*, 4th ed. (Philadelphia: J. B. Lippincott, 1976), 263; see also idem, "The Founding Period of the U. S. Pharmacopeia: III. The First Edition," *Pharmacy in History* 36 (1994): 104-105, 109, and 112, and Lee Anderson and Gregory J. Higby, *The Spirit of Voluntarism, A Legacy of Commitment and Contribution: The United States Pharmacopeia, 1820-1995*

(Rockville, Md: United States Pharmacopoeial Convention, 1995), 22-23.

5. USP (1820) (n. 3).

6. *Pharmacopoeia of the United States of America* (New York: William Wood, 1882), xxi.

7. Anderson and Higby, *Spirit of Voluntarism* (n. 4), pp. 167-168 (quote is on p. 167, from 1890 Circular 22, 22 September 1890).

8. Anderson and Higby, *Spirit of Voluntarism* (n. 4), 180; Higby cites as examples asafetida, myrrh, and musk, as well as pharmaceutical necessities such as lemon oil and licorice root.

9. Anderson and Higby, *Spirit of Voluntarism* (n. 4), 205, 207, 215.

10. Anderson and Higby, *Spirit of Voluntarism* (n. 4), 212.

11. Anderson and Higby, *Spirit of Voluntarism* (n. 4), 224-227, which includes discussion of some of the problematical issues associated with including proprietary pharmaceuticals in the USP.

12. Anderson and Higby, *Spirit of Voluntarism* (n. 4), 290-292, 341-342, and 366-367.

13. James Harvey Young, *The Medical Messiahs: A Social History of Health Quackery in Twentieth-Century America* (Princeton: Princeton University Press, 1967; 1992), 66-67.

14. *Annual Report of the Surgeon General of the United States Public Health and Marine Hospital Service*, 1906: 233; 1909: 76.

15. Arnold Thackray, et al., *Chemistry in America, 1876-1976* (Dordrecht: D. Reidel Publishing, 1985), 130. Harvey Wiley's *Report of the Chemist for 1899, U. S. Department of Agriculture*, p. 30, reports that the Postmaster General submitted an article marked "rauchsault" on 6 April 1897, and his division was able to report that it was not poisonous, dangerous, or explosive, and in no way unsuitable for the mails.

16. Young, *Medical Messiahs* (n. 13), 69-72.

17. Young, *Medical Messiahs* (n. 13), 73.

18. *Federal Food, Drug and Cosmetic Law: Administrative Reports, 1907-1949* (Chicago: Commerce Clearing House, 1951), 101 (Report of the Bureau of Chemistry, from Annual Reports of the Department of Agriculture, 1909, p. 433).

19. Young, *Medical Messiahs* (n. 13), 86-87.

20. Lyman F. Kebler, "Public Health Conserved through the Enforcement of Postal Fraud Laws," *Am. J. Public Health* 12 (1922): 678-683.

21. The labeling provision did not enter the regulations until 1919. See Eugene A. Timm, "75 Years Compliance with Biological Product Regulations," *Food Drug Cosmetic Law J.* 33 (1978): 226, and United States Public Health Service, Treasury Department, *Regulations for the Sale of Viruses, Serums, Toxins and Analogous Products in the District of Columbia and in Interstate Traffic*, Misc. Publication No. 10 (Washington, D. C.: Government Printing Office, 1919), 11: "each package shall be marked with the date beyond which the contents can not be expected beyond reasonable doubt to yield their specific results."

22. U. S. Public Health and Marine-Hospital Service, Treasury Department, *Regulations for the Sale of Viruses, Serums, Toxins, and Analogous Products in the District of Columbia, Etc.*, Misc. Publication No. 4 (Washington, D. C.: Government Printing Office, 1903), 5-7, and Laurence F. Schmeckebier, *The Public Health Service: Its History, Activities and Organization*, Institute for Government Research: Service Monographs of the United States Government, No. 10 (Baltimore: Johns Hopkins Press, 1923), 131.

23. Ramunas A. Kondratas, "Biologics Control Act of 1902," in *The Early Years of Federal Food and Drug Control* (Madison: American Institute of the History of Pharmacy, 1982), 20, 27. Under the Public Health Service Act of 1944, which consolidated the 1902 act along with other laws under the PHS's jurisdiction, a biologic product was, by definition, a serum, toxin,

etc. "applicable to the prevention, treatment or cure of diseases or injuries of man;" see 12 *Fed. Reg.* 6218, 16 September 1947.

24. "Mixed Vaccines," *Journal of the American Medical Association* 65 (1915): 720.

25. *Regulation of Sale of Viruses, Serums, Toxins and Analogous Products, etc.*, Hearings before the Subcommittee of the Committee on the District of Columbia, House of Representatives, 68th Congress, 1st Sess., on H. R. 5845, H. R. 7366, and H. R. 8618, 21 and 25 February 1924, 3 and 24 March 1924, 30 April 1924, and 6 May 1924 (Washington: Government Printing Office, 1924), 19.

26. G. W. McCoy, "Official Methods of Control of Remedial Agents for Human Use," *J. Am. Med. Assoc.* 74 (1920): 1554.

27. According to McCoy, "to secure the data by controlled clinical experiments, save in most exceptional cases, is impossible;" "Official Methods" (n. 26): 1554.

28. McCoy, "Official Methods" (n. 26): 1554-1555 (cf. *Regulation of Sale of Viruses*, 53); A. M. Stimson, *A Brief History of Bacteriological Investigations of the United States Public Health Service*, Supp. No. 141 to *Public Health Reports* (Washington, D. C.: Government Printing Office, 1938): 21-23; and meeting of the Advisory Board, Surgeon General's Office, Washington, D. C., 2 January 1925, 64-page transcript (file 0240, box 34, PHS Records, RG 90, National Archives, Washington, D. C.), p. 4: "For a number of years acting under a ruling made by the Surgeon General's office and approved by the Secretary, we have declined to issue a new license for biologic products unless there was a reason and proof of their worth and it has led to some rather peculiar situations." Perhaps one such situation was that of Friedmann and von Ruck's alleged tuberculosis cure, discussed by Stimson above.

29. Victor H. Kramer, *The National Institute of Health: A Study in Public Administration* (New Haven, Conn.: Quinnipiack Press, 1937), 31.

30. *Regulation of Sale of Viruses* (n. 25): 7 (includes quote), 18, 53, and 55, and *Drug Industry Antitrust Act*, Hearings before the Subcommittee on Antitrust and Monopoly of the Committee on the Judiciary, U. S. Senate, 87th Congress, 1st Sess., pursuant to S. Res. 52 on S. 1552, 13 and 15 September 1961 and 12-13 and 18-29 December 1961, Part 5 (Washington, D. C.: Government Printing Office, 1962), 2582-2583 (*A Legislative History of the Federal Food, Drug, and Cosmetic Act and Its Amendments* 20: 324-325).

31. *Regulation of Sale of Viruses* (n. 25): 9-11, 21-22, 32-33, 48, 66-67, 113, 144, and 158-221 (which reproduces the many letters and editorials that poured in from groups of physicians opposed to the bill).

32. *Regulation of Sale of Viruses* (n. 25), 48-68 *passim*.

33. "New Amendment for Serum Act," *J. Am. Med. Assoc.* 83 (1924): 1270.

34. "New Amendment" (n. 33); "The Rathbone Bill on Serums and Vaccines," *J. Am. Med. Assoc.* 82 (1924): 886-887; and *Regulation of Sale of Viruses* (n. 25), 158-221.

35. Compare the concerns voiced by McCoy's colleagues Ralph Dyer and Walter Harrison, *Regulation of Sale of Viruses* (n. 25), 140 and 226, with McCoy's earlier testimony.

36. Kramer, *National Institute of Health* (n. 29), 32-33.

37. Food and Drugs Act of 1906, Public Law 59-384 (34 *U. S. Stat.* 768), 30 June 1906, Sec. 8.

38. James Harvey Young, "Drugs and the 1906 Law," in John B. Blake, ed., *Safeguarding the Public: Historical Aspects of Medicinal Drug Control* (Baltimore: Johns Hopkins Press, 1970), 148-149, and Ashley Sellers and Nathan D. Grundstein, "Administrative Procedure and Practice in the Department of Agriculture under the Federal Food, Drug, and Cosmetic Act of 1938," 308-page typescript in 2 Parts, Part I: 12 (FDA History Office files).

39. Mastin G. White and Otis H. Gates, *Decisions of Courts in Cases under the Federal Food and*

Drugs Act (Washington, D. C.: Government Printing Office, 1934), 267-269 (quotes are from p. 268).

40. Quoted in Young, "Drugs and the 1906 Law" (n. 38), 149.

41. Sellers and Grundstein, "Administrative Procedure and Practice" (n. 38), I: 14-15 n. 31.

42. Sherley Amendment of 1912, Public Law 62-301 (37 *U. S. Stat.* 416), 23 August 1912.

43. Young, "Drugs and the 1906 Law" (n. 38), 150, and Sellers and Grundstein, "Administrative Procedure and Practice" (n. 38), I: 13-14 n. 30.

44. White and Gates, *Decisions of Courts* (n. 39), 1240 ff.

45. Ruth deForest Lamb, *American Chamber of Horrors* (New York: Farrar and Rinehart, 1936), 64-68

46. Quoted in Harry Milton Marks, "Ideas as Reforms: Therapeutic Experiments and Medical Practice, 1900-1980," Ph. D. diss., Massachusetts Institute of Technology, 1987, 51.

47. Austin Smith, "The Council on Pharmacy and Chemistry and the Chemical Laboratory," in Morris Fishbein, *A History of the American Medical Association, 1847 to 1947* (Philadelphia: W. B. Saunders, 1947), 865.

48. The above relies principally on James G. Burrow, "The Prescription-Drug Policies of the American Medical Association," in John B. Blake, ed., *Safeguarding the Public: Historical Aspects of Medicinal Drug Control* (Baltimore: Johns Hopkins Press, 1970), 112-122. See also Jeffrey Bishop, "Drug Evaluation Programs of the AMA, 1905-1966," *JAMA* 196 (1966): 122-123; "Fiftieth Anniversary of the Council on Pharmacy and Chemistry," *J. Am. Med. Assoc.* 159 (1955): 1368; and Young, *Medical Messiahs* (n. 13), 129 ff.

49. Fishbein, *History of the AMA* (n. 47), 226-227 and 235-236, and Burrow, "Prescription-Drug Policies" (n. 48), 113-114.

50. Smith, "Council on Pharmacy and Chemistry" (n. 47), 876-877, and Fishbein, *History of the AMA* (n. 47), 884-885.

51. Paul Starr, *The Social Transformation of American Medicine* (New York: Basic Books, 1982), 133 (this rule was instituted in 1924).

52. Marks, "Ideas as Reforms"(n. 46), p. 45 n. 65.

53. Smith, "Council on Pharmacy and Chemistry"(n 47), 870 ff., and Austin E. Smith, "The Council on Pharmacy and Chemistry," *J. Am. Med. Assoc.* 124 (1944): 434 ff.

54. Harry F. Dowling, "The American Medical Association's Policy on Drugs in Recent Decades," in John B. Blake, ed., *Safeguarding the Public: Historical Aspects of Medicinal Drug Control* (Baltimore: Johns Hopkins Press, 1970), 126-127. The association's defense against antitrust violations around this time was much more expensive than the fine it incurred, according to Dowling. For elaboration on the AMA's abandonment of the seal of acceptance program, see idem, *Medicines for Man: The Development , Regulation, and Use of Prescription Drugs* (New York: Alfred A. Knopf, 1970), 170-177.

55. This was exactly the case with Clarin (heparin potassium), advertised in the 14 January 1961 issue of the *Journal* as being useful in postcoronary management, yet the 1961 edition of *NNR* said there was no convincing evidence that this product prevents or ameliorates cardiovascular disease; see *Drug Industry Antitrust Act* (n. 30), 2587-2588 (*Legislative History* 20: 329-330).

56. On some of the problems associated with organizing clinical research on therapeutic products around this time, see Harry M. Marks, "Notes from the Underground: The Social Organization of Therapeutic Research," in Russell C. Maulitz and Diana E. Long, eds., *Grand Rounds: One Hundred Years of Internal Medicine* (Philadelphia: University of Pennsylvania Press, 1988), 297-336.

57. Bishop, "Drug Evaluation Programs of the AMA" (n. 48), 123-124; "New Program of Operation for Evaluation of Drugs," *J. Am. Med. Assoc.* 158 (1955): 1170-1171; and Harry F. Dowling, "The Impact of the New Drug Laws on the Council on Drugs of the American Medical Association," *Clin. Research* 13 (1965): 162-165.

58. Smith, "Council on Pharmacy and Chemistry"(n. 47), 437-438 (note that the council authorized publication of this article).

59. Austin Smith to Robert P. Herwick, 25 April 1945, reproduced in Report No. 702, "Providing for Certification of Batches of Drugs Composed Wholly or Partly of Any Kind of Penicillin or Derivatives," Committee on Interstate and Foreign Commerce, House of Representatives, 79th Congress, 1st Session, 7 June 1945, p. 12 (*Legislative History* 7: 445).

60. Quoted in Dowling, "AMA's Policy on Drugs"(n. 54), 128; see Louis S. Goodman, "The Problem of Drug Efficacy: An Exercise in Dissection," in Paul Talalay, ed., *Drugs in Our Society* (Baltimore: Johns Hopkins Press, 1964), 65-66 ("The average practicing physician, and for three decades I have helped to train many, many hundreds of them, does not have the time, the facilities, the skill, nor the training to be able to determine drug efficacy"). See also Hearings before the Subcommittee on Antitrust and Monopoly of the Committee on the Judiciary, U. S. Senate, 87th Congress, 1st Session, 13 and 15 September 1961, 12, 13, 18-20 December 1961, Part 5: 2587-2588 (*Legislative History* 20: 329-330).

61. Quoted in Dowling, "AMA's Policy on Drugs"(n. 54), 128.

62. Trade Correspondence 13 (1 December 1939), 343 (13 December 1940), and 376 (10 December 1941; quote), in Vincent A. Kleinfeld and Charles Wesley Dunn, *Federal Food, Drug, and Cosmetic Act: Judicial and Administrative Record, 1938-1949* (Chicago: Commerce Clearing House, n. d.), 574, 705-706, and 721, respectively. I am indebted to Marks, "Ideas as Reforms"(n. 46), 90-91, for alerting me to these cases.

63. Insulin Amendment of 1941, Public Law 77-366 (55 *U. S. Stat.* 851), 22 December 1941, Sec. 3.

64. See *Congressional Record*, 18 December 1941, pp. 9988-9989 (*Legislative History* 7: 92-93).

65. Penicillin Amendment of 1945, Public Law 79-139 (59 *U. S. Stat.* 463), 6 July 1945, Sec. 3.

66. Watson B. Miller to Sam Rayburn, 15 May 1945, reproduced in Report No. 702, "Providing for Certification" (n. 59), p. 10 (*Legislative History* 7: 443).

67. Miller to Rayburn, 15 May 1945.

68. H. R. 8904, 21 June 1950, p. 2, 81st Congress, 2d Session, and H. R. 3298, 16 July 1951, p. [5?], 82d Congress, 1st Session (*Legislative History* 11: 5, 268). The companion legislation in the Senate was worded similarly.

69. "Hearings before the Committee on Interstate and Foreign Commerce, House of Representatives, Eighty-Second Congress, First Session, on H. R. 3298," 1-5 May 1951, pp. 32-33 (*Legislative History* 11: 60-61); *Congressional Record*, 1 August 1951, pp. 9334 ff. (*Legislative History* 11: 337); David F. Cavers, "The Evolution of the Contemporary System of Drug Regulation under the 1938 Act," in *Safeguarding the Public: Historical Aspects of Medicinal Drug Control*, ed. John B. Blake (Baltimore: Johns Hopkins Press, 1970), 161-163; and Harry M. Marks, "Revisiting 'The Origins of Compulsory Drug Prescriptions,'" *Am. J. Public Health* 85 (1995): 109-115.

70. *Congressional Record*, 1 August 1951, p. 9335 (*Legislative History* 11: 338); ironically, the person who said this was Rep. Oren Harris of Arkansas, whose name would be forever linked with federally mandated drug efficacy in the 1962 amendments.

71. See Marks, "Ideas as Reforms"(n. 46), 70-80.

72. Mostafa S. Mohamed and David M. Greenberg, "Liver Arginase, I: Preparation of Extracts of

High Potency, Chemical Properties, Activation-Inhibition, and pH-Activity," *Arch. Biochem.* 8 (1945): 349.

73. David M. Greenberg and E. Norberg Sassenrath, "Lack of Efficacy of High Potency Arginase on Tumor Growth," *Cancer Res.* 13 (1953): 709.

74. The Electronic Medical Foundation was the successor to the College of Electronic Medicine, an institution that sought to perpetuate the doctrines of Albert Abrams. Abrams was a pathologist at Cooper Medical College (which was incorporated by Stanford University) when he developed his theory known as the Electronic Reactions of Abrams, or ERA, that claimed body parts emit electrical impulses of different frequencies, depending on whether the patient was sick or well.

Illness and personal characteristics such as sex, age, and religion could be identified by tuning in to the relevant frequency. By inserting into one apparatus a sample of dried blood—or even a signature—from a patient, and then hooking up another part of his machinery to a healthy person—a sort of proxy patient, Abrams claimed he could diagnose the disease. It did not matter whether the patient was on the other side of the room or the other side of the world. Having thus identified the patient's complaint, the therapeutic component of ERA, the oscilloclast, could be made to produce electrical impulses at the proper radio frequency to heal the ailing tissue or organ. Not coincidentally, Abrams devised ERA around the late 1910s and early 1920s, a time when radio was beginning to weave its way into American culture. See Young, *Medical Messiahs* (n. 13), pp. 137ff.

75. See Vrat's four articles that appeared in *Permanente Foundation Med. Bull.* 9, nos. 2 and 3 (July 1951): 49-74.

76. Both individuals suspected subterfuge on Vrat's part; on this and the clinical tests at the Permanente Foundation, see memorandum of interview between Cecil Cutting and Ralph W. Weilerstein (FDA), 30 November 1955, NDA 9214, "Mfr. No. 460, vol. 1;" memorandum of telephone conversation between Eaton MacKay and Ralph W. Weilerstein, 13 March 1957, NDA 9214, "Hepasyn—General Material;" memorandum of interview between Eaton MacKay and Ralph W. Weilerstein and Stanley J. Gilmore, 20 June 1952, NDA 9214, "Weilerstein's Material;" and Milton Silverman, "'Cancer Treatment' Discounted in Bay Area Tests," *San Francisco Chronicle*, 26 April 1952. Cutting reported ten patients in the arginase study, whereas Silverman mentions that there were five; both sources report the same outcome of the trial. I am grateful to Paul Peterson of FDA's San Francisco office for unearthing many of the Hepasyn papers I used.

77. Irons charged Vrat with pilfering his laboratory notebooks, and sued Vrat to that effect; how the lawsuit was resolved is not clear. See memorandum of interview between McKay and Weilerstein and Gilmore, 20 June 1952; Eugene Eno and Richard M. Stalvey, Factory Inspection Report: W. G. Irons Laboratory, San Francisco College of Mortuary Science, 12 December 1951, NDA 9214, "Mfr. No. 460, vol. 1," p. 7; and Silverman, "Cancer Treatment Discounted"(n. 76).

78. "The Treatment of Cancer with Arginase: A Report by the Cancer Commission of the California Medical Association," *California Med.* 79 (Sept. 1953): 248; memorandum of interview between Michael B. Shimkin and Barbara Moulton, 8 March 1957, NDA 9214, "Misc. File IV;" Van W. Smart, "Memorandum for the File: Summary of the Hepasyn Investigation," 10 March 1958, NDA 9214, "Hepasyn—General Material;" and Wesley G. Irons, "Arginine-Arginase Relationship in Regeneration, Repair and Development of Neoplasms," *J. Dental Research* 25 (December 1946): 497-499. There seems to be some confusion on exactly when Irons began working with arginase; one of his own publications said he began investigating

the enzyme in 1939, whereas the new drug application for this product stated that his work began in 1941. There is no doubt, though, that the bulk of his work began at UCSF.

79. Memorandum of interview between Wesley G. Irons and Alfred Barnard, Barbara Moulton, Van Smart, Stanley J. Gilmore, and William C. Hill, 19 December 1957, NDA 9214, vol. IB, and agreement between Dr. Wesley G. Irons and the San Francisco College of Mortuary Science, 28 August 1950, NDA 9214, vol. I' of II'.

80. Smart, "Summary of Hepasyn Investigation"(n. 78), 3.

81. Memorandum of interview between E. Forrest Boyd and Barbara Moulton and Van W. Smart, 12 December 1957, NDA 9214, vol. IB; Eno and Stalway, Factory Inspection Report, 12 December 1951, pp. 3, 7; and "Treatment of Cancer with Arginase"(n. 78), 248. Boyd was not the first clinician to use Hepasyn for the San Francisco college; George Chapman of San Francisco administered the drug to a handful of patients beginning in early November. Less than a half-dozen other physicians were involved at the beginning of the clinical stage, but Boyd was by far the most involved clinician. See above and Stanley J. Gilmore, Paul S. Jorgensen, and Joseph Bottini, Factory Inspection Report: Charles E. Irons Memorial Cancer Foundation, 30 April 1953, p. 10, NDA 9214, "Mfr. No. 460, vol. 1."

82. Eno and Stalvey, Factory Inspection Report, 12 December 1951, p. 3.

83. "Treatment of Cancer with Arginase"(n. 78), 248-249.

84. Eventually the FDA checked with the Laboratory of Biologics Control at the National Institutes of Health to see if arginase fell under the 1944 Public Health Service Act as a biological agent, and the Laboratory said it did not (memorandum of telephone conversation between William G. Workman and M. L. Yakowitz, 21 September 1954, NDA 9214, Misc. File IV).

85. Isabel M. Wason (NRC) to E. Forrest Boyd, 22 October 1951, and Isabel M. Wason to Erwin E. Nelson, 22 October 1951, attached to Division of Field Operations to San Francisco District, 27 November 1951, NDA 9214, "Mfr. No. 460, vol. 1," and Ainslie H. Drummond, Jr. and Robert G. Brandenburg to Chief, Los Angeles District, 28 August 1951, NDA 9214, "Weilerstein's Material."

86. W. G. Irons and E. Forrest Boyd, "Arginase as an Anti-Carcinogenic Agent in Mice and Human Beings," *Arizona Medicine* 9 (March 1952): 39-45.

87. Virginia Dennison, "'Doomed' Victims Test New Cancer Treatment," *Oakland Tribune* 12 March 1952.

88. "Treatment of Cancer with Arginase"(n. 78), 254, and "Sloan-Kettering Report, Parts I, II, and III," n. d., NDA 9214, "Mfr. No. 460, vol. 1" (this document, by agreement of 24 February 1953, includes a preliminary report by the San Francisco college, the Sloan-Kettering report, and a response to the Sloan-Kettering Report by the college). The experiments were done at the Sloan-Kettering laboratories in side-by-side experiments conducted by Irons and Sloan-Kettering staff. Irons objected strenuously to the Sloan-Kettering conclusions, claiming their methodology violated the prior agreement.

89. "The Facts Show 'Arginase' Drug Won't Help Cancer," 25 April 1952; "'Cancer Treatment' Discounted in Bay Area Tests," 26 April 1952; "L. A. Hospital Halts Cancer Experiment," 27 April 1952; and "'Cancer Treatment' Called Total Failure by Doctors," 28 April 1952. Hosford considered the articles "libelous," though I have seen no evidence to suggest he pursued this opinion in the courts; see J. Bottini to Milton P. Duffy, 30 April 1953, NDA 9214, "Mfr. No. 460, vol. 1."

90. Leo W. Hosford, President, San Francisco College of Mortuary Science, New Drug Application: Hepasyn, 25 June 1953, NDA 9214, vol. I; Michael F. Markel to New Drug Section, 11 December 1953, *ibid.*; and Earl L. Meyers to Ralph W. Weilerstein, 7 March 1957, NDA

9214, Misc. File IV, in which Meyers postulates that key damaging clinical cases may have been removed from the NDA during the long interim between completion and filing of the NDA, based on later statements made by the sponsor.

91. Gilmore, Jorgensen, and Bottini, Factory Inspection, 30 April 1953, and memorandum of interview between Boyd and Moulton and Smart, 12 December 1957.

92. Boyd was definitely in charge of the clinical investigation of Hepasyn and treated the vast majority of the patients, though four other California physicians had a handful of clinical cases involving Hepasyn; see Gilmore, Jorgensen, and Bottini, Factory Inspection Report, 30 April 1953, p. 10. One Phoenix physician treated one patient with Hepasyn that had been mailed to Arizona, but the agency did not feel warranted to pursue any action based on this limited movement in interstate commerce; see McKay McKinnon, Jr. to Administration, 4 May 1953, NDA 9214, "Mfr. No. 460, vol. 1."

93. E. Forrest Boyd, "Report on Clinical Applications of Arginase as an Anticarcinogenic Agent in Ten Patients with Malignancies," 19-page typescript, in Hosford, New Drug Application: Hepasyn, 25 June 1953 (quote from p. 15).

94. Ernest Q. King to San Francisco College of Mortuary Science, 26 January 1954, NDA 9214, vol. I (first quote), and Geoffrey Woodard, "For Comment," 18 January 1954, NDA 9214, Misc. File IV (second quote).

95. Memorandum of interview between George H. Hauerken and Michael F. Markel (attorneys for the San Francisco College of Mortuary Science) and George P. Larrick, 30 March 1954, NDA 9214, Misc. File IV; cf. Donald M. Counihan to Melvin W. Snead, 10 May 1954, *ibid.*

96. Memorandum of interview between Irons and Barnard, Moulton, Smart, Gilmore, and Hill, 19 December 1957, and Barbara Moulton to Regulatory Management, 21 September 1957, NDA 9214, vol. IB. Irons himself, though, was characterized as extremely hostile and suffering from a persecution complex; see memorandum of interview between Shimkin and Moulton, 8 March 1957.

97. They used 2 drops of arginase in a 500 cc solution of glucose or sodium lactate by intravenous drip, twice a week (the strength of the arginase drops was unknown); see C. A. Wayne, Factory Inspection Report: Arenac Osteopathic Clinic, 25-26 August 1954, NDA 9214, "Mfr. No. 460, vol. 1," pp. 4-5.

98. Stanley J. Gilmore, Factory Inspection Report: Charles E. Irons Memorial Cancer Foundation, 3-4 August 1954, NDA 9214, "Mfr. No. 460, vol. 1," pp. 1-2, and Wayne, Factory Inspection Report, 25-26 August 1954.

99. Agreement between Irons and the San Francisco College of Mortuary Science, 28 August 1950.

100. Fred Maggiora, vice mayor of Oakland, California, and Leon Raesly, an aide to a Congressman from Pennsylvania, delivered the application to the FDA; Raesly apparently died shortly after the submission. It is not clear what interest these men had in the application or the sponsors, but Maggiora remained a champion of NDA 9999 for some time, at one point trying to enlist the assistance of the National Association of Retail Druggists to speed the evaluation along. See Arenac Laboratories, NDA 9999 (Acutalyn), 12 May 1955, (original application), records, Food and Drug Administration, Rockville, Maryland, and memorandum of telephone conversation between George Frates (NARD) and Barbara Moulton, 15 February 1956, NDA 9999.

101. NDA 9999 (original application), 12 May 1955; memo of interview between Norman M. Littell, W. G. Irons, and W. W. Harper, and E. L. M., Dr. Granger, and [Ralph G. Smith], 22 September 1955, NDA 9999; W. W. Harper et al. to Ralph G. Smith, 2 February 1956, (NDA

Supp.), NDA 9999; Herbert Blumenthal to New Drug Section, 23 March 1956, NDA 9999; and "Before the Department of Health, Education and Welfare, Food and Drug Administration, Washington 25, D. C.," 10-page typescript, n. d., attached to Cyril Saunders to Ralph G. Smith, 25 May 1956, NDA 9999.

102. NDA 9999 (original application), 12 May 1955.

103. Ralph G. Smith to Fred Maggiora, 20 July 1955, NDA 9999.

104. Memo of interview between Littell, Irons, and Harper, and E. L. M., Granger, and Smith, 22 September 1955, and W. W. Harper and H. G. Henry to Ralph G. Smith, 11 August 1955, NDA 9999.

105. "Before the Department of Health," attached to Saunders to Smith, 25 May 1956.

106. Ralph G. Smith to Metabolyn Laboratories, 11 June 1956, NDA 9999, and W. G. Irons to Ralph G. Smith, 3 October 1956.

107. *Interagency Coordination in Drug Research and Regulation*, Hearings before the Subcommittee on Reorganizations and International Organizations of the Committee on Government Operations, U. S. Senate, 87th Congress, 2d Sess., Part 2, pp. 461 and 466; "San Leandro Drugmaker Arrested, Accused of Violating State Health, Safety Code," *Oakland Tribune*, 17 July 1960; and "Last Services Held for Dr. Wesley G. Irons," *ibid.*, 18 January 1967. I am indebted to Steven Lavoie of the *Oakland Tribune* for the last two sources.

108. Gilmore, Factory Inspection Report, 3-4 August 1954, and Stanley J. Gilmore and Maurice L. Strait, Inspection Report: San Francisco College of Mortuary Science, 12, 13, and 16 December 1955, NDA 9214, "Mfr. No. 460, vol. 1."

109. Gilmore, Factory Inspection Report, 3-4 August 1954, p. 3; Gilmore and Strait, Inspection Report, 12, 13, and 16 December 1955, pp. 2 and 15; and Smart, "Summary of Hepasyn Investigation," pp. 4-5.

110. The quotation is from the report of a conversation with Leon S. Utter, in Gilmore and Strait, Inspection Report, 12, 13, and 16 December 1955, p. 16.

111. See John L. Harvey to San Francisco District, 2 September 1954, NDA 9214, "Mfr. No. 460, vol. 1." On the Hoxsey case, see Young, *Medical Messiahs* (n. 13), 362 ff.

112. Geoffrey Woodard to Dr. Moulton, 5 May 1955, NDA 9214, Misc. File IV.

113. E. Forrest Boyd to The Administrator, Federal Security Agency, Food and Drug Administration, 14 March 1955, NDA 9214, vol. I' of II', and Barbara Moulton to San Francisco College of Mortuary Science, 13 May 1955, NDA 9214, "Mfr. No. 460, vol. 1."

114. George P. Larrick to San Francisco College of Mortuary Science, 11 October 1955, NDA 9214, Mfr. No. 460, vol. 1."

115. Gordon A. Granger to Ralph W. Weilerstein, 14 October 1955, NDA 9214, Misc. File IV.

116. For example, see memorandum of telephone conversation between Gordon B. Wood, Ralph W. Weilerstein, and James R. Cribbett, 3 November 1955, NDA 9214, Misc. File IV.

117. For example, see James R. Cribbett to Los Angeles District, NDA 9214, "Misc. File IV;" William H. Kessenich to Ralph W. Weilerstein, 28 October 1955, *ibid.*; James R. Cribbett to Chiefs of Districts, 28 October 1955, NDA 9214, "Mfr. No. 460, vol. 1;" memorandum of telephone conversation between James R. Cribbett, Ralph W. Weilerstein, and Gordon R. Wood, 2 November 1955, *ibid.*; Ralph W. Weilerstein to William H. Kessenich, 18 November 1955, *ibid.*; Ralph W. Weilerstein to William H. Kessenich, 21 November 1955, *ibid.* (evidence that some patients had other treatment options but opted for Hepasyn instead, possibly with encouragement from Hepasyn clinicians); and memorandum of interview between Cutting and Weilerstein, 30 November 1955.

118. George P. Larrick to San Francisco College of Mortuary Science, 23 December 1955, NDA

9214, vol. I' of II'.

119. Memorandum of telephone conversation between McKay McKinnon to James R. Cribbett, 10 January 1956, NDA 9214, "Mfr. No. 460, vol. 1B," and memorandum of interview between Leo W. Hosford, Leon S. Utter, Hilario G. Marquez, and Stanley J. Gilmore, 10 January 1956, NDA 9214, "Hepasyn—General Material." The NDA was withdrawn on 3 January 1956; see Gordon A. Granger to Dr. Garland, 3 April 1956, NDA 9214, Misc. File IV.

120. Leo W. Hosford to George P. Larrick, 3 May 1956, NDA 9214, vol. I' of II'; Leo W. Hosford, President, San Francisco College of Mortuary Science, New Drug Application: Hepasyn, 10 October 1956, NDA 9214, vol. II' of II'; Barbara Moulton to San Francisco College of Mortuary Science, 10 December 1956, NDA 9214, "Hepasyn—General Material;" Leo W. Hosford to Food and Drug Administration, 7 January 1957, NDA 9214, vol. II' of II'; and John L. Harvey to San Francisco College of Mortuary Science, 17 January 1957, NDA 9214, "Hepasyn—General Material."

121. Dr. Holland to Ralph G. Smith, 13 November 1956, NDA 9214, Misc. File IV (first quote), and Albert H. Holland to John L. Harvey, 8 February 1957, *ibid.* (second quote).

122. Barbara Moulton to Mr. Goodrich, 20 February 1957, NDA 9214, Misc. File IV.

123. Frank McKinley to Chief, Los Angeles District, 23 August 1957, NDA 9214, "Hepasyn—General Material."

124. F. D. Clark to Chiefs of Districts, 18 February 1957, NDA 9214, "Hepasyn—General Material;" Meyers to Weilerstein, 7 March 1957; memorandum of interview between George K. Wharton and Ralph W. Weilerstein, 12 March 1957, NDA 9214, "Hepasyn—General Material;" and Stanley J. Gilmore, Inspection Report: San Francisco College of Mortuary Science, 23-24 April 1957, NDA 9214, "Investigation by Stanley Gilmore."

125. Notice of Hearing FDC-D-42, in the matter of "Hepasyn," [8 April 1957] NDA 9214, vol. II' of II'. The grounds for the hearing were: 1) "The methods, facilities and controls used in the manufacture, processing, and packing of Hepasyn are inadequate to produce a drug of standardized identity, strength, and purity...," 2) "The results of the clinical trials of the drug reported in the application show that Hepasyn is unsafe, because... there is no reliable scientific evidence reported which would establish that Hepasyn has any therapeutic value whatever in the management of malignancies....," 3) "The information in the application is inadequate to support a conclusion that the drug is safe for use under the conditions prescribed, recommended, or suggested...," and 4) "The proposed labeling fails to contain information adequate for the use of the drug in that it fails to contain adequate indications for use...."

126. Ralph W. Weilerstein to Arthur Dickerman, 30 April 1957, NDA 9214, "Hepasyn—General Material."

127. Barbara Moulton to Dr. Weilerstein, 20 September 1957, NDA 9214, "Hepasyn Records—Case Histories," and Albert H. Holland to Allen E. Rayfield, 13 May 1957, NDA 9214, Misc. File IV.

128. George P. Larrick to San Francisco College of Mortuary Science, 1 May 1957, NDA 9214, Misc. File IV.

129. Though some evidence suggested, according to Moulton, that he may have practiced medicine without a license (Moulton to Regulatory Management, 21 September 1957). Hosford indeed had a license on his wall—from a bogus diploma mill posing as a legitimate representative of the Homeopathic Examining Board of Maryland; see Kenneth R. Lennington to Chiefs of Districts, 28 September 1956, NDA 9214, Misc. File IV; Stanley J. Gilmore to San Francisco District, 10 October 1956, *ibid.*; James W. Skipper to Baltimore District, 23 April 1957, NDA 9214, "Hepasyn—General Material;" and "Reddick Case Findings to Be Circu-

lated," (Baltimore) *Sun*, 23 August 1956.

130. Moulton to Regulatory Management, 21 September 1957.

131. M. R. Stephens to San Francisco District, 10 July 1958, NDA 9214, "Hepasyn—General Material."

132. Walter Sneader, *Drug Prototypes and their Exploitation* (Chichester: John Wiley, 1996), 248-249; Louis S. Goodman and Alfred Gilman, eds., *The Pharmacological Basis of Therapeutics*, 3d ed. (New York: Macmillan, 1965), 1043-1044; and Gary L. Nelson, ed., *Pharmaceutical Company Histories*, vol. 1 (Bismarck, N. D.: Woodbine Publishing, 1983), 114-116.

133. Paul F. MacLeod to New Drug Branch, 1 May 1959, and Jerome H. Epstein to Paul F. MacLeod, 26 June 1959, 14 July 1959, and 9 September 1959, NDA 11-965, vol. I, FDA Records, Rockville, Maryland; the NDA was made conditionally effective on July 14th pending FDA approval of Altafur labeling.

134. Paul F. MacLeod to Jerome Epstein, 21 October 1959, *ibid.*

135. Alfred W. Wagner, "New Allergic Reaction to Furaltadone," *J. Am. Med. Assoc.* 173 (1960): 363.

136. Memorandum of telephone conversation between Paul F. MacLeod and David S. Davis, 22 June 1960, NDA 11-965, vol. I; memorandum of telephone conversation between Paul F. MacLeod and Ralph G. Smith and Julius Hauser, 1 July 1960, *ibid.*; memorandum of meeting between Paul MacLeod and P. J. Christenson and Ralph G. Smith, Julius Hauser, David S. Davis, and Irwin Siegel, 6 July 1960, NDA 11-965, vol. V (quote).

137. Press Release HEW-N47, 24 June 1960, files, FDA History office; "NDA Files Received from FDA for Use of Special Committee," n.d., 3-page typescript, "MED: Com to Review Policies Procedures & Decisions of Division of Antibiotics and New Drug Branch of FDA... ," Archives, National Academy of Sciences, Washington, D.C.; Herbert N. Gardner to Special Committee, 22 June 1960, *ibid.*; "Notes for Meeting of FDA Committee, 28 June 1960," n.d., 1-page typescript, *ibid.*; Minutes of Meeting, [Special Committee on the Food and Drug Administration,] 28 June 1960, *ibid.*; "NRC Special Committee on FDA," [30 August 1962?], 1-page typescript, "Organization: NAS: Com Adv to HEW on FDA," NAS Archives. "Statement by the Commissioner of Food and Drugs Regarding Charges Made by John O. Nestor, M. D.," Exhibit 144, Hearings before the Subcommittee on Reorganization and International Organizations of the Committee on Government Operations, U. S. Senate, 88th Congress, 1st Sess., Part 3, p. 1019; Richard E. McFadyen, "FDA's Regulation and Control of Antibiotics in the 1950s: The Henry Welch Scandal, Félix Martí-Ibáñez, and Charles Pfizer & Co.," *Bull. Hist. Med.* 53 (1979): 168-169; and National Academy of Sciences-National Research Council, "Report of Special Committee Advisory to the Secretary of Health, Education, and Welfare to Review the Policies, Procedures, and Decisions of The Division of Antibiotics and the New Drug Branch of the Food and Drug Administration," exhibit 1, *Drug Industry Antitrust Act*, Hearings before the Subcommittee on Antitrust and Monopoly of the Committee on the Judiciary, U. S. Senate, 87th Congress, 1st sess. (Washington, D. C.: Government Printing Office, 1961), p. 459 (*Legislative History* 18: 219).

138. Memorandum of meeting between MacLeod and Christenson and Smith, Hauser, Davis, and Siegel, 6 July 1960, and memorandum of telephone conversation between MacLeod and Smith and Hauser, 1 July 1960. On chloramphenicol see Thomas Maeder, *Adverse Reactions* (New York: William Morrow, 1994).

139. Memorandum of interview between L. E. Daily, Paul MacLeod, Paul R. Dohl, and Vincent Kleinfeld and David S Davis, Ralph G. Smith, and Julius Hauser, 20 July 1960, NDA 11-965, vol. V, and P. F. MacLeod, "Dear Doctor," 21 July 1960, attached to David S. Davis to Paul F.

MacLeod, 25 July 1960, *ibid.*: the indications were revised to read: "Because this is a new drug and because of the possibility of certain side effects, the use of Altafur should be confined to infections that are not amenable to other drugs now available to the physician."

140. Paul F. MacLeod to David S. Davis, 18 October 1960, NDA 11-965, vol. XV, and David S. Davis to Paul F. MacLeod, 16 November 1960, *ibid.* During the interim period FDA contacted Maxwell Finland, a clinical researcher at Harvard who had been studying Altafur; he strongly advised the agency to withdraw Altafur; see William R. Kessenich to Office of the Commissioner, 5 December 1960, *ibid.*

141. Kessenich to Office of the Commissioner, 5 December 1960.

142. See, e.g., William R. McCabe et al., "Furaltadone: A Critical Evaluation of Clinical and Laboratory Studies," *New England J. Med.* 263 (10 November 1960): 927-934.

143. "Text of HEW Dept. Hearing Examiner's Findings on Altafur," *Drug Research Reports* 4 (8 November 1961): 424-S.

144. "Text of HEW Hearing" (n. 143), pp. 430-S and 431-S; cf. the editorial, "Furaltadone," *New England J. Med.* 263 (10 November 1960): 975: "This [advertising-driven] use of the drug and the results thereof are clear evidence of the benefit that manufacturers may derive from the testimonial type of evidence for the effectiveness of preparations as presented by uncritical observers. The very careful and critical clinical and laboratory evaluation of the drug presented elsewhere in this issue of the *Journal* not only failed to provide evidence of the type of activity that is claimed for it but also showed clearly that such activity cannot even be expected. The authors also indicated that the few favorable reports... will not stand critical analysis."

145. Edward F. Turkel to George P. Larrick, 1 December 1961, AF 9-700, vol. 9, FDA Records; Alvin L. Gottlieb to John L. Harvey, 16 January 1962, *ibid.*; and John L. Harvey, "In the Matter of 'Altafur Tablets,'" 33-page typescript, 16 August 1962, AF 9-700, vol. 10. For Lloyd Cutler's assessment of Eaton's chances going into this hearing vis-à-vis the construction of the hearings system, see Lloyd Cutler, "Practical Aspects of Drug Legislation," in Paul Talalay, ed., *Drugs in Our Society* (Baltimore: Johns Hopkins Press, 1964), 153-154.

146. J. V. Sladek to Alan T. Spiher, Jr., 11 May 1962, AF 9-700, vol. 10; James H. Mark to Harold D. B. Roberts, 19 May 1962, 25 May 1962, 6 July 1962, and 22 August 1962, *ibid.*; and E. T. Wulfsberg to Alan T. Spiher, Jr., 8 August 1962, *ibid.* A summarized version of the Altafur story can be found in "Food and Drug Administration Chronology with Respect to Actions on the Drug Altafur," exhibit 78, *Interagency Coordination in Drug Research and Regulation* (n. 107), pp. 504-508.

147. Arthur H. Hayes, Jr., "Safety Considerations in Product Development," *Drug Safety* 5, Supp. 1 (1990): 25.

Historical Perspectives on the Marketing of Medicines

by Mickey C. Smith

In this presentation it is my intention to describe and delineate some of the most important elements in the marketing of medicines in this century, following a brief look at earlier marketing developments and preceding a timid bit of forecasting.

A definition or two and a discussion framework are probably necessary before the details are presented. While there is no "Bible" of marketing, some eleven editions of McCarthy's *Basic Marketing* certainly attest to its durability and essential correctness. I will use materials from that text to lay a marketing foundation.

McCarthy differentiates between micro-marketing and macro-marketing, and his is a useful differentiation.[2] "Micro-marketing is the performance of activities which seek to accomplish an organization's objectives by anticipating customer or client needs and directing a flow of need-satisfying goods and services from producer to customer or client".[3]

On the other hand, and often overlooked ... "Macro-marketing is a social process which directs an economy's flow of goods and services from producers to consumers in a way which effectively matches supply and demand and accomplishes the objectives of society".[4]

Over the years McCarthy (and many others) have used a "4 - P's" framework for discussion of the functions of marketing. One can find a variety of definitions but those of the originator do nicely:

- "Product—the needs-satisfying offering of a firm"
- "Price—what is charged for 'something'"
- "Place—making products available in the right quantities and locations when customers want them"
- "Promotion—communicating information between seller and buyer to influence attitudes and behavior"[5]

It is the 4-P's framework on which much of the following will be based, although the legal, social and political environment will not be ignored.

"Ancient History"

Certainly marketing functions have been a part of the entire history of medication use. First, there was the need for a *product*, however primitive or irrational. It was necessary to deliver it somehow, although place concerns were much less important in a village society. Price was often an issue of barter. As Edmond Crispin wrote in his contemporary mystery story, *Beware of Trains*, "the solicitor pays for his groceries by giving legal advice to the grocer; the grocer pays for his medicines by supplying sugar to the chemist."

In their fascinating book, *Advertising in America: The First Hundred Years*, Goodrum and Dalrymple credit *patent* medicine activity with three developments in the history of advertising: [6]

- Because producers wanted to place their ads in every community, advertising agents were forced to identify media and regularize rates.
- Because of the often outrageous claims of the patent medicines, the advertising business began to consider self-regulation.
- When it became clear that some of these products were genuine threats to health, government regulation became a serious consideration.
- They led to the invention of the magazine in America.

One cannot identify a certain year, or even a decade, in which pharmaceutical marketing as we know it today began. Surely the expansion of what were once the pharmacies of the Squibbs, Lillys, and others and the development of transportation facilities allowing widespread distribution were two of the major early factors, but the development of the industry in all its aspects was thrust into modern times by the developments surrounding World War II. We shall use that as a starting point for this historical survey.

•

The discussion which follows will focus on what the author believes to be the five most important historical developments in each of the four "P's"

Mickey Smith is F.A.P. Barnard Professor of Pharmacy Administration at the University of Mississippi where he has taught for thirty years. His text *Principles of Pharmaceutical Marketing* was first published in 1968 and is now in the fourth edition. He is founding Editor of *The Journal of Pharmaceutical Marketing and Management*, which has just seen its tenth anniversary issue. Smith's interest in pharmacy history and the subject of his publications in the field have centered on pharmacy on the radio and the role of pharmaceuticals in World War II.

and in the marketing environment. The limitation to five in each category is arbitrary and the author will be very surprised if readers do not have their own lists that they judge to be equally important.

Product

When considering this category the immediate temptation is to list individual medications, e.g., penicillin. But here (**Table 1**) is my list beginning with the transfer of the compounding function from pharmacists to pharmaceutical manufacturers. From today's perspective this is a natural evolution, but from an historical perspective it was a revolution. An entire profession built upon a special knowledge of product preparation was relieved of that function and faced with the challenge of discovering and justifying new reasons to be. It is only recently that challenge appears to have been met.[7]

Table 1. Major Developments in Pharmaceutical Products

Transfer of Compounding to Drug Manufacturers
"The Pill"
Psychotropic Medications
Dosage Form Developments
Generic Pharmaceuticals
Other Possibilities
• Antibiotics
• Vaccines
• AIDS Medications
• Services as "Products" at Retail

I have chosen "the Pill" for my next product candidate. There are, of course, many "pills," but the oral contraceptive as a social concept required much more than pharmacology and chemistry to reach the market place and to stay there. Surely, this class of drugs which really do not "treat anything," fits the *macro*-marketing definition provided above. Carl Djerassi, in his very personal survey of the state of contraception published nearly twenty years ago, quoted an Aldous Huxley from more than twenty years earlier: "Most of us choose birth control—and immediately find ourselves confronted by a problem that is simultaneously a puzzle in physiology, pharmacology, sociology, psychology and even theology".[8]

The next class of product is the result of two individual drugs, one a clear medical breakthrough and the other a (probably) fortuitous case of mistaken identity. The first of these, chlorpromazine, changed both the length of and character of hospitalization for mental illness.[9] The second, meprobamate, was responsible for the public awareness of the possibility of legal use of mind-altering substances. New terminology was necessary with the ultimate term, "tranquilizer," the result.[10] With Prozac the latest center of attention, the debate on the costs and benefits of such medications will surely continue for the foreseeable future.

The fourth class of product developments I have grouped under "dosage forms," but could as well have called delivery systems, and saved for the discussion of the future. In any case, sustained release oral medications, patches, implants, and the like have totally and forever changed drug administration and set the stage for even more dramatic developments in the future.

Generic pharmaceuticals, the fifth on the list, belong in the pricing discussion as well. As a product issue they represent a trend toward commodity status for both prescription and nonprescription medications. Everyone is familiar with Robert Thom's series of illustrations on the history of medicine and pharmacy. It was no accident that a depiction of Terra Sigillata the first brand name (?) found its way between Hippocrates and Galen. Brand names, without the possibility of "substitution" were the backbone of the industry for many years. The existence of generic divisions in dozens of what were once brand-name manufacturers attests to this total change in the generic market.

Other possibilities (and the reader will certainly be eager to add more) include the entire field of antibiotics, vaccines which have measurably improved life expectancy in this century, AIDS medications which may do so, and the redefinition of the product of retail pharmacy to include services and outcomes.

Price

As **Table 2** indicates, the first development considered under price is that of pharmacists' professional fee. That fee is at the heart of negotiations with third-party payers today, but this was not always the case by any means. As recently as 1962, McEvilla and others were advocating adoption of the professional fee concept in the pages of the *Journal of the American Pharmaceutical Association*.[11] Over time the fee concept was adopted and now serves, along with a confused jungle of product reimbursement procedures, as the basis for most pharmacist payment systems.

Fair trade is listed next because the issue occupied the time and attention of pharmacy (especially NARD) for so long and eventually failed. Fair Trade or "Resale Price Control" had its legislative beginning in 1931 in California with a Fair Trade Act that required wholesalers and retailers to observe prices set by the manufacturer.[12] Subsequently nearly every state enacted such laws. Although the market rationale for such legislation is complex fair trade clearly protected the independent pharmacists from price competition. Support for enforcement of these laws ultimately failed as any shopper now knows.

The pricing pattern change listed in **Table 2** refers to a shift in prescription drug pricing. For years, beginning in 1960, Professor John Firestone of the City College of New York calculated and published a price index for prescription drugs.[13] Supported, or at least encouraged by the (then) Pharmaceutical Manufacturers Association, the Index uniformly showed little increase and sometimes a decline in prices. Without exploring the technicalities of Firestone's calculations the results did reflect a pattern called "skimming" in the marketing literature. This means that new products were initially offered at what would be their highest price with price decreases following in response to competition and other factors. Inflation and other alterations in market strategy have resulted in a reversal of this practice such that many products, some of them rather old, have experienced a pattern of continuing price increases. This pattern may be altered, however, by the development to be described next.

Table 2. Major Developments in Pharmaceutical Pricing

Professional Fee
Fair Trade
Rx Pricing Patterns Change
Development of Oligopsony
Focus on Economic Outcomes/Price vs. Value

For most of this century, a comparatively few drug companies developed, patented, manufactured and sold pharmaceutical products to retailers, at prices of their own determination. Pharmacists could, in effect, "take it or leave it." Inasmuch as the demand for the product was already developed they tended to "take it," McEvilla described this oligopoly in terms of a "kinky" demand curve.[14] Today, and increasingly in the future, because the patients' drug costs are paid by comparatively few buyers, the power has greatly shifted. A company representing perhaps 20 million patients and 100 million prescriptions annually can now often tell the manufacturers "take it or leave it."

In response to the foregoing and because of some innovative economic research the focus has shifted to an appreciable degree from the price of a drug, to the costs of treatment and often to the ratio between that cost and its benefit. Quality of life issues, cost-effectiveness, and cost-utility analyses have made simple price comparisons a thing of the past.

Place

Among the many effects of World War II was a shortage of person-power in the work force. With (mostly) men in the service and women filling jobs heretofore unthinkable, some things had to change. One of these was the tradition of personal service in retail stores, including drug stores. Once people became accustomed to making their own selections there was no turning back and this was closely tied to the next two developments.

In his twenty-five-year review of the development of drug chains Godfrey Lebhar, Editor-in-Chief of *Chain Store Age*, described the genesis in these words:

> The fact is that when the chains first came into the picture the competition of the established corner druggist was hardly of the aggressive type. The retail druggist of those days was essentially a professional man, interested primarily in compounding prescriptions accurately and selling proprietary and other medicines and medical supplies. He expanded into other lines not by choice or any particular desire to become a merchant but by force of economic circumstances.

> The result was that although the druggist of those days performed an essential service and did a satisfactory job on the professional side, he left himself wide open for the kind of competition which the chains introduced.[15]

The dominance of the chains in pharmacy today has changed the profession into one of employees from what was largely entrepreneurial in the first half of this century.

Paralleling the growth of the chains and in part due to mutual interests by large retail corporations was the incursion of food stores into the non-prescription drug market place. To a generation today who expect at least one aisle in any major food store to be devoted to health and beauty aids it would seem impossible that at one time many drug manufacturers had a strict drug-

---

Table 3. Major Devlopments in Pharmaceutical Distribution (Place)

Self Service
Rise of Chains and Decline of the Corner Drug Store
Shift of Non-Prescription Medications out of Pharmacies
Impact of Hospital Pharmacy Practices
Clozaril/Methadone Incidents
Other Possibilities
• Mail Order Prescriptions
• Wholesale vs. Direct
• Drive-In Pharmacies

---

store-only distribution policy. Pharmacists' objections when such products as Contac® and Sucaryl® began to be sold in food stores were understandable given the history but unrealistic given the times. By 1991 food stores had gained more than 50 per cent of the non-prescription drug business.[16]

The changes at retail have been dramatic but in many ways exceeded by those in the hospital (which is really a retail institution as well). Hospital pharmacy has changed dramatically in the past forty years at least, moving out of its traditional basement location often to the patient's bedside. From a marketing point of view the hospital pharmacy administration has moved into a position of prominence and power among drug company customers and The American Society of Health-System Pharmacists Clinical Midyear Meeting has become one of the most successful drug marketing events in all of pharmacy.

The final point on this list is less a development than a possibility. In the case of Methadone the government and in the case of Clozaril a manufacturer have attempted to limit the distribution of a specific medication to certain pharmacies. Traditionally a pharmacy license assured free access to all legal medications. While neither of these efforts to restrict distribution was successful, some believe that there is merit in the idea and feel that more will follow.[17]

Certainly any list of place developments could also include: mail order prescriptions which are making an impact; drive-in pharmacies; and the *current* continued importance of wholesalers after some period of decline.

Promotion

The basic marketing literature suggest that promotion be the last of the "p's" to consider as the function of promotion is to inform the customer about the *other "p's"*. Promotion, in the form of advertising, has a rich history in the field of pharmaceutical marketing. It has also, along with pricing, received a great deal of criticism.

First on our list of developments is the media. While drugs had long been advertised it remained for radio to make truly national promotion possible, and drug promotion helped make the expansion of radio possible. When television followed it, pharmaceuticals could be visually portrayed in a dramatic, if sometimes tasteless, way as a necessary part of life.

The second item on the list may be a bit of a surprise—it surprised me when I really thought of it—*The Physicians Desk Reference*. The year 1996 marks the 50th edition of this remarkable book. This quasi-official reference text has proved to be indispensable to hundreds of thousands of health professionals most of whom are unaware that the drug companies pay to have their information included. That apart, there is nothing like it available from either the public or private sector.

Describing promotion as medical education is meant in two ways here. In one sense is meant the long-standing practice of drug company financial sponsorship of educational programs for physicians and other health professionals. Certainly the subject matter is virtually always related in some way to a company product, but the audience (possible bias not withstanding) is afforded an educational experience.

Table 4. Major Developments in Pharmaceutical Promotion

Media Development
Physicians Desk Reference
Promotion as Medical Eduction
Direct to Consumer Promotion of Legend Drugs
Changing Appeals
Other Possibilities
• Changing Targets
• Sampling Changes
• Supreme Court Decision

Advertising, in journals especially, contributes in two ways to the educational process. First there is whatever information of value is gained from the advertisement itself. Second is the real, but unofficial subsidy of the non-promotion editorial material which the readers might not otherwise receive. Criticism aside (although there is plenty of it), if it were not for pharmaceutical advertising a new system of education about medications would have to be invented immediately.

The direct-to-consumer (DTC) promotions of prescription drugs is the next item. By most accounts the phenomenon was first noticed when, in October 1981, Merck, Sharp and Dohme promoted their pneumonia vaccine, Pneumovax, directly to consumers in several publications including *Modern Maturity* and *Reader's Digest*. The advertisement, which was addressed primarily to the elderly, alerted readers to the availability of the product, noted the product's benefits, indicated that Medicare would reimburse the cost of the product, and suggested that readers mention the product to their physicians.

It may be interesting to know, however, that in the 1940s Squibb was using the following text in a radio commercial.

Just as thrilling as tracking down some fabulous treasure is the search for the unknown which goes on unceasingly in the Squibb Research Laboratories. For that is the search that leads to new discovery of new life-saving drugs and new-life uses for existing drugs. Streptomycin is one of the newest products of research. In the new field of medicine opened up by penicillin, Streptomycin, still in the testing stages whose great promise against additional enemies of mankind. That is why Squibb scientists are working night and day to unlock the secrets of Streptomycin, to improve the strain, to find and test all the ways in which it may be used in the conquest of disease. It is this same questing spirit, this refusal to stop anywhere short of perfection, that inspires all endeavors of the house of Squibb. It is one reason why, wherever you come across it in the service of human health, Squibb is the name you can trust.

The eventual effects of direct-to-consumer promotion of prescription drugs are potentially enormous.

The appeals/messages used in drug advertising, especially to physicians, have changed considerably over the past 50 years, partly due to regulation and partly to market forces. In either case the messages still contain needed information on safety, effectiveness and use, but now to a much greater extent they tend to focus on economics, quality of life and other "non-clinical" issues. This change suggests a greater concern with the socio-economic aspects of selling drugs than with the clinical concerns of the prescriber. It also suggests a much greater interest in influencing different targets, i.e., pharmacy benefit managers.

Sampling, long a favorite and presumably effective, promotional technique has undergone serious regulation and no longer is treated in the sometimes cavalier fashion that was the case in the past. Also a consideration under Promotion, but probably under Environment as well, was the U.S. Supreme Court decision in the 1970s that prohibition of advertising of professional services under professional codes of ethics was a violation of First Amendment rights.

Environmental Developments

In the section to be discussed with the items in **Table 5** the temptation to list a hundred or so was almost overwhelming, but a few examples should suffice to show that pharmaceutical marketing is and will be a victim and a product of the environment. The evolution of the Food and Drug Administration under the various amendments to the Food, Drug and Cosmetic Act is well known. For marketing students two of these deserve special attention. The Durham-Humphrey Amendment created a retail-prescriber monopoly, something not often seen in a free market and it gave to a Federal regulatory agency the power to determine which products were to be so regulated. It created a prescription drug industry. The so-called 1962 Amendments gave the FDA even more power including greater strength in regulating promotion.

The Congressional Investigations item covers a multitude of events with the first, famous series of hearings being those conducted by Senator

Kefauver. Ostensibly to investigate pricing, but fueled by the Thalidomide tragedy, the Hearings resulted in the 1962 Amendments, but also forever raised America's consciousness about an industry that was just about the realize its importance in the health history of this country. Other names—Montoya, Kennedy, Pryor—are associated with similar investigations.

Table 5. Major Environmental Developments in the Pharmaceutical Marketplace

---

Durham-Humphrey Amendments/1962 Amendments
Congressional Investigations
Public Interest and Knowledge/Muckrakers
Waxman-Hatch/Patent Extension
Third-Part Payment Programs
Rx-to-OTC shift
Evolution of Pharmacy Education/Practice

In part because of the investigations just mentioned and also because of professional critics the environment includes much more interest and awareness by the general public of workings of the pharmaceutical industry. When the first effective antibiotics (led by tetracycline) appeared they were referred to as "wonder drugs." The members of the public were excited by the prospects of future research. Today there seems to be both hope and skepticism when the industry is discussed.

The Waxman-Hatch Patent Extension Act is included for two reasons. First, it is the only example of a commodity for which a patent extension is even a legal possibility. Second, it is a classic example of political action in which both interested parties got something they wanted. The generic manufacturers had easier access through the FDA and the research companies had at least the possibility of longer market life for their patented products.

Third-party payment prescription programs are essentially a phenomena of the second half of this century. The prescription drug marketplace was *already* an anomaly. One must see *one* professional (prescriber) to go to *another* professional (pharmacist) to obtain needed goods. Insurance, government, and employee benefit programs have added another layer of complexity, so that this particular market bears little resemblance to any other.

The prescription to non-prescription shift is a comparatively recent development with enormous potential impact. Drugs for which a prescription were once required are now available in increasing numbers, without a prescription. Once two or three of these switches were effected the product planning strategies in the drug companies had to include such possibilities in the future. Further, those third party payers, considering their own budgets, also now think in terms of how shifted drugs may be deleted from their benefits package.

Finally, a word about the efforts of pharmacy education and practice to construct a future. Many people do not know that the 6-year Doctor of Pharmacy degree which will soon be the only degree awarded by schools of pharmacy was proposed in 1950. A half century later this will be realized. During that interim the profession has undergone many changes that have not been uniformly positive nor uniform throughout all segments of practice. Nevertheless, pharmacy *is* and pharmacists *are* different from our perspective on marketing.

The Future

Goodrum and Dalrymple tell us that: "There is general agreement that there are few things advertising does as well as introducing new inventions to the community."[18] Such terms as "tranquilizer,"[19] antibiotic, and genetic engineering must somehow be explained to the public who must accept and use them. This function has evolved into a partnership between the mass media and commercial promotion. Both will have their hands full in the future.

From a product perspective we see an almost limitless range of developments in drug delivery systems. These will require education of both patients and prescribers.

Disease management, quality of life enhancement and other terms are currently being used to describe the products of what we once thought of as the *drug* industry. A redefinition of the product must result in a redefinition of the industry.

Continued pressure on prices is almost guaranteed as is industry response. Capitation is included in **Table 6** because a number of providers are

Table 6. Future Prospects in the Marketing Mix

Product
  Dosage Form Developments
  Quality of Life and Other Outcomes
Price
  Capitation
  Portland Case and 1996 Case
Distribution
  Verticle Integration
  Limitation of Access
Promotion
  Information Technology—Internet and Beyond
Environment
  Health Care Reform
  GATT/NAFTA

already using it. While not a new concept (a trial of the concept was conducted in Iowa in the 1970s)[20] the rationale is sufficiently compelling that additional trials are almost certain.

The 1996 settlement out of court of the pharmacy pricing suit is evocative of earlier challenges to industry pricing practices and suggest that more challenges may follow. In a recent report on the case *F-D-C Reports* suggested that those companies involved in the settlement acceded in order to "preserve a range of pricing options."[21] This portends further conflict in the pricing area.

In distribution the vertical integration activities that have recently joined merger acquisitions as part of an overall pattern of industry consolidation seem likely to continue. Limitation of access to some pharmacists to drug distribution programs seems a real possibility but in the future various "*credentialing*" initiatives by drug benefit providers may serve the same purpose.

The story of the future in promotion will surely be written by communications technology. The internet and similar media will transform information transfer as the industry attempts to balance the many target audiences that are developing and to exploit the databases that make marketing more sophisticated.

Environmentally we can expect domestic pressure to continue for some kind of health care reform. The nature and degree of success of those efforts is, of course, a function of social, economic and political developments. Internationally it is quite easy to predict a smaller world with continuing integration and accommodation of formerly international differences.

Conclusion

It has been my long-standing position that good marketing makes good medicine. The logic seems inescapable. Find a medical need and fill it with a product that has the best possible balance between safety and efficiency. Produce and *price* the product such that the ultimate user by some means can afford to use it. Assure that the product is in the *place* where it is needed when it is needed. Through *promotion,* supply to all parties who need to know the information necessary to use the product properly.

At the outset of this essay McCarthy was quoted as describing marketing as a "social process . . , which effectively matches supply and demand and accomplishes the objectives of society."

A quarter of a century ago Paul Stolley described a "cultural lag" in health care. As he put it:

Sociologists have long observed that changes do not occur in a coordinated way even in closely related parts of our culture. Technological advances commonly outstrip the ability of society to adapt to and utilize these advances. This delay is called "cultural lag" by sociologists.[22]

Perhaps the twenty-first century will find society better able to define its objectives. If that occurs marketing will play a major role in meeting them.

References

1. E. J. McCarthy, W. D. Perreault, *Basic Marketing: A Managerial Approach*, 8th ed. (Homewood, IL: R. D. Irwin, 1984).
2. McCarthy, *Basic Marketing* (n. 1), p. 10.
3. McCarthy, *Basic Marketing* (n. 1), p. 11.
4. McCarthy, *Basic Marketing* (n. 1), p. 13.
5. McCarthy, *Basic Marketing* (n. 1), p. 816-18.
6. C. Goodrum, H. Dalyrymple, *Advertising in America, The First 200 Years* (New York: Harry N. Abrams, 1990), p. 29.
7. *Pharmacists for the Future* (Ann Arbor: Health Administration Press, 1975), pp. 10-12.
8. Quoted in C. Djerassi, *The Politics of Contraception* (New York: W. W. Norton, 1979), p. 227.
9. A. Caldwell, *Origins of Psychopharmacology from CPZ to LSD* (Springfield: Charles C. Thomas, 1970).
10. M. C. Smith, *Small Comfort* (New York: Praeger, 1985), pp. 64-82.
11. J. D. McEvilla, "Pharmacy and the professional fee," *Journal of the American Pharmaceutical Association* ns2 no. 9 (1962): 520-24.
12. P. C. Olsen, *Marketing Drug Products* (New York: Topics Publishing, 1964), p. 34.
13. J. M. Firestone, "A price index for drugs,"*Drug and Cosmetic Industry* 87, no. 4 (1963): 470.
14. J. D. McEvilla, "Price determination theory in the pharmaceutical industry,"*Drug and Cosmetic Industry* 82, no. 1(1958): 34.
15. G. M. Lebhar, "The story of drug chains," *Chain Store Age* 25, no. 6 (1950): 2.
16. E. T. Kelly, H. A. Palmer, "Increasing OTC market share: Strategies for pharmacists," *Pharmcy Business* 4, no. 1 (1993): 6-9.
17. C. D. Helper, "Clozapine and the outmoded drug use process," *American Pharmacy* N530, 12 (1990): 739.
18. Goodrum, *Advertising in America* (n. 6), p. 173.
19. Smith, *Small Comfort* (n. 10), p. 65.
20. C. E. Yesalis, et al. "Use and costs under the Iowa capitation program," *Health Care Financing Review* 3, no. 1 (1981): 127-39.
21. Anon., "Price suite settlement," *F-D-C Reports* 58, no. 5 (January 29, 1996): 1-2.
22. P. Stolley, "Cultural lag in health care," *Inquiry* 8 (1971): 71-76.

Suggested Readings

Home Medication and the Public Welfare, Annals of the New York Academy of Sciences, vol. 120, art. 2, pp. 807-1024, July 1965.

Pharmacists for the Future, The Report of the Study Commission on Pharmacy (Ann Arbor: Health Administration Press, 1975).

Bandelin, F. J., *Our Modern Medicines* (Hankinson, ND: Woodbine Publishing, 1986).

Engel, L. *Medicine Makers of Kalamazoo* (New York: McGraw-Hill Book Company, 1961).

Kedersha, R. G., ed. *Pharmaceutical Marketing Orientation Seminar* (Newark, NJ: Rutgers, n.d., ca. 1964).

Keller, B. G., and Smith, M. C. *Pharmaceutical Marketing, An Anthology and Bibliography* (Baltimore: Williams and Wilkins, 1969).

Liebenau, J., Higby, G. J., and Stroud, E. C., *Pill Peddlers: Essays on the History of the Pharmaceutical Industry* (Madison, WI: American Institute of the History of Pharmacy, 1990).

Nelson, G. L., ed. *Pharmaceutical Company Histories* (Bismark, ND: Woodbine Publishing, 1983).

Olsen, P. C. *Marketing Drug Products* (New York: Topics Publishing Company, 1964),

Smith, M. C. *Pharmacy and Medicine on the Air* (Metuchen, NJ: Scarecrow Press, 1989).

Smith, M. C. *Small Comfort: A History of the Minor Tranquilizers* (New York: Praeger, 1985).

Smith, A., and Herrick, A. D. *Drug Research and Development* (New York: Revere Publishing Co., 1948).

Physician-Pharmacist-Patient Interaction

by Paul L. Ranelli

MEDICINES are a major tie that binds pharmacists, patients, and physicians. A dynamic, sometimes strained relationship, due to discordant agendas, perceptions, and priorities, has been the circumstance between physicians and pharmacists from the beginning of the nineteenth century. Years of friction aside, the blossoming of medical and pharmaceutical information in the twentieth century has spawned greater cooperation between the professions and injected squarely the patient into the dyad. Cowen argues that as cooperation increases between physicians and pharmacists and as professional tensions ease, patient care should benefit.[1]

The shift from a physician-pharmacist professional dyad to a patient-included triad represents more accurately the relationship and interactions among contemporary physicians, pharmacists, and patients about medicines. Interestingly, formation of the trio comes when the cooperative relationship between physicians and pharmacists has not had much time to congeal. In fact, the American Medical Association recently adopted a position that only physicians should have the authority and responsibility to determine the drug of choice for a patient.[2] Evidently, hundreds of years of friction does not dissolve easily.

The purpose of this essay is to discuss the contemporary nature of interactions among physicians, pharmacists, and patients about medicines and how those interactions can affect the health-related outcomes of medical and medication-related therapy. I submit that the earnest incorporation of patients into the partnership accelerates, rather than obstructs, the congealing process because a person's long-term partnership with his or her physician and pharmacist is a bond of trust, as posited by Leopold, Cooper, and Clancy,[3] that can

277

lead to healing in and of itself; that trust also is essential to help guide patients through the health system.

Background and Significance

Pharmaceutical care is the responsible provision of drug therapy for the purpose of achieving definite outcomes that improve a patient's quality of life.[4] Pharmaceutical care, also known as patient-care pharmacy, is the synthesis of the traditional distributive and informational responsibilities into a *responsibility for drug therapy*. Pharmacists practicing in this model would (1) advise and consult physicians and patients, (2) accept responsibility for implementing therapeutic plans, including the supply of drug products, and (3) monitor patient progress and drug-related outcomes. The pharmacist's primary relationship is with the patient as a therapist; the relationship with the physician is collegial, as a co-therapist.[5]

If the quality of care for patients under a patient-care model is to improve, it will be necessary to modify or bridge communication gaps between pharmacists and physicians. Generally, pharmacists and physicians communicate only with a written or telephoned prescription order. When this is the case, pharmacists have a limited amount of information with which to evaluate a patient's drug therapy. In addition, physicians are unable to benefit from a pharmacist's suggestions about drug therapy. Bridging the gap would facilitate the transfer of information to patients about drug effectiveness, drug interactions, and cooperation with medication regimens.

Research Findings

A review of the literature reveals strong evidence for the value of an open, communicative relationship among patients, pharmacists, and physicians. Overall, an examination, known as a meta-analysis, of 61 published

Paul L. Ranelli is an Associate Professor of Social and Behavioral Pharmacy at the University of Wyoming School of Pharmacy, Laramie, a position he has held since 1995. He received his Ph.D. in social and behavioral pharmacy from the University of Wisconsin at Madison, M.Sc. in pharmaceutical administration from Wayne State University, and B.S. in pharmacy from the University of Rhode Island. While in Wisconsin, he was pharmacy director at the Menominee Tribal Clinic and a pharmacist with the Cuban-Haitian Resettlement Task Force in 1980. At Wyoming, he teaches strategies of patient-professional communication and a sociological and policy-oriented course in public health. Dr. Ranelli studies medication-use behavior, specifically, the medication-information needs of family caregivers and the elders they care for, and the experiences and expectations of urban and rural elders with medication-related communication.

studies about direct provider-patient communication showed that the strongest predictor of patient satisfaction was the amount of information provided by the health professional and that patient cooperation with treatment also was associated with more information.[6]

Providing patients with information on treatments has beneficial effects on recovery; the effect may result, possibly, as much from the interpretation of the communication as from an increase in knowledge. More information has an additional benefit, too. Providers who more fully inform patients are seen by patients as more sincere, more concerned, more interested, and more dedicated.[7]

The prescription, figuratively and literally, is an integral part of the physician-pharmacist-patient triad. In one study of physician-patient communication about prescriptions written during an office visit, 17% of the encounters had no discussion of the medication, in only 10% of the encounters was the duration of therapy discussed, and patients who received more explicit instructions had better understanding and higher levels of cooperation with therapy.[8] An advantage of a more verbal approach was shown likewise by Street.[9] In his study, patients who asked more questions of providers received more information beyond answers to the questions and more practical information. And, as Roter and Hall point out, patients who are more verbal are seen by providers as more interested in their own health.[10]

Implications for the value of verbal discourse about medication therapy are great. For example, patients who are allowed to tell their own story in their own words about medical complaints and beliefs about treatment rate their providers as more "warm" and report higher feelings of trust, confidence, and freedom to express themselves.[11] Statistical associations were found only with the number of open-ended questions asked by providers, not with the number of closed-ended questions. The wording of a question and extent of the answer sought determines whether it is labeled as open or closed. Generally, open questions are used to stimulate answers or comments that are more than a few words. Closed questions, on the other hand, are constructed to elicit a "yes,""no," or very brief answer.

Again, the influence of questioning style remains clear in a study by Frankel and Beckman.[12] An "indirect" questioning style was significantly less successful in identifying medication use problems than a "direct" style. As an example, an indirect approach such as, "Everything okay with your medications?" was less effective than a direct approach when the provider reviewed each medication and the patient told the name of the drug, dosage, number of times taken during the day, and problems with taking the medication.

Beckman and Frankel also studied the level of openness between provider and patient as a function of the number of interruptions.[13] Tape recordings of office visits with primary-care physicians were analyzed. In this study, seventy percent of initial statements by patients about health concerns were interrupted by physicians. Interruptions occurred after an average of eighteen seconds and most interruptions occurred after the patient mentioned their first concern. Specifically, physicians asked closed questions about the first concern and no further opening was provided for the patient to give other concerns. Yet, for patients who were allowed to speak without interruption, statements averaged thirty-eight seconds. The longest statement lasted two and a half minutes and those concerns expressed first were no more serious or medically important than those expressed later.

Research specifically on pharmacist-patient communication indicates that pharmacists seldom ask questions of patients to assess understanding, use, or problems with treatment. The communication that does exist is largely the provision of information by the pharmacist, often in response to a patient question.[14] Even though information seeking by pharmacists, that is, question asking, of patients is minimal, this finding may still benefit the building of a relationship since patients are more likely to ask questions when providers have first given them information.[15]

Furthermore, what occurs during or is recalled from a visit with a provider is instructive. During interviews conducted by Tuckett and his col-

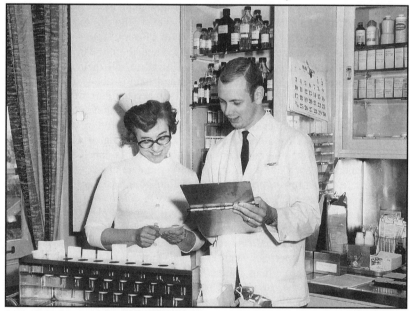

Pharmacy Resident Harold St. Clair and Nurse J. Manning review patient medication orders at the Veterans Adminstration Hospital, in Cincinnati, Ohio, 1970. (Courtesy AIHP Collection, Kremers Reference Files, F. B. Powers Pharmacy Library, University of Wisconsin-Madison.)

leagues with patients immediately after they had seen their physician, patients were asked if they had questions or concerns during the medical visit that they did not mention.[16] Seventy-five percent of the study participants said yes. When asked why they did not voice their concerns the following three reasons surfaced regularly: fear of being humiliated, it takes time away from more needy patients, and the doctor was too busy and the visit too hurried. Patients have cited the pharmacist appearing too "busy" as a deterrent to asking questions or raising concerns about treatment.[17]

Preparing patients for provider visits is supported by four well-controlled studies. The researchers prepared patients for medical visits immediately before they went into their physicians. The patients were randomly assigned to treatment and control groups. The experimental group patients were found to take more control of the communication, ask more questions, and express more feelings and concerns about treatment. They also obtained more information from physicians and had improved health outcomes at follow-up interviews; that is, the subjects with diabetes had better blood glucose control and the patients with hypertension had better blood pressure control.[18]

Discussion and Summary

The research evidence presented reinforces the notion that the provider-patient relationship should be a helping relationship, which has as its professional purpose, especially within the context of this paper, to help patients manage medication. Physician-pharmacist-patient interaction cannot be standardized since communication depends on patient need. Nevertheless, providers have the burden of responsibility for improving relationships with patients. Physicians and pharmacists must convey their purpose in patient care to patients and express that purpose in terms of benefit to the patient. If the purpose of a treatment plan or medication therapy goes unexplained, patients will still try to guess why a physician or pharmacist is doing what she or he is doing, thereby leaving open the chance for misunderstanding.

As this review illustrates, a more active involvement by providers in the communication process with patients is related to greater patient satisfaction with care and improved patient outcomes. And, a more active involvement by patients in the communication process with health professionals is related to greater patient satisfaction with care and improved patient outcomes. In turn, patients must have the opportunity to tell their story about medical treatment in their own words. Since patients generally do not do a good job of being assertive in communication with providers, pharmacists and physicians must take it upon themselves to make more active patient involvement possible. This can be done by teaching patients what questions to ask and how to ask them.

References

The assistance of Carole L. Kimberlin is acknowledged.

1. D. L. Cowen, "Changing relationship between pharmacists and physicians," *American Journal of Hospital Pharmacy* 49(1992): 2715-21.
2. J. Breu, "Pharmacists clucking over some new AMA measures," *Drug Topics* 140, no. 13 (1996): 31.
3. N. Leopold, J. Cooper, C. Clancy, "Sustained partnership in primary care," *Journal of Family Practice* 42 (1996): 129-37.
4. C. D. Hepler, L. M. Strand, "Opportunities and responsibilities in pharmaceutical care," *American Journal of Hospital Pharmacy* 47 (1990): 533-43.
5. C. D. Hepler, "Pharmaceutical care as a goal," in *Challenges in Pharmaceutical Care: Where, When and How to Begin* (Princeton, NJ: Bristol-Myers Squibb Company, 1993), pp. 1-5.
6. D. Roter, "Which facets of communication have strong effects on outcome—a meta-analysis," in M. Stewart, D. Roter, eds. *Communicating with Medical Patients* (Newbury Park, CA: Sage, 1989), pp. 183-96.
7. D. L. Roter, J. A. Hall, N. R. Katz, "Patient-physician communication: a descriptive summary of the literature," *Patient Education and Counseling* 12 (1988): 99-119.
8. B. L. Svarstad, "Patient-practitioner relationships and compliance with prescribed medical regimens," in L. H. Aiken, D. Mechanic, eds. *Applications of Social Sciences to Clinical Medicine and Health Policy* (New Brunswick, NJ: Rutgers University Press, 1986), pp. 438-59.
9. R. L. Street, "Information-giving in medical consultations: the influence of patients' communication styles and personal characteristics," *Social Science and Medicine* 32 (1991): 541-48.
10. D. Roter, J. A. Hall, *Doctors Talking with Patients/Patients Talking with Doctors: Improving Communication in Medical Visits* (Westport, CT: Auburn House, 1992).
11. W. B. Stiles, S. M. Putnam, M. H. Wolf, S. A. James, "Interaction exchanges structure and patient satisfaction with medical interviews," *Medical Care* 17 (1979): 667-779.
12. R. M. Frankel, H. B. Beckman, "Conversation and compliance with treatment recommendations: an application of micro-interactional analysis in medicine," in B. Dervin, L. Grossberg, B. J. O'Keefe, and E. Wartella, eds. *Rethinking Communication* (Newbury Park, CA: Sage, 1989), pp. 60-74.
13. H. B. Beckman, R. M. Frankel, "The effect of physician behavior on the collection of data," *Annals of Internal Medicine* 101 (1984): 692-96.
14. D. H. Berardo, C. L. Kimberlin, C. W. Barnett, "Observational research on patient education activities of community pharmacists," *Journal of Social and Administrative Pharmacy* 6 (1989): 21-30; C. L. Kimberlin, D. H. Berardo, J. F. Pendergast, L. C. McKenzie, "Effects of an education program for community pharmacists on detecting drug-related problems in elderly patients," *Medical Care* 31 (1993): 451-68.
15. S. M. Putnam, W. B. Stiles, "Verbal exchanges in medical interviews: implications and innovations," *Social Science and Medicine* 36 (1993): 1597-1604.
16. D. Tuckett, M. Boulton, C. Olson, A. Williams, *Meetings Between Experts: An Approach to Sharing Ideas in Medical Consultations* (London: Tavistock, 1985).
17. R. S. Beardsley, C. A. Johnson, G. Wise, "Privacy as a factor in patient compliance," *Journal of the American Pharmaceutical Association* NS17 (1977): 366-68.

18. D. L. Roter, "Patient question asking in physician-patient interaction," *Health Psychology* 3 (1984): 395-409; S. H. Kaplan, S. Greenfield, J. E. Ware, Jr., "Assessing the effects of physician-patient interactions on the outcomes of chronic disease," *Medical Care* 27 Suppl. 3 (1989): S110-S127.

Bibliography

Albro, W. "How to communicate with physicians." *American Pharmacy.* NS33 (1993): 59-61.

Almy, T. P., K. K. Colby, M. Zubkoff, D. S. Gephart, M. Moore-West, L. L. Lundquist. "Health, society, and the physician: problem based learning of the social sciences and humanities." *Annals of Internal Medicine.* 116 (1992): 569-74.

Angaran, D.M., D. B. Brushwood, D. J. Tennenhouse. *Risk Prevention Skills: Communication for Pharmacists.* Corte Madera, CA: Tennenhouse Professional Publications, 1995.

Anon. "How is your doctor treating you?" *Consumer Reports.* Feb. (1995): 81-88.

Anon. *Schering Report V: Pharmacists and Physicians: Attitudes and Perceptions of Two Professions.* Kenilworth, NJ: Schering Corporation, 1983: 1-12.

ASHP Research and Education Foundation. "Understanding and preventing drug misadventures." *American Journal of Health-System Pharmacy.* 52 (1995): 369-416.

Brody, H. *The Healer's Power.* New Haven: Yale, 1992.

Delbanco, T. L. "Enriching the doctor-patient relationship by inviting the patient's perspective." *Annals of Internal Medicine.* 116 (1992): 414-18.

DeYoung, M. "Research on the effects of pharmacist-patient communication in institutions and ambulatory care sites, 1969-1994." *American Journal of Health-System Pharmacy.* 53 (1996): 1277-91.

DiMatteo, M. R. *The Psychology of Health, Illness, and Medical Care: An Individual*

Perspective [out of print]. Pacific Grove, CA: Brooks/Cole, 1991: 186-223.

Hitchens, K. "Talking to docs." *American Druggist.* Nov. (1995): 24-27.

Kaplan, S. "Patienthood." In: Kaplan, A. K., ed. *Improving Patient-Physician Relations. Proceedings of The Future of the Patient in Emerging Approaches to Quality Assurance; 1991 Dec 3-4; Washington, DC.* Washington, DC: Public Policy Institute/ American Association of Retired Persons, 1991: 8-13.

Katz, J. *The Silent World of Doctor and Patient.* New York: Free Press, 1984.

Landis, N. T. "Lessons from medicine and nursing for pharmacist-patient communication." *American Journal of Health-System Pharmacy.* 53(1996): 1306-14.

McCallum, D. B., S. L. Yenney. *Communicating the Benefits and Risks of Prescription Drugs* [monograph 106]. Washington, DC: Institute for Health Policy Analysis, Georgetown University, 1989.

Mechanic, D. "Health and illness behavior and patient-practitioner relationships." *Social Science and Medicine.* 34 (1992): 1345-50.

Meldrum, H. *Interpersonal Communication in Pharmaceutical Care.* New York: Haworth Press, 1994.

Ranelli, P. L. "Patient communication." In: Gennaro, A. R., ed. *Remington: The Science and Practice of Pharmacy* [nineteenth edition]. Easton, PA: Mack, 1995: 1779-85.

Segal, R., and D. S. Pathak. "Influencing physician acceptance of consultant pharmacists' recommendations." *The Consultant Pharmacist.* Jul./Aug. (1986): 129-33.

Sherman, S. E., S. M. Putnam, M. Lipkin, A. Lazare, J. Stoeckle, V. Keller, J. G. Carroll, eds. *Annotated Bibliography of Doctor-Patient Communication of the Task Force on Doctor and Patient* [second edition]. West Haven, CT: Miles Inc. Pharmaceutical Division, 1992.

Tindall, W. N., R. S. Beardsley, C. L. Kimberlin. *Communication Skills in Pharmacy Practice.* Philadelphia: Lea & Febiger, 1994.

Vree, T. B. "Pharmacist-physician interaction: a battle of genes." *DICP, The Annals of Pharmacotherapy.* 25 (1991): 1132.

Wiederholt, J. B., B. R. Clarridge, B. L. Svarstad. "Verbal consultation regarding prescription drugs: findings from a statewide study." *Medical Care.* 20 (1992): 159-73.

Zellmer, W. A. "Transforming the work of the pharmacist: the need for historical perspective." *Pharmacy in History.* 33 (1991): 159-63.

Zellmer, W. A. "Searching for the soul of pharmacy." *American Journal of Health-System Pharmacy.* 53 (1996): 1911-16.

The Global Impact of Medicines

by William H. Foege

A class of four-year-olds was receiving instructions on their first day of school. The teacher told them that anyone needing to use the bathroom should raise their hand. A perplexed four-year-old-boy asked, "But how does that help?"

We have heard, over the past two days, of chance observations, of the systematic gathering of information, scientific breakthroughs, medicines found in nature, medicines from the body, and medicines synthesized in the laboratory. We have heard of inspired conclusion and heroic tenacity. And we are led to ask, "But how does that help?" How does it make a difference to people? What is the impact on an individual? On a family? On a community? On the world?

Steven Hawking reminds us that the history of science is to gradually see that things do not happen in an arbitrary fashion. This is a cause-and-effect world. To go from observations, that fermented beverages could lead to drunkenness, or that some actions were associated with problems of health, such as eating spoiled food, is one thing. But even harder has been the step of associating activities or the ingestion of substances with strength or health. Indeed it is only now, with large studies, that we can come to understand the benefits of Vitamin A or folic acid. It is quite another thing altogether to experiment with medicines, to give some substance in the hope of preventing or curing an illness, and to do that with enough frequency that the observations add up to a conclusion.

When we look at the entire spectrum of medicines, including therapeutics for cure, prevention, or diagnosis, one can only be astonished and intrigued by the courage, the insight, and the persistence that drove people to find useful ways of medicating.

An example of the difficulties involved in this process is found in the history of variolation, which preceded our current vaccines. In variolation, the material from a smallpox pustule is inoculated into a susceptible individual to provide protection against smallpox disease. It was used in Africa, Afghanistan, India, and China and perhaps was developed independently in several places. The practice was introduced to England from Turkey and was widely used in the United Kingdom in the eighteenth and early nineteenth centuries. It was introduced to the United States from Africa by slaves. And yet it is difficult to understand how it could have started. It is based on the observation that the mortality from smallpox was lower when the virus was transmitted from person to person through the cutaneous route, rather than through the usual respiratory route. Mortality might be only one percent instead of twenty, thirty, or forty percent. But how did people discover that? Who had the courage to try it? And how did they accumulate enough volunteers to have a series large enough to draw conclusions?

The later stages in the development of variolation are more understandable. When Lady Montegu, wife of the British ambassador to Turkey, wrote home about her observations regarding variolation, the royal family tried it on prisoners. They were so impressed that they next attempted the same ex-

---

William H. Foege is an epidemiologist who is widely recognized as a key member of the successful campaign to eradicate smallpox in the 1970s. After serving as a medical missionary in Nigeria, Dr. Foege became Chief of the CDC Smallpox Eradication Program, and was appointed director of the U.S. Centers for Disease Control in 1977.

In 1984, Foege and several colleagues formed the Task Force for Child Survival, a working group for the World Health Organization, UNICEF, The World Bank, the United Nations Development Program, and the Rockefeller Foundation. Its success in accelerating childhood immunization led to an expansion of its mandate in 1991 to include other issues that diminish the quality of life for children. Now called The Task Force for Child Survival and Development, the group works with its sponsoring agencies to achieve the broad health goals of the 1990 World Summit for Children.

Dr. Foege joined The Carter Center in 1986 as its Executive Director, Fellow for Health Policy, and Executive Director of Global 2000. In 1992, he resigned as executive director of The Carter Center, but continues in his role as a Fellow, and as Executive Director of the Task Force for Child Survival and Development. Two areas of special interest to him are the disease eradication and agricultural projects of Global 2000. By ridding the developing world of the crippling diseases of Guinea worm and River Blindness, and by teaching basic, easily implemented planting techniques, Global 2000 projects enable communities and villages in the developing world to become self-sufficient.

periment on their own children. Again the results were so good that the practice was introduced to the general public and various variolators, including the Sutton family did hundreds of thousands of variolations. At the time of the Battle of Quebec, British troops were variolated while US troops were not. A smallpox outbreak selectively decimated US troops and decided the outcome of the Battle of Quebec. But the question remains. How can one understand the events that started the long and widespread process of using variolation?

It is easier to understand the use of cowpox by Edward Jenner to protect James Phipps against smallpox. Jenner's observations had convinced him that cowpox was protective, and based on those observations he had the courage to prove the protective power of cowpox.

My plan is to look briefly at the impact of medicines on individuals, the impact on society, the groups of medicines with the highest impact, the gap between public health and medicine, and finally, what we might expect in the future.

The Impact on Individuals

We have heard speakers relating their own health experiences before various drugs were available. It makes us wonder how many of us would have lived to our current age, if held to the rules of 200 years ago, 100 years ago, or 50 years ago? Some of you owe your lives to the availability of insulin, or antihypertensives, or chemotherapy. We can speculate about others. I can say with some certainty that I would not be here had I not been successfully treated for septicemia with penicillin in the 1940s, an antibiotic that had not been available for civilian use two years earlier. Therefore I credit my last 50 years to the availability of a specific medicine.

Perhaps most people my age carry such a debt and do not recognize it. Examine several generations, and you will find that a significant percentage owe their lives to medicines, directly or indirectly. For example, while I can be quite confident in crediting my adulthood to penicillin, my children will never tie their very existence to that successful therapeutic episode, unless I tell them. And within another generation there will be no memory at all that a medicine of the right kind, at the right time, changed forever a family tree.

If we knew the secret history of all, we would be surprised by the close calls, the chances missed, the events dependent on the use of a medicine or the availability of a medication that for some reason was not used. Some quick examples:

The Chronicle of St. Augustine relates, around 1633, the miraculous cures from fever felt to be due to a powder taken from the bark of a tree—one of the first specific treatments for a given disease. Catholic missionaries observed and brought the bark itself from South America to Europe by the 1640s. In 1658, Oliver Cromwell became ill with malaria, and quinine was available for his treatment. The understanding existed to know this would be an appropriate treatment and yet he refused to take quinine, because he regarded it as a Catholic or Jesuit plot.

Gary Wills has written of the importance of the Gettysburg address in changing the history of the United States. Wills maintains that Lincoln, using all of his experience and insight into our history, changed the United States from a plural to a singular noun. Less well known is the fact that Lincoln gave the address while incubating smallpox. Indeed he developed symptoms while on the train returning to Washington, D. C. A twenty-four hour change in the time of exposure or the length of the incubation period could have forced him to forego that significant address.

Princes and Peasants, by Donald Hopkins, tells how history changed, even after smallpox vaccine was available, because people either were or were not protected by the use of that vaccine.

West Africa has often been described as the "White man's grave." The book, *Ladder of Bones*, by Ellen Thorp, tells the story of the short lives of the early Europeans in West Africa. They faced many diseases, but especially the lethality of malaria and yellow fever. The odds changed when quinine became available, and then again with yellow fever vaccine. What is forgotten is that it was also the "Black man's grave," keeping whole societies at a subsistence level as large numbers were compromised by malaria, yellow fever, intestinal helminths, diarrhea, iron deficiency, and malnutrition.

We understand the individual stories, but we can only barely understand what this means in the aggregate as health improves.

The Impact on Society

The World Development Report 1993, issued by the World Bank, describes the improvement of health in the world in the past four decades as being greater than in the entire previous history of the world. Infant mortality rates (IMR) have declined by fifty percent in the world in the past thirty-five years. Life expectancy for the entire world has increased by fifteen years during that same time period. The threats are still great, but vastly improved over earlier generations. What is the impact on society when people in the aggregate are healthier?

There are, of course, changes just because many are healthy. For example, there is a more efficient economy where individuals contribute more because they spend less time unable to work and they require less care from others. In addition to being healthy there is the inestimable value of improved quality of life.

What is the effect of iodine in salt? It is not just the productivity of healthier people directly helped, but also a released energy of those not directly treated. For example, with iodine deprivation a child may be retarded. Prevent that and society gets the services of parents, especially the mother, who need not spend the extra strength required for a retarded child, the planning which requires arrangements for such children when parents die, the requirement to plan all activities around that child, and so forth.

Vitamins in bread provide benefits not fully understood in preventing some conditions at low cost. Likewise, the effects of polio vaccine are very clear for the millions of persons who in 40 years have not been paralyzed. But there are also benefits for everyone else. Efforts not spent on medical care release resources for other health conditions. Society has been able to forego the costs of maintaining iron lungs and special care for those paralyzed for life.

What is the point? The benefits of medicines go beyond the sum total of each person made healthy. Society benefits in both obvious and hidden ways.

What are the Medicines with the Highest Impact?

In the interest of time we are forced to choose, to condense, to summarize. What are some of the most important medicines from the perspective of impact on worldwide society? I vote for seven, heavily influenced by their impact on developing countries.

1. Vaccines—This is a category of medicines that need be developed but once in the entire history of the world. Unlike antibiotics which are eventually faced with organisms that have developed resistance, vaccines could retain effectiveness for all time. In addition they are relatively inexpensive and have in many cases been made available to all, thereby changing the world.

The eradication of smallpox provides the first case of a disease having been eliminated from the world by the plan of people, and this event was possible because of a vaccine. Even thirty years ago millions died each year because of the smallpox virus and now the world has gone almost twenty years without a case!

Measles virus, only fifteen years ago, was the world's single most lethal agent. Measles accounted for over three million deaths a year. Now measles is a rarity in this hemisphere and mortality rates are estimated to have declined by eighty-five percent worldwide.

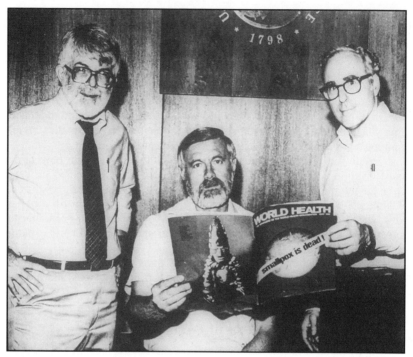

Three former directors of CDC's smallpox eradication efforts (J. Donald Millar, William H. Foege, and J. Michael Lane, l. to r.) pose together to hold up the copy of World Health magazine announcing "Smallpox is Dead." (Courtesy National Library of Medicine.)

Polio conjures up a picture of iron lungs, 50,000 cases a year in this country alone, beggars around the world, and now on the threshold of eradication. These are not simply interesting examples, they are miracles with major impacts, all because our science has been able to develop inexpensive, effective and safe vaccines.

2. Antibiotics—Throughout history there have been two principle causes of premature mortality, infections and violence. Antibiotics have changed the power of the infectious diseases. There will always be new infectious diseases and those unresponsive to antibiotics, but a significant start has been made. Pneumonia, septicemia, typhoid fever, and other once fatal conditions have yielded. To the antibiotics, add the impact of oral rehydration salts (ORS), one of the simplest medications we have in our portfolio, and millions of deaths are averted each year.

3. Analgesics and Anesthetic agents—Albert Schweitzer once pointed out that, "Pain is a greater burden on humankind than death itself." From headaches and arthritis, which can dominate your day, to the pain of injury and surgery, life quality has been improved immeasurably. We can no longer imagine what it was like, even 135 years ago, during the American civil war, to have limbs amputated while conscious.

4. Contraceptives—The current and future impact of contraceptives on individuals and on society has changed everything. It has changed the ability to plan the number and spacing of children and thereby has made it possible for individuals and societies to plan rational futures.

5. Antihypertensive medicines—While it is still not clear how many cases of hypertension could be effectively treated by means of diet, exercise and other non-medication approaches, there is no question that this category of medicines has had a marked impact in reducing the number of strokes, early death, disability, and compromised life quality.

6. Insulin—We have forgotten the stark difference between what could be provided to patients in 1920 versus 1996. The talk yesterday helped us to remember what it was like to gradually starve to death because of diabetes. As with antibiotics, this is a life-saving medication for many.

7. Mental Health Drugs—In recent decades new life has been offered to many who were thought to be beyond the help of conventional medicine. Society is reaping the benefits of people finding relief from depression, bipolar disease, and schizophrenia.

Gaps—The Great Divide Between Medicine and Public Health

Our demand for medicines is greater than it should be because we have not learned how to adequately fund and deliver prevention. An article in the *Journal of the American Medical Association* has looked at generic causes of death in this country rather than at the organ system that failed. Three problems are responsible for forty percent of all deaths—tobacco, with over 400,000 deaths per year; diet, which accounts for over 300,000 deaths per year; and alcohol, responsible for over 100,000 deaths per year. Proper prevention could reduce our need for lung cancer surgery, coronary intensive care units, and treatment for the complications of diabetes or chronic obstructive respiratory disease.

Why inject this into a symposium on medicines? Dr. Koop mentioned yesterday that the pharmacists of tomorrow must also be the health educators. Kipling once said that words constitute the most powerful drug known to humankind. We must learn to improve our health education by the creative use of words, a drug grossly underutilized in the prevention of illness. Prevention should be our first reaction.

Medicine has the responsibility to provide the best knowledge to each patient. Public health has the problem of providing that knowledge to everyone. In trying to do that we find that our science is ahead of everything—our humanity, ethics, law and sociology.

The market place simply does not solve all health problems. It may be the best system in general but as Francis Fukiyama points out, we get to a point where we need trust and the knowledge that a system exists to take care of those who are not benefiting from the market place.

How do we make medicines available to all? At least four quandaries have not been solved, especially in the developing countries.

Price—This has been solved for vaccines by providing a subsidy for vaccines given to the poor within a society or by having rich countries subsidize programs in poorer countries. Could such a system work for other medicines?

Availability—Primary health centers around the world lack needed medicines. One approach, the "Bamako Initiative," attempts to employ a revolving fund, better prices through volume purchase and the recovery of some funds from those receiving the medicines.

Development of drug resistance—How do we control the use of a drug so as to make it effective for as long as possible? That is part of the public health concern for social justice that involves even those who will be born in the future. We have not figured out how to handle the next therapeutic drug against malaria or bacteria, in order to be sure we can balance demand, the need for profit and the need to control inappropriate use to avoid early development of resistance. What we do know is that the market system alone, without any controls, favors profit, which may lead to inappropriate use and the early development of drug resistance.

Research—The challenge, in this age of science, is to apply the awesome research capacity of pharmaceutical companies to problems of the developing world, even if the solution of those problems will not necessarily provide the greatest profit. Is there a way for global health committees to develop a list of priority needs and a mechanism to encourage and subsidize the development of medicines that would be of great benefit to the poor of the world?

One of the most intriguing stories of modern medicine is the decision by Merck to provide Mectizan free for human use in the case of onchocerciasis. The drug is now being given to about fifteen million people a year, provided by Merck and distributed through a consortium of UN agencies, Ministries of Health, medical mission groups, non-government organizations and foundations. Now, the World Bank has started a program to raise $120 million over ten years to assist countries in the distribution of the drug. The program is one of the most important coalitions in global health today, so successful as to raise the possibility of actually eradicating onchocerciasis.

What can we look forward to?

Vaccines—The future will simplify the present confusing schedule that requires multiple visits by each child with multiple injections, a different age window for each antigen, a requirement for refrigeration, and a low level of adverse effects. In the future there will be fewer visits required, eventually providing protection against all vaccine-preventable diseases with one, two or three visits. Booster doses will be a memory and vaccines will be given orally or by aerosol rather than by needle and syringe. The number of antigens will increase to several dozen and adverse effects will decline.

Cancer drugs—An increasing sophistication will provide extremely specific poisoning of cancer cells without harm to adjacent normal cells. Combined with genetic screening for predispositions and early diagnostic tests, medicines provide new hope for those with cancer.

Correction of genetic defects—Early approaches to such problems as cystic fibrosis has led to the expectation that both prenatal and postnatal treatments for genetic problems will increase the power of medicines in the near future.

Preventive micronutrients—The history of iodine supplementation in salt and vitamin additions to bread and cereal has been so successful in this country, and increasingly in the world, that it offers a model for the use of preventive medicines. It should be possible to neutralize the impact of vitamin A deficiency, folic acid, zinc, and other deficiencies by carefully defining the therapeutic range of the micronutrient and providing it as a hidden benefit in the preferred diet of a population.

Where will it stop? Mae West once said that too much of a good thing is just fine. The improvements in medicines will not stop and that is just fine. The power of medicines to improve life is only now beginning to be understood.

It was once feared that the computer would reduce people to a social security number or similar identifier. Instead the computer has freed individuals to benefit from science. Not only do we have "medicines for all," in addition, we have a new power that can harness the products of science for each individual, to tailor-make an approach. Such an individual approach would include:

    1. Identification of risks

2. Screening those at highest risk

3. Preventive drugs or vaccines

4. Specific therapy—for a wide spectrum of conditions from infectious diseases to cancer.

As we sympathize with those who had a paucity of medicines available a century ago, so will people entering the twenty-second century pity our current lack of tools in medicine. What is the bottom line? The history of medicines is rich but the impact has just begun.

C. P. Snow doubted that there would ever be a bridge between science and the humanities. The history of medicines shows us that bridge every day.

Chairman's Conclusion

by Gregory J. Higby

At the end of the two-day symposium at the Carter Center, I scheduled myself ten minutes for closing remarks. I had hoped to pull together some of the themes of the previous two days. As is so often the case, however, we had run out of time and I had no opportunity to say much more than thank you and good bye. After reading the presentations in this volume, I have decided to conclude with what I actually said that day. Thanks for reading.

T HANK you, Dr. Foege. Since we are running out of time, I will forego my prepared remarks. Instead, I wish to thank again all our speakers, Michael Harris, the Medicines staff, the Task Force for Child Survival and Development, and the Carter Center. Special thanks go out to Dr. Elaine C. Stroud, for her efforts to put this all together. And, of course, appreciation goes out as well to our sponsor, Glaxo Wellcome, and their representative, Elliott Sogol.

I wish to conclude by reiterating the questions posed by Dr. Koop yesterday. As we all return to our offices, labs, and class rooms next week, perhaps we can keep them in mind: In what areas of health have medicines had their greatest impact? And in what areas have they seemed to fail? Do the chronic diseases of the industrialized West attract more research attention than the acute illnesses afflicting much of the developing world? Are there limits to what medicines can do in theory, and if so, what are they? And what is the long-term future for medicines research and what can be done to improve its prospects?

Thank you all for coming and have a safe trip home.

Gregory J. Higby is a third-generation pharmacist, receiving his B.Sc. in Pharmacy from the University of Michigan in 1977. In 1984, he received his Ph.D. in the History of Pharmacy from the University of Wisconsin-Madison. His research and publications have centered on the history of American pharmacy. Since 1988, he has served as Director of the American Institute of the History of Pharmacy and as an adjunct faculty member at the University of Wisconsin School of Pharmacy.

Name Index

1-fluoroadenosine, 187
acetazolamide, 125
Ackerknecht, Erwin, 51
Acosta, Cristoval, 23
Acutalyn, 241
Adams, Samuel Hopkins, 233
adrenalin, 225
Adson, A. W., 129
Afovirsen, 180
agar, 24-25
Albertson, N. F., 151
alcohol, 38
Alexander of Tralles, 69
aloe, 19-21, 23
Altafur, 224, 246-250
anakinra, 176
Andromachus, 18
anticholerin, 67
antipyrine, 86
Antril, 176
Archer, Sydney, 151-152
arginase, 237-246
aspirin, 225
atoxyl, 88
Avicenna (ibn Sina), 18, 20-21
AZT, 204, 222

Baer, John, 125
Baines, Eric, 106, 108
balsam of Peru, 9
Banbar, 232
Banting, Frederick, 93-96
Barker, Lewellys 96
Barton, Joe, 223
Becher's Tonic Pills, 43
Beckman, H. B., 279
Bedford, D. Evan, 101, 102, 112
Beecher, Henry K., 149-150

belladonna, 225
Bernard, Claude, 38, 47, 65-67
Best, Charles, 94-95
Beyer, Karl, 125-126, 130
Bigelow, Jacob, 45
Billon, Jacques, 105
bismuth salicylate, 68
black hellebore, 43
black snake root, 225
Black, James, 186
Blaise, Edmond, 105, 113
Blake, James 81-83
blessed thistle, 43
Bliss, Eleanor, 110
Boerhaave, Hermann, 32, 34, 37
Boyd, E. Forrest, 238, 240, 242-245
Boyle, Robert ,81
bran, 24-25
Broussais, F., 59
Brown, John, 35-37, 56-57
Brunton, Thomas Lauder, 85-86
Buchheim, Rudolf, 47
buckthorn, 20-21
Buttle, G. A. H., 101, 105
Byar, David, 206

Cabanis, Pierre, J. G. 57
calomel, 24, 43
camomile flowers, 38
Campbell, Walter, 232
camphor, 225
captopril, 186, 191
carbolic acid, 68
Caroid Laxative, 20
carrot, 225
cascara sagrada, 20-21, 23
cassia, 18, 25
castor oil, 23, 24

Caventou, Joseph, 81
Celsus, A. C., 21
chaparral, 167
Chiang Kai-shek, 101
chloral hydrate, 65
chlorothiazide, 125, 126-133
chlorpromazine, 265
Churchill, Winston, 75, 101-102, 111,
    112, 114
cider, 40
cimetidine, 186
cinchona, 225
Cinnamomum cassia, 18
cinnamon, 38, 225
cladribine, 187
Clancy, C., 282
Clark, A. J., 185
Clowes, G. H. A., 96
Clozaril, 269
Clusius (Charles de L'Ecluse), 18
Collip, J. B., 95-96
colocynth, 23, 24
coltsfoot, 167
comfrey, 167
Contac, 269
Cooper, J., 282
Cordus, Valerius, 26
Cowen, D. L., 277
Cramp, Arthur, 233
cream of tartar, 43
Crellin, John, 86
Crispin, Edmond, 264
croton oil, 23, 25
Crum Brown, Alexander, 83-86, 185,
    190
Cullen, William, 32, 37, 55, 57
Cushman, David, 186
Cushney, A. R., 185
cyclosporin, 189
cytarabine, 187

Dagenan, 109
Dakin, Henry D., 237
Darvon, 177
De Kruif, Paul, 78, 229
Denton, Jane, 149
desomorphine, 144-146

DeStevens, George, 126
Diamox, 125
Dietl, Joseph, 63-64
digitalis 9, 40, 41-44, 46
Dioscorides, 19-21, 23, 25
diphtheria antitoxin, 123, 229
Diuril, 125, 128-129
Djerassi, Carl, 265
Domagk, Gerhard, 104
Double, François, 59-60
Dover's powder, 43
Dowling, Harry F., 16, 234
Duncan, Andrew, 44-45

echinacea, 167
Eddy, Nathan, B., 143-147, 150-
    153
Ehrlich, Paul, 78-79, 87-89, 142, 159,
    171-173, 185
Eisenhower, Dwight, 101
Eisleb, O., 147
elaterin, 23
elixir vitriol, 40
ephedra, 165-166
Erasistratus, 26
Esidrix, 126
Estes, J. Earle, 130
etorphine, 154
eucalyptus, 68
Evans, G. M., 109, 114
Ewing, Oscar, 236
Ewins, A. J., 105-106, 108-109,
    112-115
Ex-Lax, 20

feverfew, 167
Finland, Maxwell, 249
Firestone, John, 267
Fischer, Emil, 185
Fisher, Ronaly Aylmer, 205
fludarabine phosphate, 186
fludarabine, 187
Foege, William H., 2, 292
Ford, R. V., 126
Fourcroy, Antoine, 34
Frampton, John, 23
Frankel, R. M., 279

Franklin, Benjamin, 36
Fraser, Thomas, 83-86, 185, 190
Freis, Edward D., 126, 131
Fukiyama, Francis, 294
furaltadone, 246-250

Gaisford, Wilfrid, 109, 114
Galen, 19-21, 25
ganciclovir, 192
Ganellin, Robin, 186
garlic, 166
Gay-Lussac, Joseph, 80
Geber (Jabir ibn Haiyan), 24
ginkgo, 167
Girtanner, Christoph, 34
Gold, Harry, 202
Goldstein, Avram, 153
Goodell, Helen, 149
Goodrich, William, 243
Grandel's Liver and Gallbladder
    Tablets, 19
Greenwood, Major, 205
Gregory, James, 56
Grillet, Nicholas, 105, 113

Habitina, 228
Hacking, Ian, 206
Hahnemann, Samuel, 60-61
Hales, Stephen, 38
Hall, A. J., 279
Hapgood, Norman, 229
Hardy, James, 149
Harris, Louis, 151-152, 154
Hart, E. Ross., 148, 150
Hart, L. E., 106, 108
Harvey, William, 37, 55
Hatcher, Robert, 144, 148
Havens, James 97
Hawking, Steven, 287
Henderson, L. J., 16
Heparamine, 242
Hepasyn, 224, 237-246
heroin, 141, 228
Hill, Austin Bradford, 201, 202, 205,
    221
Himmelsbach, Clifton K., 145-146
Hippocrates, 16

Hoffmann, Friedrich, 32, 37, 61
Holland, Albert, 244
Hollander, W., 126
Holmes, Oliver Wendell, 231
Hopkins, Donald, 290
Hopkins, F. Gowland, 86
Hosford, Leo, 238-239, 241, 245
Howson, Colin, 206
Hughes, Charles Evans, 97, 231
Hughes, Elizabeth, 97
Hunt, Reid, 142
Huxley, Aldous, 265
Huxley, Thomas, 78
hydralazine, 129
hydrochlorothiazide, 126
Hydrodiuril, 126

ibn Masawaih, 18
idoform, 68
insulin, 93-99, 236, 293
iron, 38
Irons, Wesley G., 237-239, 241-
    242
Isbell, Harris, 149-150

Jackson, George, 249
jalap, 23, 24
Jefferson, Thomas, 36, 46-47
Jenner, Edward, 289
Joslin, Elliott, 98, 232

Kämpf, Johann, 36
Kannel, William, 123
Keats, Arthur D., 149
Kefauver, Estes, 272
Kessler, David, 164
Kipling, Rudyard, 294
Klebs, Edwin, 67
Kleiner, Israel, 95
Kleinfeld, Vincent, 249
Kneipp Herbal Tablets, 19
Knorr, Ludwig, 86
Koch, Roert, 66-67
Kolbe, A. W. H., 65
Kondremul, 20
Koop, C. Everett, 294
Kossell, Albrecht, 237

Kosterlitz, Hugh, 153

L-Dopa, 180-181
Laennec, R., 58
Lane, J. Michael, 292
Langley, James Newport, 88, 185
Larrick, George, 240, 244
Lasagna, Louis, 149
Lavoisier, Antoine, 34, 79
Laxagel, 18
Leake, Chauncey, 148
Lebhar, Godfrey, 268
lemons, 40
Leopold, N., 277
Liebreich, Oscar, 65
Lincoln, Abraham, 290
Lind, James, 40, 202, 203
linseed, 21
Lister, Joseph, 66, 86
Locke, John, 81
Long, Perrin H., 110
Louis, Pierre, 59-60

M & B 693, 75, 102-120
M & B 760, 102, 112
Macleod, J. J. R., 94-96
Magendie, François, 59, 79-81
magnesia magma, 24
magnesium salts, 24
Major, Randolph, 148
Maren, Thomas, 124
Martin, William, 154
Mattioli, Pietro, 18, 25
May, Everette, 151-154
McAnnulty, J. M., 227
McCarthy, E. J., 263, 274
McCawley, Elton, 148, 150
McCoy, George, 228-229
McEvilla, J. D., 266
Mectizan, 294
Mendeleev, D. I., 83
meperidine, 147, 150-151
meprobamate, 265-266
Merck, George, 124
mercurous chloride of calomel, 24
Mesmer, Franz Anton, 36
Metamucil, 21

methadone, 150-151
metopon, 146
Milk of Magnesia, 20, 24
Millar, J. Donald, 292
Miller, Phillip, 248
mineral oil, 20, 24, 25
mineral waters, 38
Minkowski, Oskar, 93
Molitor, Hans, 124
Monardes, Nicolas, 23
Mondino, De' Luzzi, 24
Moran, Lord, 101, 102, 112
morphine 65, 80, 140-147, 151, 228
Mosettig, Erich, 143, 151
Moskowitz, Milton, 128
Mosteller, Frederick, 149
Moulton, Barbara, 244-245
Moyer, J. H., 126
musk, 225
myrrh, 43

nalorphine, 148-152
naloxone, 150
naphthol, 68
Needham, Elsie, 97
Newbery, George, 105-106, 113
nicotiana, 43
nitrofuran, 248
Norplant, 198
Novasurol, 125
Novello, Frederick, 125
Novrad, 177

oak bark, 38
olive oil, 225
Ondetti, Miguel, 186
opium, 9, 38, 46, 55, 80, 140, 147, 225
oranges, 40
Osler, William, 68-69, 103

Paracelsus, 55
Parran, Thomas, 146
Pasteur, Louis, 66-67, 176
Paul of Aegina, 19

Paulesco, N. C., 95
Peet, M. M., 129
peldesine, 189
Pelletier, Pierre-Joseph, 81
penicillin, 89, 102, 121, 236,
    289, 270
pentazocine, 152
Perdium Granules, 18
Pert, Candace, 153
Peruvian bark, 37-38, 46, 56
phenacetin, 86
phenolphthalein, 20
Phillips, Montague, 106-108,
    114-115
Phipps, James, 289
Pinel, Philippe, 57-58
Pitts, Robert, 125
Pliny, 20-21
Pneumovax, 270
podophyllium, 23
Popper, Karl, 210
potassium and sodium tartrate, 24
Priessnitz, Vincent, 61-62
probenecid, 126
Prontosil, 103, 104, 105
propoxyphene, 177
Prostalin, 9
Prozac, 266
Pseudo-Mesue, 24-26
psyllium seed, 21, 24, 26
Pulvertaft, R. J. V., 102
purple foxglove, 40

quinine 37, 65, 80, 86

Radol, 226-227
Rayburn, Sam, 236
Reichel, John, 228
Reilly, David, 209
reserpine, 129
rhubarb, 18-19, 23, 25-26
Ribicoff, Abraham, 229
Rice, Charles, 225
Richards, Alfred N., 124
Richardson, Benjamin Ward 82-
    83, 85
Robinson, Edward G., 78

Robiquet, Pierre, 80
Roblin, Richard, 125
Roosevelt, Theodore, 101, 250
Rosenau, Milton, 97
Roter, D., 279
Rounds, William, 98
Rush, Benjamin, 36, 60
Ryder, Theodore, 97

salicylic acid, 65
Salvarsan, 78, 89, 229
Sarton, George, 16
saw palmetto, 167
Schaumann, O., 147
Scheele, Carl, 80
Schmidt, J. A., 161
Schreiner, Robert, 127
Schwartz, William, 125
Schweitzer, Albert, 293
Scott, E. L., 95
sea water, 40
senna, 23, 165
Sertürner, Friedrich, 80
Shapiro, Arthur K., 16
Sherley, Swagar, 231
Silverman, Milton, 239
Simon, Eric, 153
Skoda, Josef, 63
Small, Lyndon F., 143-147, 150-151,
    154
Smith, Adam, 15
Smithwick, R. H., 129
Snow, C. P., 296
Snyder, Solomon, 153
Sollmann, Torald, 232
Sonokot, 18
Spink, Wesley, 248
Sprague, James, 125
Spurr, C. L., 126
Squibb, Edward R., 224
squill, 43
St. Clair, Harold, 280
St. John's wort, 167
Stahl, G. E., 37
Stalin, 101
Stamler, Jeremiah, 130
Stedman, Edgar, 185

Stickings, R. W. E., 108-109
Stolley, Paul, 274
Street, Ellis, 242
Street, R. L., 279
streptomycin, 201, 205, 207, 270
Sucaryl, 269
sulfanilamide, 9, 103-104, 125, 126
sulfapyridine, 75, 102-120
sulfathiazole, 102, 112
Swann, John, 123
Sydenham, Thomas, 55

Taft, William, 231
Terenius, Lars, 153
Terra Sigillata, 266
tetracycline, 272
Thalidomide, 201, 272
Thom, Robert, 266
Thomas, Lewis, 51
Thompson, Leonard, 95, 97
Thorp, Ellen, 290
tragacanth, 24-25
Tschirch, Alexander, 20, 25
Tuberclecide, 227-228
tuberculin, 67
Tuckett, D., 280-281
Turkel, Edward E., 249
turpentine oil, 68
typhoid vaccine, 229

Urbach, Peter, 206

Valsyn Gel, 250
Vichow, Rudolf, 64-65
vidarabine, 187
Vogl, Alfred, 124
Vrat, Ved, 237-239

Wanko, A., 126
water, 17
Welch, Henry, 248
Welford, Ron, 108
Whitby, Lionel, 106-112, 114
Wieland, Heinrich, 143
Wien, Richard, 108
Wikler, Abraham, 149

wild lettuce, 225
Wiley, Harvey, 232
Wilkins, Robert, 126-27
Wilkinson, William, 126
Wills, Gary, 290
Wilson, I. M., 126
Wistar, Caspar 36
Withering, William 40-42
Wolff, Harold, 149
Woods, Donald, 185
Wunderlich, Carl 64-65

Young, James Harvey, 227

zidovudine, 204, 222
Zinsser, Hans, 15
Zuelzer, Georg L., 95